T0177528

BE THE CHANGE

BE THE CHANGE

Putting Health Advocacy, Policy, and
Community Organization into Practice in
Public Health Education

EDITED BY

KEELY S. REES, PHD, MS, MCHES®, FESG

JODY EARLY, PHD, MS, MCHES®

CICILY HAMPTON, PHD, MPA

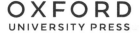
OXFORD
UNIVERSITY PRESS

OXFORD
UNIVERSITY PRESS

Oxford University Press is a department of the University of Oxford. It furthers the University's objective of excellence in research, scholarship, and education by publishing worldwide. Oxford is a registered trade mark of Oxford University Press in the UK and certain other countries.

Published in the United States of America by Oxford University Press
198 Madison Avenue, New York, NY 10016, United States of America.

Library of Congress Cataloging-in-Publication Data
Names: Rees, Keely S., editor. | Early, Jody, editor. | Hampton, Cicily, editor.
Title: Be the change : putting health advocacy, policy, and community
organization into practice in public health education /
[edited by] Keely S. Rees, Jody Early, Cicily Hampton.
Description: New York, NY : Oxford University Press, [2023] |
Includes bibliographical references and index.
Identifiers: LCCN 2022018803 (print) | LCCN 2022018804 (ebook) |
ISBN 9780197570890 (hardback) | ISBN 9780197570906 (paperback) |
ISBN 9780197570920 (epub) | ISBN 9780197570937 (online)
Subjects: MESH: Health Promotion—methods | Policy Making |
Community Participation—methods | Public Health—education
Classification: LCC RA427.8 (print) | LCC RA427.8 (ebook) | NLM WA 590 |
DDC 362.1—dc23/eng/20220727
LC record available at https://lccn.loc.gov/2022018803
LC ebook record available at https://lccn.loc.gov/2022018804

DOI: 10.1093/oso/9780197570890.001.0001

We dedicate this book to the incredible change-makers,
past, present, and future.

CONTENTS

FOREWORD

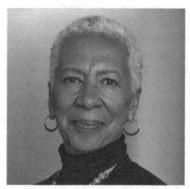

Angela Glover Blackwell
Founder in Residence at PolicyLink

Ms. Blackwell is an American attorney, civil rights advocate, and author. In 1999, she founded the research and advocacy nonprofit organization, PolicyLink, and currently serves as its Founder in Residence after 20 years as president and chief executive officer. Blackwell regularly provides expert commentary in a variety of news media, is author of *Uncommon Common Ground: Race and America's Future*, and hosts the podcast *Radical Imagination*.

As I consider the importance of this text, and why policy and advocacy are so vital to public health, my thoughts go back to where it all started for me. I actually came to policy and advocacy after years of only thinking of myself as a justice advocate. I started off as an organizer, then wanted to have more skills and went to law school and did public interest law for a decade, which was advocacy, which was a step more sophisticated than organizing, but definitely in the realm of being an advocate for change. It was while I was at Public Advocates doing class action litigation in areas that had to do with consumers and employment that I began to understand something about policy: We were often looking for policy solutions rather than just monetary solutions for the clients that we represented because we represented whole classes of people who were being victimized by systems and policies. So that introduced me to policy.

In doing this early work, I engaged with policy organizations. Some of these groups we were representing and some we sought for the expertise we needed. I realized that this was a pretty powerful platform. I leaned into trying to think about systems and the big changes and the sustainable changes that would reach into the future and impact people at a level of scale that the problem required. My first real policy work was at the Urban Strategies Council, which I founded in 1987, to try to inform policy from the best practices that were going on across the country to reduce persistent urban poverty.

One of the things that I learned while I was working with the Urban Strategies Council was how important it is to create policy that is informed by the wisdom, voice, and experience of people who are working for change in their local communities. I had figured out from getting to know the national policy scene that most national policy organizations were based in Washington, D.C., and sort of moved with the rhythm of Congress. They attracted people who were trained in policy schools but weren't necessarily trained in being proximate to problems. It seemed to me that there was real wisdom and opportunity to do policy in such a way that we could hold ourselves accountable for what the people who were ultimately going to be impacted by the policy needed and wanted. So I thought there was space for a new kind of policy institute that was really working from the community-building sensibility and doing policy from the point of view of those who needed the change and were working in partnership with people in place. I also understood that place was a powerful predictor of opportunity. That's part of what the community building work was based on. Within place, you see the dynamics of race. Race and place very much work together. A policy institute that really understood the power of place and could put policies in place that would improve the possibility for change within the places where people were living in concentrated, persistent urban poverty was needed. This led me to establish PolicyLink.

PolicyLink explores the impact of place and race on opportunity. It approaches policy development through a lens of interconnectedness, acknowledging factors that impact place, such as housing, transportation, education, health, and the environment. This was something novel: We felt that we could step into any policy arena and bring a point of view that could both help people who were experts in that area to see what they were doing in a different light and connect it in a different way. Over time, we have seen that what we are doing is accomplishing that objective by doing deep data work to understand the impact of place, race, and opportunity. PolicyLink analyzes those data and connects the analysis to what people are doing in a community. Not only were we influencing the traditional policy people and institutions, but also we had a whole new policy framework to bring forward.

PolicyLink has been growing and evolving over the past 23 years. It's gained more expertise, has a broader constituency, and understands the policy work and the politics. Communication strategies are a critical part of doing the work. Narrative is important. Making sure that people who are elected officials understand what they ought to be doing in the policy realm is important, and so is staying connected to those who are working for change. This is why it's so important for us to be connected to the advocates and to their movements that are in place.

Public health was ahead of the curve in terms of the kinds of things that PolicyLink was wanting to do. If we stand on the shoulders of any discipline, we stand on the shoulders of public health; more specifically, we stood on the shoulders of the environmental justice movement from the beginning. The environmental justice movement was the first to start talking about health and place. What was happening in the places where poor, low-income people of color were living and how the environmental impacts were particularly impacting their health. They had the "place in health" narrative down but they hadn't really lifted it up for the health community because they saw themselves so much as environmental justice advocates. We definitely felt that we were standing on their shoulders.

Whether it was something that was contagious, whether it was something that was happening in a place, like buildings that were full of lead, public health stakeholders understood the urgency and importance of the issues. The demands of people who live in these communities, the education of people who live in these communities, and the agency that you want to help strengthen in people who live in the community are all important for public health and for environmental justice wins. You can't just impose a public health agenda. You have to understand the values, the customs, and the relationships that people in a community have to be able to really develop an effective strategy. You have to really understand the power dynamics of why it is that low-income communities are the dumping grounds for toxins. Once you understand the power dynamics, you have to push back against that power. This push-back requires the advocacy and the movement building and the organizing that are essential. This is why a book like this (*Be the Change* . . .) is so essential. It contains collective wisdom about what's involved with creating change through effective advocacy and how to go the distance.

My advice to advocates is to study the history of public health because it hasn't always been a good history. Come to fully understand how it's been influenced by the racism and the hierarchy of human value that controls so much in society rather than trying to defend against it or say that it hasn't been that. It *has* been that. Understand how these mistakes happened and embrace the need to be antiracist, to try to work on structural issues and to hold in high regard, not just as charity, not just as someone who believes in the humanity of all, but hold the value of the wisdom and the strivings of the people for whom you serve. Finally, be able to see yourself as a leader—and as a motivating force within a movement to create an equitable society where all can reach their full potential.

ACKNOWLEDGMENTS

As co-editors, we would like to acknowledge and extend our love and gratitude to our families and loved ones who supported us through this journey. We also thank our incredible chapter coauthors, who despite a global pandemic and the world (literally) aflame, somehow found the passion and drive to persevere and make this text possible. And to the advocates, who have inspired us and/or mentored us, whose words, work, and example contributed to this text and to the advocates we have become, we lift you up in gratitude.

We would also like to acknowledge the artist who designed our cover art, Gina Rivas-Velasquez, who uses her art to advocate on behalf of marginalized communities. Kirsten (KJ) Newkirk, CHES®, and Dr. Casey Tobin, LPC dedicated their time to creating ancillary materials to accompany this textbook. We are grateful to all who contributed their time, talents, and energy to this text.

ABOUT THE EDITORS

Keely S. Rees, PhD, MS, MCHES®, FESG is Professor and Chair of the Department of Public Health and Community Health Education at the University of Wisconsin-La Crosse and now Past-President of National Eta Sigma Gamma. Dr. Rees was formerly an annual trustee for the Society for Public Health Education (SOPHE) and has planned and participated in statewide advocacy experiences for students in Wisconsin and at the SOPHE Advocacy Summit for over eighteen years. Her research and teaching focuses on health policy and advocacy, grant seeking, and women's health and she has taught internationally with universities, researchers, and organizations to identify ways to better prepare public health educators in Ireland, Spain, and Costa Rica.

Jody Early, PhD, MS, MCHES®, is a Professor in the School of Nursing and Health Studies at the University of Washington Bothell. Her teaching, scholarship, and public health praxis focus on the intersections between education, health, and human rights and applying community-based participatory approaches to co-design and evaluate tailored health education programs. Dr. Early serves as co-founder and co-director of the program, Mental Health Matters of Washington (La Salud Importa) and is a principal investigator and co-author of the award-winning workplace training and video, Basta! Prevent Sexual Harassment in Agriculture. In addition to her scholarship and public service, Dr. Early is also passionate about teaching and mentoring emerging public health advocates and strengthening their capacity to change oppressive systems and eliminate barriers that impede health for all.

Cicily Hampton, PhD, MPA is the Professor of Practice in Applied Healthcare Research at the Virginia University of Lynchburg. There she teaches the next generation of public health researchers how to conduct research ethically in historically underserved populations. Dr. Hampton targets social determinants of health to eliminate health disparities using research. Dr. Hampton began her career advocating on behalf of patients enrolled in federal health programs as well as leading development and execution of advocacy strategies around delivery system and payment reform in what later became the Affordable Care Act. She has more than 10 years of experience in health policy and advocacy on behalf of nonprofit organizations to advance progressive causes.

CONTRIBUTORS

Kathleen G. Allison, PhD, MPH, MCHES®, is a health education specialist and professor of community and public health education in the Department of Health Science at Lock Haven University. Her research and teaching interests include cultural aspects of health, health literacy, and community health methods and strategies, including advocacy. She has served on the national SOPHE Board of Trustees and NCHEC's Board of Commissioners.

Angela Glover Blackwell is Founder in Residence at PolicyLink, the organization she started in 1999 to advance racial and economic equity for all. Under Angela's leadership, PolicyLink gained national prominence in the movement to use public policy to improve access and opportunity for all low-income people and communities of color, particularly in the areas of health, housing, transportation, and infrastructure. Angela is also the host of the Radical Imagination podcast and Professor of Practice at the Goldman School of Public Policy, University of California, Berkeley.

Alexis Blavos, PhD, MCHES®, is currently an associate professor in the Health Department at the State University of New York Cortland. Dr. Blavos's academic and work experiences include 15 years of service in the public health field as a practitioner and researcher. As an elected Division Board director for the National Commission for Health Education Credentialing, she served as the national director of advocacy for Eta Sigma Gamma for more than 5 years, and co-chaired the Society for Public Health's Advocacy Committee for 3 years. Among her many research interests are college health, advocacy, and health policy.

Jean M. Breny, PhD, MPH, is a professor in the Department of Public Health at Southern Connecticut State University in New Haven. Her scholarship aims to eliminate health disparities through an antiracism lens using Photovoice research and a community-based participatory research paradigm that informs public health practice.

Jodi Brookins-Fisher, PhD, MCHES, FESG, is director and professor in the Division of Public Health, School of Health Sciences at Central Michigan University, a former national president of Eta Sigma Gamma, and a past SOPHE Advocacy Committee co-chair. She is passionate about everything advocacy and achieving health equity among all.

Aditi Srivistav Bussells, PhD, MPH, is faculty and director of research at the Children's Trust of South Carolina in the Arnold School of Public Health at the University of South

Carolina. She is a mixed-methods researcher that specializes in the areas of risk behavior prevention, health equity, health communications, and adverse childhood experiences.

Anders Cedergren, PhD, CHES®, is an Assistant Professor in the Department of Public Health & Community Health Education at University of Wisconsin-La Crosse. Dr. Cedergren has studied the role of health education in healthcare and value-based benefits. He is interested in upstream approaches in public health relying on advocacy and ethics to change systems, most recently related to social and emotional learning. Dr. Cedergren tries to provide opportunities for and assess experiential learning and collaboration across professional responsibilities, as well as partner with community organizations for wise utilization of resources in translational projects.

Julie Colehour is a partner at C + C, a 90-person social marketing agency with offices in Seattle, Boston, and Portland. She has spent her career working to motivate people to alter their behaviors for social good in the areas of the public health, environment, and safety.

Breanna De Leon, MPH, is an epidemiology student at the Johns Hopkins Bloomberg School of Public Health and a research coordinator/program evaluator at Lake County Tribal Health Consortium. She strives to dismantle health and racial inequities that create a disproportionate burden of disease through multisector action and translational epidemiology research and medicine.

Jennifer Disla, MA, is the co-executive director of Detroit Action. She has over 10 years of experience with labor organizing and coalition building to bring about change within communities. She is a member of Organization for Black Struggle, Missouri Jobs With Justice, and Missouri Immigrant & Refugee Advocates. She also sits as an advisory board member for the Leadership Center for Democracy and Social Justice and instructs the Social Justice Early Career Cohort.

Molly Fleming, MS, is the founding executive director of the Missouri Organizing and Voter Engagement Collaborative (MOVE) and MOVE Action, c3 and c4 coordinating tables catalyzing political transformation in Missouri through an antiracist, multiracial movement. Under Molly's leadership, MOVE and MOVE Action member organizations have won major ballot initiatives through grassroots voter engagement, including an increase in the minimum wage, major ethics and redistricting reform, defense of collective bargaining rights, and Medicaid expansion.

Sara Finger is the founder and executive director of the Wisconsin Alliance for Women's Health. She works to advance comprehensive women's health in Wisconsin by engaging, educating, empowering, and mobilizing individuals and organizations. Sara has received numerous awards for her leadership and advocacy efforts, including being named a Woman to Watch by *BRAVA Magazine* and awarded a Champion of Change by the White House for her work related to the Affordable Care Act.

Heidi Hancher-Rauch, PhD, MCHES®, is a professor and director of the Public Health Program at the University of Indianapolis, where she teaches courses at the graduate and undergraduate level regarding health advocacy and health policy. She is highly engaged in health advocacy through her work with the Society for Public Health Education as a former Advocacy & Resolutions Committee co-chair, Advocacy & Resolutions Board trustee, and the Indiana SOPHE advocacy director for two terms. She provides advocacy training for others regularly and engages in advocacy herself at the national, state, and local levels.

Amy Hedman-Robertson, PhD, MCHES®, is a full professor in public health and health promotion at the University of St. Thomas in St. Paul, Minnesota. She earned CHES® certification in 2004 and MCHES® in 2011. Currently, she is vice coordinator and director for DBCHES with the National Commission for Health Education Credentialing. She is passionate about educating future public health educators and devotes her research efforts to studying community-based suicide prevention and mental health help seeking.

Kristen Hernández Ortega, MPH, is a public health consultant and native southwest borderland resident. Her experience coordinating public health programming in diverse communities has focused on advancing health equity by improving the environments in which we live, learn, work, and play so that all people have a fair and just opportunity to reach their full health potential.

Christina Jones, PhD, is an assistant professor of health education and promotion in the College of Health at Ball State University. Dr. Jones's expertise and accompanying research program in health disparities and health advocacy span across community-based research, social justice and health, and mass media influences on health behaviors.

Dianne Kerr, PhD, MCHES®, is an emeritus professor from the Health Education and Promotion Program, School of Health Sciences, at Kent State University. Her scholarship foci include HIV, LGBTQ health, and advocacy. She currently serves as the coordinator for the Division Board of Certified Health Education Specialists for the National Commission for Health Education Credentialing and as secretary of their Board of Commissioners.

Holly Mata, PhD, MCHES, CPH, is a public health specialist and health equity advocate in Southern New Mexico and El Paso, Texas. With her colleagues in the Paso del Norte region, she loves providing internship experiences for emerging public health professionals in diverse community settings. As deputy editor of Health Promotion Practice, she enjoys supporting practitioners in sharing their advocacy and scholarship.

E. Lisako J. McKyer, PhD, MPH, FAAHB, is a professor and Vice Dean for Faculty Affairs and Diversity, Equity, and Inclusion at the Alice L. Walton School of Medicine Sciences. Formerly, Dr. McKyer was the senior associate dean for climate and diversity and a professor in the Department of Health Promotion and Community Health Sciences in the School of Public Health at Texas A&M University. Dr. McKyer's research foci include (1) social–ecological determinants of health inequities and minority health issues and (2) health education research methods (measurement and data analytical strategies). Her pedagogical interests are in child health issues, as well as cultural competency training and development.

Montrece McNeill Ransom, JD, MPH, ACC, is the director of the National Coordinating Center for Public Health Training within the National Network of Public Health Institutes and the president of the American Society for Law, Medicine, and Ethics. A prolific speaker and author, Ms. Ransom is also the lead editor of the Springer-published textbook, *Public Health Law: Concepts and Case Studies.*

Selina A. Mohammed, PhD, MPH, MSN, RN, is a professor and associate dean of the School of Nursing and Health Studies at the University of Washington Bothell. Her scholarship centers on social justice and social determinants of health. She examines the impact of racialized discrimination and other structural disadvantages on health and uses critical theories to explore how historical, sociocultural, political, and economic contexts contribute to health inequities, particularly for American Indians.

Holly T. Moses, PhD, MCHES®, FESG, is an instructional assistant professor in the Department of Health Education and Behavior at the University of Florida, where she serves as the internship coordinator and the coordinator for the online MS degree program. Dr. Moses is a former president of National Eta Sigma Gamma and currently serves on the National Commission for Health Education Credentialing (NCHEC) Division Board for Professional Preparation and Practice. Among her many interests are school and youth health, advocacy, and professional preparation and career development for health education students.

Elizabeth J. Schwartz, MPH, is a lecturer of public health at Southern Connecticut University and manages a COVID-19 and flu education, outreach, and vaccination program. She sits on the Executive Board of the Connecticut Public Health Association and is a cofounder of the Connecticut Society for Public Health Education. When not knee deep in the world of public health, Elizabeth is an avid baker, a learner of languages, and a passionate globe trekker.

Amy J. Thompson, PhD, CHES, FESG, is the Provost and Sr. Vice President of Academic Affairs at Wright State University. She has published numerous peer-reviewed studies on advocacy and has devoted her efforts to train future public health advocates. She has served as the SOPHE national president from 2022 to 2023 and also as the national advocacy trustee.

Emily Whitney, PhD, is an associate professor in the Department of Public Health and Community Health Education at the University of Wisconsin–LaCrosse as well as a master certified health education specialist. Dr. Whitney's research aims to explore the use of theoretical frameworks in addressing the determinants of health in relation to college student health, youth health issues, and underage/adolescent drinking. Additionally, she teaches motivational interviewing and health literacy as tools to help students learn about, engage in, and advance health advocacy.

INTRODUCTION

The impetus to write this text originated from working alongside dedicated health advocates working on issues at local to global levels. Students, faculty, researchers, health education specialists, and others working in public health are seeking education, training, and resources to help them strengthen their capacity to advocate: for our communities, our profession, and ultimately our health and quality of life. The term *change* is woven throughout this textbook, and as you progress through the chapters, case examples, and activities, you will continue to explore its meaning. You will further your own advocacy understanding and skills and learn more about who you are as an advocate.

As public health students you are engaged in advocacy in your courses and/or student organizations such as Eta Sigma Gamma, and local chapters of state or national organizations. If you have tabled an event on your campus, marched in a walk or vigil, attended a forum on your campus—you have engaged in advocacy efforts. For the public health professionals using this textbook, it will deepen your advocacy skill set when working at a county or state level or in a nonprofit organization or leading change in your healthcare setting. Advocacy is at the heart of what we do in this field.

As editors, we saw the need to create a user-friendly, comprehensive, and affordable tool for those working or pursuing careers in public health. We offer this as a guide, with historical perspectives, practical steps, and examples that illustrate how community organization and policy work accompanies advocacy.

Objectives

The primary aims of this text are to

- Address a gap in the field: Although there are several textbooks available on health policy, most are written at a graduate level and do not focus heavily on *advocacy*.
- Offer an affordable resource that can inspire and guide emerging and established health professionals to engage in advocacy at any level.
- Provide an overview of the purpose, strategies, and tactics used in successful advocacy in public health and amplify the important advocacy work being organized and led by health professionals around the United States.
- Present examples of advocacy campaigns along with concrete and strategic recommendations for implementing the advocacy strategies discussed in the text to advocate for change at the local, state, and federal levels.

Keely S. Rees, Jody Early, and Cicily Hampton, *Introduction*. In: *Be the Change*. Edited by Keely S. Rees, Jody Early, and Cicily Hampton, Oxford University Press. © Oxford University Press 2023. DOI: 10.1093/oso/9780197570890.001.0001

- Highlight the work of traditional and emerging regional or national voluntary health organizations as well as the mighty work of grassroots, public health departments, and community-based health nonprofits.
- Speak to and engage an undergraduate audience using a narrative and conversational style. This text is a great complementary textbook to an upper division or graduate course or for a guidebook for the working professional.

FORMAT AND ORGANIZATION

There are 14 chapters in this text, and each chapter is coauthored by advocates holding a variety of titles working in a wide range of settings, including nonprofits and nongovernmental organizations, federal and state agencies, schools and universities, corporations, law, government, and private practice. Collectively, our experience spans over three decades.

Each chapter begins with learning objectives that guide the content topics and subtopics and map to the end-of-chapter activities. The chapter content that addresses each objective/question not only provides key terms and concepts but also is designed to help you understand those concepts as they are applied in real-world settings.

Within each chapter you will find *Advocacy Spotlights*, and *Advocacy in Action* boxes. These provide vignettes, tips, checklists, reflective activities, and examples that complement and expand on the chapter content and enhance your learning.

The end-of-chapter activities include *discussion questions, application activities, and additional resources. Discussion questions* promote critical thinking and spark group dialogue about content and issues presented in the chapter. *Application activities* contain instructions for recommended activities that can be undertaken on your own if they are not assigned by the instructor. Some application activities can occur totally within the confines of a classroom. Others may require you to engage with community stakeholders, visit organizations or agencies, or listen to advocates. *Application activities* are designed for learners to apply concepts within the text to address advocacy situations in real time. Additional resources are links to websites, organizations, articles, or media that provide additional information about concepts and examples mentioned in the chapter. These resources allow the reader to expand their exploration of a particular topic or concept.

A TOOL FOR CHANGE

We invite you to view this book as more than required reading in a college course. Ultimately, we hope this book serves as a resource to you and is something you will want to keep in your personal library throughout your career. We hope the information, stories, advice, and tools shared within these pages inspire you to "be the change" and catalyze your involvement in health advocacy in a way that works for you.

Why Advocacy and Policy Matter

JODY EARLY AND KEELY S. REES

Change will not come if we wait for some other person,
or if we wait for some other time. We are the ones we've been waiting for.
We are the change that we seek.

—BARACK OBAMA, Super Tuesday (February 5, 2008)

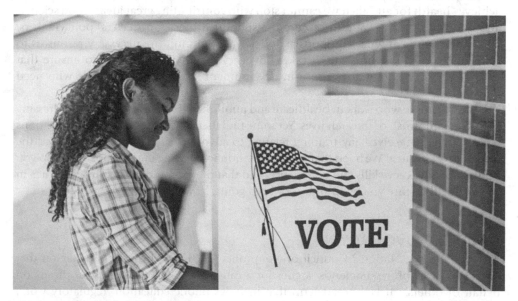

FIGURE 1.1 Voting is a form of advocacy.
Photo byiStock.com.

Objectives

1. Explain why advocacy and policy are important tools for improving health for all.
2. Distinguish how "advocacy," "lobbying," and "activism" are related but distinct.
3. Examine historical and contemporary examples of how advocacy and policy have impacted public health.

Jody Early and Keely S. Rees, *Why Advocacy and Policy Matter*. In: *Be the Change*. Edited by Keely S. Rees, Jody Early, and Cicily Hampton, Oxford University Press. © Oxford University Press 2023. DOI: 10.1093/oso/9780197570890.003.0001

4. Apply the World Health Organization's "Health in All Policies" approach to addressing a particular health issue.
5. Create a compelling argument for how everyone can play a role in advocacy.

INTRODUCTION

Have you ever witnessed or experienced something and thought: "This isn't right! Someone needs to do something about it!"? This is exactly how advocacy begins. Even if you've never considered yourself an advocate, advocacy is for everyone. If you have ever signed a petition to show your support for a cause or spoken out about something you felt people should better understand—that's advocacy! Advocacy can take many forms—from voting in an election (Figure 1.1), to raising awareness, to organizing a campaign for change, or leading an entire movement. It happens at multiple levels, from local to global. It's democracy in action.

In public health and healthcare, if we want to improve one's quality of life and achieve "health for all," then we cannot stop with contributing great ideas, good science, and good healthcare. We must secure the support of decision makers, policymakers, and others who can enact supportive policies and commit the necessary resources to bring these solutions to scale. It takes advocacy as well as ingenuity to ensure that existing solutions, as well as those in development, can reach the people who need them most.

Many people who work in healthcare and public health serve as leaders in addressing issues that diminish or threaten lives. Yet some find themselves thrust into these positions without having received any training relating to advocacy, or not enough. This was the impetus for this text. We hope that the information we provide in this book will help you build your advocacy skills and confidence, and that the examples shared by advocates in the field will inspire you to jump in—or keep going.

WHAT IS ADVOCACY?

According to the National Council of Nonprofits (2021), **advocacy** is "any action that speaks in favor of, recommends, argues for a cause, supports or defends, or pleads on behalf of others." It is a broad term that includes public education, regulatory work, litigation, work before administrative bodies, lobbying, nonpartisan voter registration, nonpartisan voter education, and more. Advocacy in its many forms can include large-scale efforts, such as actively working to create social movements or individual efforts such as voting.

Being a public health advocate gives you the opportunity to influence the way the public and policymakers think and act on public health policies. Professional organizations like the American Public Health Association and the Society for Public Health Education, as well as many others, engage in both education and advocacy campaigns. Public and policymaker education campaigns communicate information about specific issues, usually providing information about various sides of a particular issue, but

TABLE 1.1 Distinguishing Between Advocacy and Lobbying

Advocacy	Lobbying
Usually voluntary	Usually paid
Broad range of strategies	Narrow
Could be aimed at a variety of audiences	Aimed at specific policymakers or decision makers
Does not directly ask for a vote	Asks the person to vote in a particular way
Example activity: Writing your state representative to inform them about how a particular health issue has impacted their constituents	Example: Writing your state representative to discuss your group's position on a particular bill and to asking them to vote in favor of it
Example: Organizing a coalition to build public awareness about a particular issue	Example: Leading a special interest group that is supporting a presidential proposal and trying to convince members of Congress to vote in its favor
Example: Your nonprofit organization that works to improve children's health encourages the public to call your organization to learn more about the benefits of a new school-health nutrition initiative underway	Example: While being interviewed by a local radio station, you urge voters to support a particular piece of legislation on the ballot about school–health nutrition

Adaptation based on terms defined by National Council of Nonprofits (http://councilofnonprofits.org).

leaning toward a policy solution that the organization feels is best in order to achieve their goals (which may include improving the status quo). Advocacy campaigns also encompass efforts to engage the public, organizations, or specific groups to directly encourage policymakers to consider policy action on a particular public health issue.

Advocacy is often confused with **lobbying**. Lobbying falls within the umbrella of strategies used in advocacy. Lobbying consists of direct communication with policymakers regarding specific legislation and urging the policymakers to vote in a particular way. Lobbyists are also usually paid by organizations, groups, or corporations to represent them. Government and nonprofit organizations that have government relations staff who lobby on behalf of the organization must comply with federal laws by submitting regular reports detailing their activity and expenditures.

To better distinguish advocacy from lobbying, remember this: While *all lobbying is advocacy, not all advocacy is lobbying*. Advocacy includes a broad range of activities, inclusive of lobbying, but lobbying is very narrow. The National Council of Nonprofits (2021) provided another helpful distinction: In order for it to be characterized as lobbying *all three* of the following components are required: (1) communication is aimed at decision makers; (2) it's about a particular piece of legislation; and (3) it's asking the person to vote a particular way. Table 1.1 below provides additional tips for distinguishing between advocacy and lobbying.

GRASSROOTS TERMINOLOGY

The editors and contributors to this book share a belief that the work of community organizing, grassroots advocacy, and community building are central to public health and health promotion and to creating lasting change that improves the quality of life for our communities and nations. As a student or practitioner in public health or in social services, you will likely hear the words "grassroots" or "community-organizing" and "community building" as you engage in community activities, read or watch the news, or study the professional literature. So what do these terms mean? The terms **grassroot** (n.) and **grassroots** (adj.) indicates that something is at the most basic level, and we like to think of it as a start from the "ground up" or out of the earth, soil, and grass. A public health **grassroots movement** is a group of individuals (small or larger) taking on a health issue and mobilizing (moving) and organizing efforts to make positive changes that improve the health and safety of individuals and communities (Minkler, 2012). Grassroots efforts usually originate organically with a group of people in the community who feel passionate about creating a change of some kind, in contrast to some elite group or political forces.

Community organizing is "a process by which communities identify their assets and concerns, prioritize and select issues, and intentionally build power and develop and implement action strategies for change" (Minkler et al., 2019, p. 10S). Community organizing incorporates the combined competencies of planning, capacity and needs assessment, implementation, communication, leadership, and advocacy. The grassroots nature of community organizing is pulling together people, organizations, thought leaders, media, and advocates that can share stories and facts and then mobilize for a specific change.

Grassroots advocacy takes this one step further and brings along communities and other health-related organizations with the purpose of making a policy change, advocating for a bill or law to be changed or made at the state or federal level all while starting on a local level. Health advocates then mobilize efforts to include human re-sources, funding, media, and ultimately their voices to create energy and movement on a public health issue. Grassroots advocacy includes partnering with key stakeholders, influencers, or a thought leader in the field to garner support to make policy changes. These grassroots efforts include youth-led movements, also coined as youth organizing, and have gained significant momentum and media attention in the last 25 years. Grassroots advocacy includes protests and demonstrations, rallies, campaigns, door-to-door canvasing, signature gathering, tabling events, vigils, town hall forums, and marches (Figure 1.2).

EXAMPLES OF GRASSROOTS ADVOCACY

Examples of grassroots advocacy surround us. For example, Greta Thunberg, a Swedish teen, is one of the leading youth activists, creating a platform that has gained policy traction on climate change. Greta's grassroot leadership spawned local teens to activate climate change events, rallies, forums, media, and social media attention. Another well-known advocate, Malala Yousafzai, was born in Pakistan in 1997 and is one of the world's most famous proponents for girls' right to education. At age 11, she began to speak out against the rule of the Taliban, which stripped girls of the right to attend school. She began an anonymous blog with the British Broadcast Corporation (BBC) to detail life as a young woman under the Taliban and was soon seen as a threat. At age 15, while on a bus to school, she was shot in the face by the

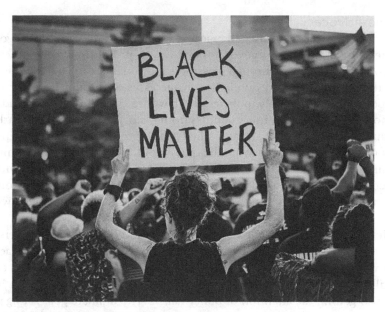

FIGURE 1.2 Black Lives Matter advocate holding up sign.

Taliban, an attempt to silence her and to make her an example. Moving to England, where she underwent many surgeries and months of rehabilitation, Malala continued her activism. She grew a worldwide movement, leading to the creation of the Malala Fund, which "invests in education activists and advocates who are driving solutions to barriers to girls' education in their communities" (https://MalalaFund.org/about). By age 17, Yousafzai became the youngest person to receive the Nobel Peace Prize for her work.

Another example of grassroots advocacy is the Black Lives Matter movement. In 2013, Alicia Garza, Patrisse Cullors, and Opal Tometi began a Black-centered movement to organize and build local power to intervene and stop state-sponsored violence inflicted on Black communities. It rose out of the acquittal of George Zimmerman, who killed young Trayvon Martin, 17, in Sanford, Florida, as he walked through the neighborhood where Zimmerman and Trayvon Martin's father lived after his trip to a nearby convenience store to grab a bag of Skittles and a few other sundries. He was unarmed. #BlackLivesMatter is now a member-led global network of more than 40 chapters and growing.

As these examples show, grassroots advocacy can start with just one person courageously taking action against injustice and crescendo into a national or even global effort to save lives. One could argue that grassroots advocacy and community organizing are the most powerful aspects of our work in public health and health promotion, as these processes can heighten social consciousness about injustice as well as lead to systems-level and policy changes that positively impact health and health equity.

Legislative Advocacy

Legislative activity leads to policy change and laws. This is the aspect of advocacy that can be the most gratifying for advocates and health professionals. Advocacy, such as speaking out about an issue through grassroots movements, can lead to policy change. Some of the nation's greatest public health successes would not have been possible without policy change. Ideally, policies and laws are created to protect and enhance lives, although there are certainly examples from history where this was clearly not the case. As public health, healthcare, and allied health professionals, many of us work to save lives or work toward improving the quality of life for individuals, communities, and populations. Some say we are in the "business of selling health or in the business of reducing morbidity and mortality (M/M)." This is the nonglamorous part of our jobs. It entails rolling up our proverbial sleeves and doing challenging work—day after day.

The legislative process will be explained further and discussed in Chapters 6 and 7; however, it is imperative that you have the big picture of the legislative advocacy process and work we engage in daily. When an individual or group starts a grassroots campaign, they usually have a goal of not only raising awareness of the issue that is impacting lives but also getting the attention of policymakers. The ultimate goal is to garner support, petitions, or the introduction of new or better legislation (laws) that addresses the health behavior. Legislative advocacy can include individuals or organizations educating policymakers on a local, state, or federal level. The ultimate goal is then to introduce new policy that would be put through the process of adoption. Getting a bill to the point of adoption is difficult; it could take years to get it to a vote in the House or Senate, and many bills never even make it to the president's desk for signature or veto. This is why advocacy and activism are so important: It takes people working together, using different strategies, to raise awareness and to garner support to help legislation come to pass. Below, we briefly introduce you to these two terms and offer you a few historical examples relating to public health.

ACTIVISM VERSUS ADVOCACY

In public health and healthcare, we need both activists and advocates. Subtle differences exist in their definitions, but these two are very intertwined and overlapping in skills and attributes. As we described previously in this chapter, **advocacy** is an umbrella term that includes many different strategies for publicly representing an individual, organization, or idea. The word **activist**, according to the *Oxford Dictionary* (2021), is a narrower term, defined as "a person who takes direct action to achieve political or social change, especially as a member of an organization with particular aims." Activism is a form of advocacy.

Another way to differentiate the two terms is that advocacy is often characterized as working *within* a system, whereas activism often involves working *outside* a system to generate change. Some definitions of activism represent it in a more negative light, which reveals more about the bias of those creating formal definitions than of the act itself. For example, the *Merriam-Webster Dictionary* (n.d.) characterizes activism as "doctrine or practice that emphasizes direct vigorous action especially in support of or opposition to one side of a controversial issue." However, what is deemed "controversial" may be viewed as a basic human right by another. The tactics that activists use to gain attention can vary; it's important to recognize that the images and video clips selected to convey stories about activism can shape the way in which people envision activism as a whole—as something extreme rather than an important part of democracy. Activists are commonly characterized as people taking action to the streets, leading marches, sit-ins/sit-outs, vigils, and mobilization efforts on a grassroots level. However, not all activism is protest. Activists bring attention to issues to further engage communities and policymakers and to enlist a variety of collaborators who can push for policy creation or change. In short, activism is an important advocacy strategy for catalyzing legislative action.

No matter if it's as an advocate or as an activist, it is important to question our role if we are speaking on behalf of a community, group, or individual and to reflect on how being a spokesperson brings with it power and responsibility. How we represent an individual, group, or issue can impact collective action, public perception, and trust from individuals we represent.

The road to change requires engagement from many individuals, communities, and organizations that may work both "inside" and "outside" the system or arenas. In public health, we need both competent advocates and activists that can take a pressing health issue and find ways to bring awareness to it, garner support, inform the public, and compel policymakers to support legislation that helps to enhance, protect, and save lives. Advocacy involves multilevel work that is needed to foster shared purpose and actions that advance health.

HISTORICAL EXAMPLES OF ADVOCACY AND POLICY

Some of the nation's greatest public health successes would not have been possible without health advocacy and policy change. The Centers for Disease Control and Prevention's (CDC's) lists of the greatest public health achievements of the 20th and 21st centuries include things that have become such a part of our everyday lives that we may take them for granted. These public health initiatives, which include things like vaccination, prevention of spread of infectious disease, and food safety and sanitation laws, demonstrate the power of effective advocacy and policy change on individual and population health. We provide a few detailed examples below for inspiration.

Vaccine-Preventable Diseases

The impact of vaccination on the health of the global society is hard to exaggerate. With the exception of safe water, no other modality has had such a major effect on mortality reduction and population growth (Association of State and Territorial Health Officials, 2016). At the beginning of the 20th century, infectious diseases such as smallpox, measles, diphtheria, and pertussis were widely prevalent. Since there were few effective measures available, death tolls were high. Both the development and promotion of vaccinations against preventable diseases have resulted in dramatic declines in morbidity and mortality and even resulted in the eradication of smallpox.

During the first decade of the 21st century, a number of new vaccines were introduced. Two of the most significant were the pneumococcal conjugate vaccine, which has prevented an estimated 211,000 serious pneumococcal infections and 13,000 deaths, and the rotavirus vaccine, which now prevents an estimated 40,000–60,000 rotavirus hospitalizations each year (CDC, 2011). Other achievements included record low reported cases of hepatitis A, hepatitis B, and chickenpox and the development of vaccines for malaria (in 2015) and Ebola (in 2019). However, the most important vaccine so far in the 21st century has been the development of the COVID-19 vaccine. Before the end of 2021, the Institute for Health Metrics and Evaluation (IHME), an independent global research center at the University of Washington, projects U.S. deaths to reach close to 1 million and close to 10 million globally (IHME, 2021). The number of deaths from COVID-19 was dramatically reduced thanks to vaccine science.

Vaccination Laws

It wasn't just the development and testing of vaccines that has led to decreased mortality—the laws that have shaped their widespread use are also to credit. State vaccination laws include vaccination requirements for children in public and private schools and daycare settings, college/university students, as well as healthcare workers and patients in certain facilities. State vaccination laws require children to be vaccinated against certain communicable diseases as a condition for school attendance. All states also establish vaccination requirements for children as a condition for child care attendance. These requirements often mirror the requirements for public school children and are often located in the same school vaccination provisions. Of course, there are some children who cannot be vaccinated due to other health issues, and for those instances states provide a waiver (Malone & Hinman, 2007).

State laws also affect access to vaccination services by determining whether providing vaccinations to patients is within the scope of practice of certain healthcare professionals. The Public Health Law Program provides selected resources on state vaccination laws for public health practitioners and their legal counsel (Malone & Hinman, 2007).

Prevention and Control of Infectious Diseases

The leading causes of death in 1900 in the United States were infectious diseases such as pneumonia, tuberculosis (TB), and diarrhea and enteritis. All of these declined throughout much of the 20th century due to sanitation and hygiene, vaccination, and antibiotics. The United States began to see a rise of chronic illnesses overtake infectious diseases as leading causes of death. In fact, by 2019, the CDC reported that the leading causes of death for adults were heart disease, cancer, unintentional injuries, chronic lower respiratory diseases, stroke, Alzheimer disease, diabetes, kidney disease, influenza and pneumonia, and suicide (CDC, 2021). However, the world saw a shift in late 2019, when the COVID-19 coronavirus began to emerge. Spread through air, COVID-19 became the leading cause of death in the United States, killing close to 800 thousand people in America and over 5 million globally (at the end of 2021). Under the Trump administration, Operation Warp Speed, a partnership between the Departments of Health and Human Services and Defense, helped to accelerate the development of the first generation of COVID-19 vaccines, based on over a decade of research that laid the groundwork

(Berg, 2021). Strengthening public health strategies and infrastructure was also key to reducing deaths. On taking office on January 21, 2021, President Biden and his administration introduced the National Strategy for the COVID-19 Response and Pandemic Preparedness, with goals such as launching a safe and equitable vaccine campaign, providing resources and relief to millions, reopening schools and businesses safely, and restoring U.S. leadership globally and strengthening the country's preparedness and pandemic response (Biden, 2021).

Food Safety and Improved Nutrition

Imagine calming your crying baby with a soothing syrup laced with moderate amounts of opium, never knowing the expiration date of the canned goods you just put in your cart, or purchasing ground meat that was left out of refrigeration for days. All of these scenarios may seem ridiculous by today's standards, but prior to the Pure Food and Drug Act of 1906, all of these were a reality for consumers. The Pure Food and Drug Act was the first legislation in the country that sought to regulate pharmaceuticals and food products. It was also the first that required truth in labeling on products, created inspectors of drug and food manufacturing processes, and required a list of dangerous drugs that had to be labeled at all times. The Pure Food and Drug Act of 1906 came about during the Progressive Era of American history. During this era, advocates as well as investigative journalists (also known as "muckrakers") sought to improve the moral and social fabric of America through prohibition, improving public services for the immigrant poor, cleaning up corruption in politics, and improving public health and sanitation (Barkan, 1985).

During the early 20th century, contaminated food, milk, and water caused many foodborne infections, including typhoid fever, tuberculosis, botulism, and scarlet fever. In 1906, author and muckraker Upton Sinclair described the harsh and unsafe practices of the meat packing industry in his novel *The Jungle*. Sinclair raised public awareness about the exploitative and unsanitary conditions under which food was produced, and this eventually led to the Federal Meat Inspection Act and the Pure Food and Drug Act of 1906 also passed the same year. Both laws required sanitary conditions for food preparation, and the Pure Food and Drug Act of 1906 prohibited adulteration, misbranding, or selling of spoiled or noxious or poisonous or spoiled foods, drugs, medicines, and/or liquors (Barkan, 1985).

In addition, healthier animal care, feeding, and processing also improved food supply safety. As a result, rates of infectious diseases, such as typhoid, sharply declined. By 1950, the incidence of typhoid had fallen to only 1.7 out of 100,000 individuals, a dramatic downturn from 1900, when the incidence was approximately 100 per 100,000 (CDC, 2011).

Historical Examples of Women's Advocacy

With few laws or regulations, and without the right to vote, the women of early 20th century America didn't let that deter them from their desire to buy food and drugs they could trust. What they lacked in political power they made up for in sheer numbers and their determination to create positive change. If the food industry couldn't regulate itself, then women found ways to get it done and pressured the government to join them in

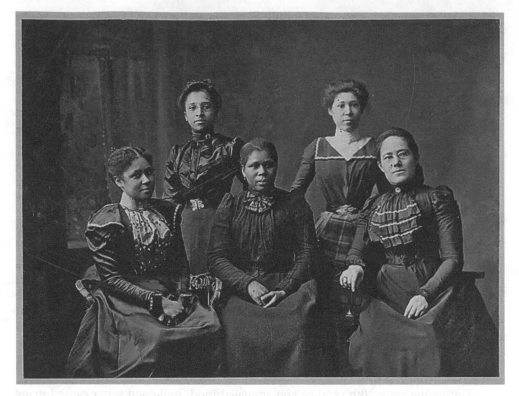

FIGURE 1.3 Five women officers of the Women's League in Newport, Rhode Island (1899).
Source: U.S. Library of Congress.

their fight. The passage of the Federal Meat Inspection Act and Pure Food and Drug Act of 1906 would not have been possible without women's advocacy, activism, and grassroots organizing. Women's clubs (also called "leagues") (Figure 1.3) began to emerge in the late 19th century and became especially popular during the women's club movement of the early 20th century (Parker, 2010). These clubs, most of which had started out as social and literary gatherings, eventually became a source of reform for various issues in the United States. Both African American and White women's clubs were involved with issues surrounding education, temperance, child labor, juvenile justice, legal reform, environmental protection, library creation, and more. As described by Parker (2010), women's clubs and leagues helped start many initiatives, such as kindergartens and juvenile court systems.

Later, women's clubs tackled issues like women's suffrage, lynching, and family planning. These women were the first consumer advocates, increasing awareness about unsanitary food storage and handling and exposing threats to health from adulterated food, medicine, and other goods. They also lobbied hard for more government involvement so that basic standards could be expected for food purity and measurements. The tenacity and resolve of these progressive campaigns eventually led to consumer rating systems and consumer protection groups that influence business practices even today!

THE IMPORTANCE OF ADVOCACY AND POLICY
FOR HEALTH PROMOTION

Many of you are enrolled in community health education, health promotion, or public health programs across the nation. The foundations of your academic programs may be preparing you to achieve national competencies in health education and promotion as established by the National Commission for Health Education Credentialing to become a certified health education specialist or master certified health education specialist. Or your degree may be preparing you to become certified in public health or achieve another certification, licensing, or credential that is promoted in your discipline. No matter the setting, our professional roles have us working in communities and organizations where we will likely engage in advocacy activities in some form or another. Working in health promotion or healthcare often requires us to communicate with stakeholders, policymakers, and leaders formally or informally to make changes. These changes can come in the form of procedures, policies, initiatives, programming, treatments, and/or laws to better serve an organization, community, and/or nation. Policy, what it is, how it's developed, and which stakeholders are involved, is further explained in Chapters 6 and 7, and strategies for engaging as an advocate and change agent are presented throughout this text.

As advocates, we must listen, learn, and then amplify voices, votes, and movements toward sustainable and meaningful changes. Ideally, these changes can be measured in some way. Measures include both quantitative and qualitative indicators, such as epidemiological data, people's lived experiences or perceived quality of life, reduction in morbidity and mortality, and individual and community-level health indicators. As we track progress, it's important to remember that positive change takes time and is usually incremental rather than grand or sweeping. Advocacy strategies, discussed in Chapters 3–14, might range from the micro to macro levels: From simply talking to someone about the benefits of proposed legislation that supports investing in renewable forms of energy to writing a policy brief that informs public opinion and garners legislator support for sponsoring a bill, there are multiple ways to engage in advocacy. As we mentioned at the beginning of this chapter, anyone can engage in advocacy. In fact, some of history's most powerful advocates have been children and young adults (read about Ryan White in Advocacy Spotlight 1.1). Also, there is no hierarchy of advocacy activities: all are necessary in order to promote and protect the health of individuals and communities and you may need to use more than one, concurrently or in succession, to achieve your goals.

THE POWER OF PERSISTENCE: THE PARABLE
OF THE MOSQUITO

Dr. Keely S. Rees, a coeditor of this text, offered an analogy about advocacy that she has provided to aspiring health educators and advocates for over a decade: When you think of yourself as a health advocate, think of yourself as a mosquito. Yes, a *mosquito*. Most of the time we think of mosquitos as useless, harmful, and annoying. They carry disease and cause itching, inflammation, and agitation. If you have ever camped, you know how much havoc one tiny mosquito can cause in your tent—in your ear. However, let's consider this also: Mosquitos provide a great source of nutrients to bats and to the ecosystem, and they are important pollinators. As advocates, we want to be tenacious mosquitos buzzing in the ears of policymakers, officers, community leaders, mayors, legislators, school boards, organizations, and think tanks. It takes a lot of advocates, activists, and mosquitos making intentional steps and actions to see changes occur. Swarms of advocates write, speak, and appear in local, state, and federal offices to voice their concerns; send letters; create campaigns and tweets; and lead political movements. Mosquitos are persistent. So are public health advocates.

HEALTH IN ALL POLICIES

It's hard to think of any kind of policy that does not impact some facet of health. The concept of Health in All Policies (HiAP) is part of Section 4001 of the Patient Protection and Affordable Care Act (2010) and is part of the National Prevention Strategy that is led by the surgeon general of the United States. **Health in All Policies** is defined as "a collaborative approach to improving the health of all people by incorporating health considerations into decision-making across sectors and policy areas" (Rudolph et al., 2013, p. 6). The National Prevention Strategy calls for increased coordination between government agencies, as well as partnerships with community organizations, businesses, healthcare providers, and others, to prioritize work around creating healthier communities and environments, empowering individuals, and integrating clinical and community preventive services to reduce and eliminate health disparities (National Prevention Council, 2011). HiAP supports the National Prevention Strategy by making health a part of decision-making at every level of stakeholder collaboration (see Figure 1.4).

Policy and advocacy work take collaborative approaches in order to effectively address the most foundational aspects that humans need to survive and thrive. The HiAP approach allows advocates (like you!) to work on the most local grassroots advocacy level to the most formal policy making with federal leaders. What determines a HiAP approach is the notion of coordinated efforts that endure the test of time to ensure outcomes for all in equitable and just ways? Solutions to our most complex and urgent health issues, locally and globally, will require collaborative efforts across many sectors and all levels, including government agencies, businesses, and community-based organizations. In your role in public health or some other health-related setting, you will likely contribute to or lead strategies that assist health agencies, organizations, and policymakers to create and/or support policies and practices that create and promote healthier, more equitable, and sustainable communities (Advocacy Spotlight 1.1).

CONCLUSION

Throughout this text we often describe advocacy as a marathon, or even an ultramarathon, rather than a sprint. Advocacy work can also harken the skills and tenacity needed to

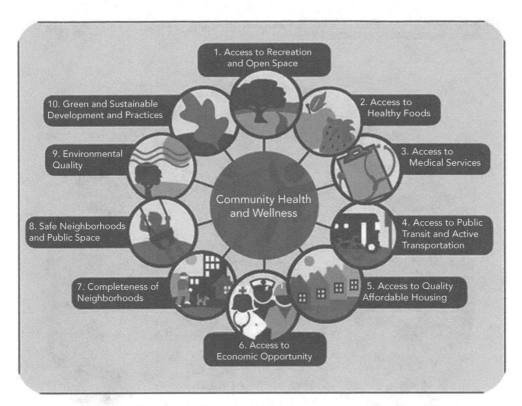

FIGURE 1.4 A HiAP approach to community health promotion.
Source: Centers for Disease Control and Prevention.

climb a large hill, bluff, or mountain. It takes bravery, courage, and willingness to fail, flail, and even fall down in order to create positive change. It also takes a united effort; one person alone cannot do this work. Many of us engage in advocacy not because it's easy or admired, but because it matters. It is likely the reason why you found your way to public health and health promotion as a career path. You want to help and serve others. You see paths leading to change. You are creative and strong, and you have lived through something or witnessed your own injustice or oppression that allows you to advocate, bear witness, empathize with others, listen, offer support, and take action. The *why* drives most of us to this work. The why is important because it helps us understand factors that influence behavior at multiple levels, from the individual, to community, to systems levels. Influencing factors might include (but are not limited) to things like socioeconomics; access to clean water, air, or fruits and vegetables; geography; experiences with discrimination; education; culture; or barriers to healthcare. Advocacy work is drilling down to the why and then helping policymakers work through the *how*. The rest of this text guides you through how to do the advocacy work. It is our hope that these pages will be a helpful resource to you as you develop your capacity and skills as a health advocate.

| ADVOCACY IN ACTION BOX 1.1 | A HiAP approach to reducing childhood obesity. |

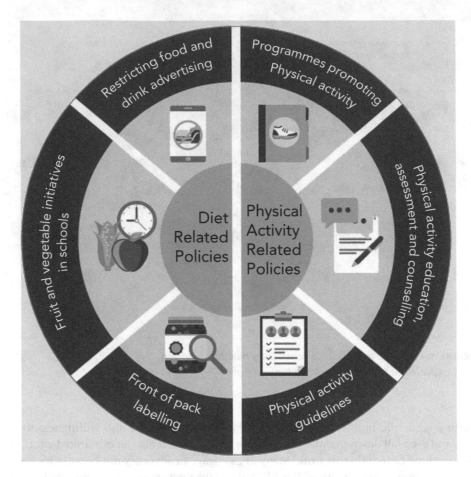

Source: World Cancer Research Fund International (2020).

REFERENCES

Association of State and Territorial Health Officials (ASTHO). (2016). Public health and its impacts. https://www.astho.org/Public-Policy/Federal-Government-Relations/Documents/Public-Health-and-Its-Impacts/

Barkan, I. D. (1985, January). Industry invites regulation: The passage of the Pure Food and Drug Act of 1906. *American Journal of Public Health*, *75*(1), 18–26. doi:10.2105/ajph.75.1.18

Berg, S. (2021, February 26). *How a decade of coronavirus research paved way for COVID-19 vaccines*. American Medical Association. https://www.ama-assn.org/delivering-care/public-health/how-decade-coronavirus-research-paved-way-covid-19-vaccines

Biden, J. (2021). *National Strategy for the COVID-19 Response and Pandemic Preparedness*. https://www.whitehouse.gov/wp-content/uploads/2021/01/National-Strat

egy-for-the-COVID-19-Response-and-Pande mic-Preparedness.pdf

Centers for Disease Control and Prevention. (2011, May 20). Ten great public health achievements in the United States, 2001— 2010. *Morbidity and Mortality Weekly*, *60*(19), 619–623. https://www.cdc.gov/ mmwr/preview/mmwrhtml/mm601 9a5.htm

Centers for Disease Control and Prevention. (2021, July 26). Deaths: Leading causes for 2019. *National Vital Statistics Report*. Vol. 70, number 9. https://www.cdc.gov/nchs/ data/nvsr/nvsr70/nvsr70-09-508.pdf

Institute for Health Metrics and Evaluation (IHME). (2021). *COVID-19 projections: Global*. https://covid19.healthdata.org/global

Malone, K., & Hinman, A. (2007). Vaccination mandates: The public health imperative and individual rights. In R. A. Goodman & R. E. Hoffman (Eds.), *Law in public health practice*. Oxford Press.

Merriam-Webster Dictionary. (n.d.). Activist. https://www.merriam-webster.com/diction ary/activist

Minkler, M. (2012). *Community organizing and community building for health and welfare* (3rd ed.). Rutgers University Press.

Minkler, M., Rebanal, R. D., Pearce, R., & Acosta, M. (2019). Growing equity and health equity in perilous times: Lessons from community organizers. *Health Education & Behavior*, *46*(1,

Suppl.), 9S–18S. https://doi.org/10.1177/ 1090198119852995

National Council of Nonprofits. (2021). *Advocacy vs. lobbying*. https://www.councilo fnonprofits.org/advocacy-vs-lobbying

National Prevention Council. (2011). National Prevention Strategy: America's *plan* for better health and wellness. U.S. Department of Health and Human Services, Office of the Surgeon General. https://www.hhs.gov/sites/default/ files/disease-prevention-wellness-report.pdf

Oxford Dictionary. (2021). *Advocacy*. https:// www.oxfordlearnersdictionaries.com/us/def inition/english/advocacy

Oxford Dictionary. (2021). *Activism*. https:// www.oxfordlearnersdictionaries.com/us/def inition/english/activism?q=activism

Parker, A. M. (2010). *Clubwomen, reformers, workers, and feminists of the Gilded Age and Progressive Era*. In C. DeLuzio (Ed.), *Women's rights: People and perspectives*. ABC-CLIO..

Patient Protection and Affordable Care Act of 2010, Pub. L. No. 111-148, 124 Stat. 119 (2010). https://www.congress.gov/111/plaws/ publ148/PLAW-111publ148.pdf

Rudolph, L., Caplan, J., Mitchell, C, Ben-Moshe, K., & Dillon, L. (2013). *Health in all policies: Improving health through intersectoral collaboration* [Discussion paper]. NAM Perspectives, National Academy of Medicine, Washington, DC. https://doi.org/10.31478/201309a

CHAPTER 1: END-OF-CHAPTER ACTIVITIES

DISCUSSION QUESTIONS

1. Why are both advocacy and policy important tools for improving the health of communities and individuals?

2. Provide a historical or contemporary example of how advocacy led to a change that benefited the public's health.

3. What are the four basic components of effective advocacy?

4. Describe an example of how the Health in All Policies approach can be applied to a health issue, such as improving air quality within a particular community.

APPLICATION ACTIVITIES

1. Research a grassroots coalition or initiative in your state or nearby that led to policy development or policy change. Prepare a 5- to 10-minute presentation for your peers about what you learned that answers the following questions:
   a. How did it begin?
   b. Who was involved?
   c. What strategies were used to build engagement and/or support?
   d. What outcomes resulted?

2. Prepare a one- to two-page written spotlight on an everyday advocate, famous or nonfamous, who is/was involved in advocacy efforts. What can we learn about advocacy from this person's example?

3. Find a contemporary example of public health advocacy in the news. What is the core issue, what are the advocacy goals, and who are the stakeholders involved?

4. Create a one-page compelling argument for how everyone can play a role in advocacy. Deliver the argument in class.

ADDITIONAL RESOURCES

American Public Health Association. (n.d.). Advocacy for *public health.* https://www.apha.org/policies-and-advocacy/advocacy-for-public-health

Centers for Disease Control and Prevention. (2016). Health in All Policies. https://www.cdc.gov/policy/hiap/index.html

Galer-Unti, R. A., Tappe, M. K., & Lachenmayr, S. (2004). Advocacy 101: Getting started in health education advocacy. *Health Promotion Practice, 5*(3), 280–288. https://doi.org/10.1177/1524839903257697

Society for Public Health Education (SOPHE). SOPHE *advocacy.* https://www.sophe.org/advocacy/

Berkley Library, University of California. *What is public health?* Public *health achievements.* https://guides.lib.berkeley.edu/publichealth/whatIsph/achievements

QUIZ QUESTIONS

1. Which of the following is true about advocacy?
   a. There are many different forms of advocacy.
   b. Advocacy is any action that speaks in favor of, recommends, argues for a cause; or defends or pleads on behalf of others.
   c. Lobbying is a form of advocacy.
   d. All of the above.

2. The act of someone communicating directly with policymakers regarding specific legislation on behalf of an organization for pay is describing what?
   a. legislation
   b. politicizing
   c. lobbying
   d. racketeering

3. Which of the following is a form of advocacy?
   a. voting
   b. lobbying
   c. community organizing
   d. all of the above

4. U.S. women's clubs or leagues of the early 20th century helped to achieve all of the following except _____?
   a. kindergartens
   b. food and safety laws
   c. prisons
   d. women's suffrage

5. A _____ is a group of individuals (small or larger) taking on a health issue and mobilizing (moving) and organizing efforts to make positive changes that improve the health and safety of individuals and communities.
   a. community
   b. grassroots movement
   c. caucus
   d. delegation

6. An example of a grassroots movement is _____
   a. COVID-19 vaccination mandates
   b. Black Lives Matter
   c. state laws
   d. Society for Public Health Education

7. _____is "a process by which communities identify their assets and concerns, prioritize and select issues, and intentionally build power and develop and implement action strategies for change."
   a. caucus
   b. delegation
   c. community organizing
   d. lobbying

8. _____ is "a collaborative approach to improving the health of all people by incorporating health considerations into decision-making across sectors and policy areas."
   a. coalition building
   b. community organizing
   c. Health in All Policies
   d. lobbying

9. The city of San Antonio has launched a statewide initiative to lower childhood obesity. An example of Health in All Policies approach is _____.
   a. providing nonsugar drinks and healthy snacks in school vending machines
   b. implementing a Let's Move program in Spanish and English pre-K and first to sixth grades
   c. involving parent associations around the state to provide caregiver and parent education about healthy meal planning on a budget
   d. all of the above

10. Which of the following is NOT a form of lobbying?
   a. writing your state representative to discuss your group's position on a particular bill and asking them to vote in favor of it
   b. casting your ballot on Election Day
   c. leading a special interest group to support a presidential proposal to convince members of Congress to vote in favor of a particular piece of proposed legislation
   d. appearing in a TikTok video on behalf of a group to urge people in a particular area to vote "no" to a particular issue on the ballot

ANSWER KEY

1. **D.** All of the above
2. **C.** Lobbying
3. **D.** All of the above
4. **C.** Prisons
5. **B.** Grassroots movement
6. **B.** Black Lives Matter
7. **C.** Community organizing
8. **C.** Health in All Policies
9. **D.** All of the above
10. **B.** Casting your ballot on Election Day

1.1 RYAN WHITE

How a Young Advocate's Short Life Led to Landmark Legislation

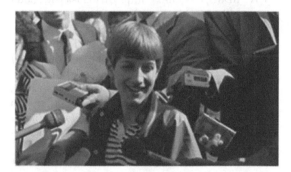

FIGURE 1A.1 Ryan White surrounded by the press, April 1986.

Source: Library of Congress.

Anyone can participate in advocacy. It's not something reserved or for those with long political careers or activists leading large coalitions or movements. Take, for example, the life of a 13-year-old boy from Kokomo, Indiana: Ryan White. At 3 days old, he was diagnosed with a condition called hemophilia, a hereditary blood coagulation disorder. For treatment, he received weekly infusions of a blood product pooled from plasma (Factor VIII), a common treatment for those with hemophilia at the time. He was healthy for most of his childhood, but then in December 1984, at the age of 13, he developed pneumonia and was diagnosed with acquired immunodeficiency syndrome (AIDS). White had apparently received a contaminated treatment of Factor VIII that was infected with HIV. At the time, little was known about HIV or its treatment. Doctors predicted White would have only 6 months to live. However, he surpassed their expectations.

By early 1985, he began to feel better and wanted to go back to his middle school. Because there was so much fear, lack of awareness, and prejudice

about how HIV was spread at the time, parents of children attending Ryan's middle school banded together, along with 50 teachers, to sign a petition that would prohibit White from returning to school. The Whites filed a lawsuit that went to the U.S. District Court in Indiana, which ruled that the school must follow the Indiana Board of Health guidelines and also allow White to return to school. However, the battle did not end there. The school board voted 7–0 to appeal the court's ruling, and Howard County upheld the ruling despite mounting opposition. Threats of violence and lawsuits persisted. White and his family moved to Cicero, Indiana, at the start of a new academic year. He attended Hamilton Heights High School, where the school administrators and a handful of students educated about AIDS welcomed him and were not afraid to shake his hand.

Ryan White's story launched him into the national spotlight, and he became THE "poster child" for the AIDS crisis, appearing in educational and fundraising campaigns. White's story helped to reduce the stigma of HIV/AIDS, then seen as a "gay man's disease." Many celebrities and public figures rallied behind him, such as Elton John; Michael Jackson; the former Surgeon General, C. Everett Coop; and athletes such as Kareem Abdul-Jabbar. In 1988, White spoke before the President's Commission on the HIV Epidemic about the discrimination he faced while trying to return to school, emphasizing the importance of education about the disease. The stark contrast between his receptions in the towns of Kokomo and Cicero was an example of the power and importance of AIDS/HIV education.

What started as a plight to defend his right to go to school led to some of the greatest health policy and legislation to pass Congress in modern times. After his death in 1990, his mother began the Ryan White Foundation, which eventually was transformed into

AIDS Action, a nonprofit, advocacy-focused organization. Ryan White inspired others, such as Elton John, to open their own AIDS Foundations to raise money for research, treatment, education, and advocacy that would help in the fight against HIV/AIDS. Just 4 months after Ryan White's death, in 1990, Congress enacted the Ryan White Comprehensive AIDS Resources Emergency (CARE) Act. Simply known as the Ryan White CARE Act, it provides funding for programs and organizations to improve the availability of care for low-income, uninsured, and underinsured individuals diagnosed with HIV. Over 30 years later (and because of long-standing advocacy efforts), Ryan White programs are still the largest provider of services for people living with HIV/AIDS in the United States. To learn more about the Ryan White Care Act and programs, visit https://hab.hrsa.gov/livinghistory/voices.

Additional Reading

Health Resources and Services Administration. (February, 2022) Who was Ryan White? Ryan White HIV/AIDS Program. https://hab.hrsa.gov/about-ryan-white-hivaids-program/about-ryan-white-hivaids-program

Ryan White HIV/AIDS Program. (2020, December 2). *Celebrating 30 years*. Encyclopedia Britannica. https://www.britannica.com/biography/Ryan-White

U.S. Department of Health and Human Services. (2020, August 18, 2020). Celebrating 30 *years* of the Ryan White CARE Act. https://www.hhs.gov/about/news/2020/08/18/celebrating-30-years-of-ryan-white-care-act.html

Advocacy Terminology

Talking the Talk

HEIDI HANCHER-RAUCH AND JODI BROOKINS-FISHER

There are two primary choices in life: to accept conditions as they exist, or accept the responsibility for changing them.

—DENIS WAITLEY

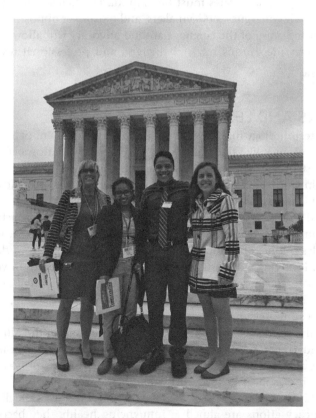

FIGURE 2.1 University of Indianapolis faculty and students at the 2018 SOPHE Health Advocacy Summit, including Heidi Hancher-Rauch, Yordanos Gebru, Shawn Schweitzer, and Megan Davish.

Heidi Hancher-Rauch and Jodi Brookins-Fisher, *Advocacy Terminology*. In: *Be the Change*. Edited by Keely S. Rees, Jody Early, and Cicily Hampton, Oxford University Press. © Oxford University Press 2023. DOI: 10.1093/oso/9780197570890.003.0002

Objectives

1. Define foundational terms such as advocacy, advocate, health advocacy, lobbying, lobbyist, stakeholder, coalition, legislative advocacy, and media advocacy.
2. Explain the difference between advocacy and lobbying.
3. Discuss examples of potential stakeholders for an advocacy initiative and how to find them.
4. Provide examples of ways advocates can connect with advocacy stakeholders at local, state, national, or international levels and communicate with them.
5. List examples of multiple advocacy organizations and agencies.
6. Consider ways to develop advocacy partnerships designed to achieve the advocacy goals.

INTRODUCTION

As discussed in Chapter 1, readers may now more fully understand the important nature of health advocacy and the professional imperative of regularly engaging in the skill. What may not have been considered, however, is the importance of utilizing the accurate and appropriate language associated with advocacy. Before it is possible to engage effectively in this space, advocates must first familiarize themselves with the common lexicon used by their colleagues, policymakers, and partner or opposition organizations. Developing a strong grasp of the language around advocacy will allow health advocates to better maneuver the various roles, challenges, and professional responsibilities of this skill.

DEFINITIONS AND LEXICON

Understanding terminology may seem like a mundane component of becoming a health advocate, but think of it like the placement of a home foundation before building the walls. The base structure (appropriate lexicon) needs to be in place in order to appropriately maintain sturdy walls (advocacy activities). One cannot provide the second part without the first—at least not for long.

As discussed in the first chapter, the term **advocacy** means "any action that speaks in favor of, recommends, argues for a cause, supports or defends, or pleads on behalf of others. It includes public education, regulatory work, litigation, and work before administrative bodies, lobbying, nonpartisan voter registration, nonpartisan voter education, and more." Health-related organizations may utilize slightly different definitions of the term, but the main components are the same. Advocacy involves trying to change something (a policy, a situation, an environment) by influencing the actions of those with the power to make the change. A very simple definition comes from the Alliance for Justice, which defined advocacy as **"making the case for your cause or mission"** (2021a, para. 1). For example, asking a course instructor to kindly review a quiz question because the student believes it was incorrectly graded would be an example of advocating. The student here is making a case (requesting the review) for their cause (a higher grade).

When advocacy efforts are aimed at influencing health, they become **health advocacy**. To bring this definition to life with a specific example, consider an advocacy task requested of students in a health policy and advocacy course. Through a partnership with a local Smoke Free chapter, students learned about the health outcomes and challenges around smoking rates in Indiana. As one of the states with the lowest tobacco taxation rate, nicotine delivery devices in the form of traditional cigarettes, electronic cigarettes, and vaping devices are low cost and relatively easy to acquire for adolescents in the state. For this reason, advocates have been seeking to raise the taxes on these devices for a number of years. Following the educational intervention, students were asked to contact their local legislators in the Indiana Statehouse to educate them about the negative health and economic outcomes associated with the high rates of tobacco use, then talk to them about the potential positive outcomes of raising the tobacco tax (fewer adolescents begin using, more people seek cessation, lower costs to state Medicaid coffers, etc.). Students were assigned the task of making a case (explaining positives of the tax increase and negatives of the current situation) for their cause (raising the tobacco tax in Indiana).

In the above explanation, the persuasive activities fall specifically into the category of advocacy because the advocates stopped at the point of educating policymakers and asking for the support of their cause. They did not ask legislators to vote a certain way on an active bill. If the advocates did take the step to request a specific vote or proposal of a specific bill, this activity would move into the category of *lobbying,* as we described in Chapter 1. The reason this distinction is important is that 501(c)(3) organizations (not-for-profit organizations) are not permitted by the Internal Revenue Service (IRS) to maintain their tax-exempt status if they spend a "substantial" amount of their time engaged in lobbying efforts, "attempting to influence legislation" (IRS, 2020, para. 1). This may seem confusing for the average person, but the difference is actually quite important for those who work within government agencies or nonprofit organizations. Though it is impossible to pin down exactly what they mean by "substantial," the definition of what the IRS includes in lobbying is quite clear: "An organization will be regarded as attempting to influence legislation if it contacts, or urges the public to contact, members or employees of a legislative body for the purpose of proposing, supporting, or opposing legislation, or if the organization advocates the adoption or rejection of legislation" (IRS, 2020, para. 3). Because of this statement, some individuals believe they are forbidden from engaging in lobbying or advocacy activities altogether. However, that is not the case at all. The IRS further states that: "Organizations may, however, involve themselves in issues of public policy without the activity being considered as lobbying. For example, organizations may conduct educational meetings, prepare and distribute educational materials, or otherwise consider public policy issues in an educational manner without jeopardizing their tax-exempt status" (IRS, 2020, para. 4). To summarize, organizations must be careful when engaging in lobbying activities, but are free to engage in as much advocacy as they wish. Individuals, working on their own time and with their own personal resources as a constituent, may legally participate in lobbying activities of their own volition unless specifically forbidden by their employers.

Now that the definitions of advocacy and lobbying are further clarified, it is helpful to define what makes someone an advocate or a lobbyist. A general misperception is that one must serve in these roles professionally or through a substantial amount of their time in order to fall into those categories. However, that is not the case. Technically, anyone engaging in the activities outlined as part of advocacy would be considered an **advocate**. The moment one signs their name to a petition requesting the university offer more mental health services for students or tries to convince a friend to stop vaping, they are serving in the role of an advocate. The same goes for acting as a lobbyist. When one calls their senator or sends them an email requesting they vote in support of the proposed bill requiring that at least 75% of the money collected from tobacco taxes be spent on public health issues, one is serving in the role of a *lobbyist*. Therefore, the definitions of the advocate or lobbyist are simply tied to the carrying out of the activities associated with advocacy or lobbying. All have the opportunity to serve in these roles, and should do so on a regular basis, regardless of whether they are part of specifically outlined job responsibilities.

FORMS OF ADVOCACY

Some, who are very passionate about their roles influencing societal change, may consider themselves activists. The difference between an advocate and an activist is somewhat limited, with some advocates unlikely to see the difference between what they do and the definition of **health activism** "efforts aimed at improving population health and challenging health inequities, whether directed at health systems or at social, economic, political, and environmental determinants of health" (Musolino et al., 2020, p. 2). The difference is that some consider activism a role involving more conflict or confrontation. For example, activism might include activities like civil disobedience, picketing, protests, or boycotts (Lee et al., 2013). Some individuals may be more comfortable in the advocacy realms of testifying before legislative committees, writing letters to policymakers, or educating decision makers on a health-related topic, but less comfortable with the more confrontational strategies of an activist. For that reason, it is important to know the difference between these two concepts.

From what has been read thus far, readers likely have picked up on the fact that health advocacy may take many different forms (Figure 2.1). For example, not all advocacy is aimed at the legislative branch of government; one may be working to encourage their employer to enforce a tobacco-free policy on organizational grounds (Figure 2.2). In this case, the advocacy is directed toward the decision makers of an individual organization. The difference between this and legislative advocacy is that **legislative advocacy** refers to "efforts to change policy through the legislative branch of government such as Congress, local statehouses, or city councils. This may include lobbying in support or opposition to a bill, the crafting of new legislative language, writing amendments to existing bills, or encouraging others to contact their legislators" (Alliance for Justice, 2021b, para 43). So, to be clear, the target of the advocacy efforts (in this case the legislative branch of government) is what determines whether the efforts are termed legislative advocacy.

Another key tool for advocacy is the use of media advocacy. Recent history has demonstrated clearly the importance of a strong media presence in helping to sway the minds of individuals, especially via the use of social media. Skilled advocates rely on both traditional mass media and the newer routes of social media to widely share their messages. The skills used in **media advocacy** blend expertise in health communication,

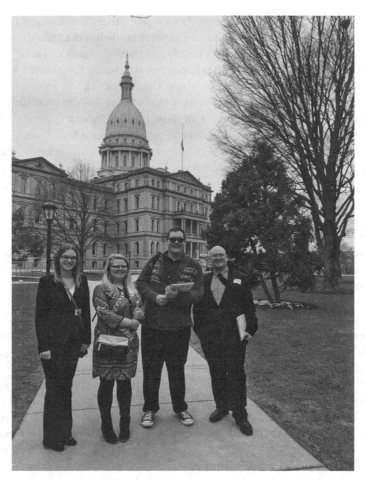

FIGURE 2.2 Central Michigan University MPH students advocating for tobacco control legislation at the Michigan State capitol.

politics, and health advocacy in order to strategically "use mass media to support community organizing and advance healthy public policy" (Dorfman & Krasnow, 2014, p. 294). Media advocacy is used by writing letters to the editor of a local newspaper, conducting interviews on the issue with a local news station, writing an op-ed for an online news service, or through posting information on social media outlets like Twitter, Facebook, TikTok, or Instagram. A combination of all these methods may be used to reach the largest audience, including the constituents advocates would like to put pressure on lawmakers or the lawmakers themselves. Just remember that the same rules that apply to in-person advocacy and lobbying also apply in the media format. Keep this in mind while learning more about media advocacy in Chapter 12.

Before beginning to practice the new advocacy skills learned in this text, there are a few more definitions to consider: coalition(s) and stakeholder(s). These were saved until last because they are two of the most important advocacy terms. Advocates are much more successful in their endeavors when they engage others and make sure to bring the most important partners to the table. Most simply, a **coalition** is a "group of two or more organizations that are working together jointly on a specific issue or cause" (Alliance for Justice, 2021b, para. 19). For example, when advocates across the country began seeking to raise the legal age for purchasing tobacco products from 18 to 21 years, they formed a broad coalition from a long list of supporters that included Campaign for Tobacco-Free Kids, the American Heart Association, American Cancer Society, American Academy of Pediatrics, and American Medical Association, just to name a few. With the support of multiple organizations, the coalition was able to successfully advocate for the passage of the nationwide Tobacco 21 bill that was signed into law on December 20, 2019. Readers will find additional details and examples of coalitions in upcoming chapters.

STAKEHOLDERS AND OPPONENTS

Finally, advocates need to know that they never will be successful without bringing the correct stakeholders to the table. In the case of advocacy efforts, a **stakeholder** is a "person, group, organization, or system who affects or can be affected by an advocacy or organizing action" (Alliance for Justice, 2021b, para. 62). Many advocates have learned the hard way that it can be deadly to the cause to overlook one or more important stakeholders potentially impacted by the changes they sought. When considering the perspectives of stakeholders, always remember to consider those who might be positively impacted by the sought public health change, but never forget those who might believe they could be negatively impacted. Those who potentially could fight against the advocacy goals are considered **opponents**, and advocates must work tirelessly to neutralize their power. For example, the Tobacco 21 advocates pulled together lists of possible opponents and their reasons for potential opposition. They were then able to try persuading opponents (e.g., convenience stores) concerned about the possible fines for selling to those underage and potential declines in their profits (Tobacco 21, n.d.). When opponents are unable to be persuaded to support an issue, advocates still must educate themselves regarding the concerns of the opponents and develop talking points designed to counter the possible attacks of those stakeholders. Remember, all stakeholders have the potential to either support or oppose the cause of the advocates, but always pay special attention to **stakeholders with power**—those who are able to quickly and efficiently organize people and organize money to support their point of view or wishes (Alliance for Justice, 2021b). For example, it took advocates years to overcome the immense power of the main stakeholders preventing serious tobacco policy change in this country–the tobacco companies themselves. Utilizing some of the strategies discussed in the next section is how advocates stayed the course and eventually had significant success.

As mentioned above, stakeholders are key to achieving advocacy efforts. Successful advocates understand how important it is to engage stakeholders from the very beginning and throughout the entire process. As advocates build their coalitions, it is helpful to brainstorm all the potential stakeholders who may either support or oppose their work. Stakeholders can be individuals, agencies, or organizations at the local, state, national, and international levels. The stakeholders engaged in any particular advocacy effort depend on the message and reach. Knowing who those stakeholders are and developing an alliance between the health advocacy organization and important community stakeholders can make the difference between success and failure of an initiative.

For example, if the advocacy goal is to change a city policy to be inclusive of LGBTQ+ individuals (lesbian, gay, bisexual, transgender, and queer; the plus sign indicates an all-encompassing representation of sexual orientation and gender identities) and offer them equal rights in a community, the advocacy effort to get this policy passed would not need to include stakeholders at the national or international levels. Perhaps state-level agencies and organizations would be used on a consultation basis, but mostly the stakeholders would be local—those most impacted by the proposed policy. Who might be included as stakeholders in this particular case? For a similar policy effort in Mount Pleasant, Michigan, stakeholders included the Mt. Pleasant Area Diversity Group; Unitarian Universalist Fellowship of Central Michigan; other local liberal faith groups; Isabella County Human Rights Commission; Spectrum (a gay/straight alliance of the local university); 35 local businesses; various community leaders; and various university student, faculty, and administration leaders. All advocacy efforts need someone who will lead the way, and this policy effort was corralled by Dr. Norma Bailey, then a local university professor and social justice activist. The opposition included several individuals who spoke against the ordinance, including representatives of local conservative faith groups. After much preparation, presentations, and debate (the ordinance was officially proposed in November 2011), the Human Rights Ordinance was passed on July 9, 2012.

Sometimes advocacy efforts are better served at the state level, in which a policy can affect all localities within the state. In this case, the many stakeholders included could come from both state and local levels to support advocacy. Even national individuals and organizations could be involved as consultants to the effort. A wonderful example of an organization working hard to change health outcomes utilizing advocacy efforts in Indiana is the Indiana Minority Health Coalition (IMHC). As of early 2021, Indiana ranked as the third-worst state in the United States for maternal mortality rates and seventh worst for infant mortality rates (World Population Review, 2021). In order to address these significant public health concerns, IMHC worked with a range of stakeholders, including the Department of Health, Family, and Social Services Administration; legislators; doulas around the state (trained coaches who provide support to women during pregnancy, labor, and/or breastfeeding); and pregnant women themselves to advocate for the coverage of doula services through Medicaid. Working with these stakeholders was key to overcoming the opposition they faced from some clinicians, hospitals, and legislators who feared an encroachment on the practice of physicians, had concerns over the financial price tag, or just lacked an understanding of doula services. As a result of their hard work, Senate Bill 416 Medicaid Coverage for Doula Services passed both chambers and was signed into law by the Indiana governor in April 2019. This was a major success, but the work of IMHC is a great example of advocates' work not being done with the signing of legislation. Into 2021, the organization continued advocacy efforts around getting funding for the bill that passed but was provided no budget for implementation. As of this writing, IMHC is working with National Health Law and the Indiana General Assembly on integrating doula services into regular maternal service options, as well as expanding Medicaid to provide a full year of postpartum coverage in order to reduce maternal and infant mortality rates in the state. Because of the incredible advocacy efforts of the IMHC policy and advocacy team to support this legislation, Indiana is being looked to as a leader in expanding doula services as a public health measure.

Since most public health laws, policies, and regulations happen at the state level due to the design of the Constitution, when advocacy efforts happen at the national level, it is a health issue that organizations and passionate individuals feel is needed due to research, assessment data, and the topic's magnitude. Firearm prevention policies often fall into this type of advocacy reach. Due to the mass shootings that have impacted families and communities across the United States, national organizations have sprung up to advocate for policy change. Organizations, such as Moms Demand Action for Gun Sense in America, the Brady Campaign, and Coalition to Stop Gun Violence, work with state and local organizations, church groups, and state- and federal-level policymakers to put forth an agenda aimed at making our communities safer from needless firearm violence. Their efforts range from supporting or opposing individual policymakers in elections, to fixing the loopholes in current legislation, and to achieving equity in who is affected most by gun violence.

An example of firearm prevention advocacy at the national level includes the organization Everytown for Gun Safety (Everytown). Everytown is a nationwide nonprofit organization that conducts gun safety research, provides education and data regarding gun violence and its prevention, promotes policy for evidence-based common sense gun safety, and coordinates the volunteer and mobilization areas of the group: Moms Demand Action, Students Demand Action, and the Everytown Survivor Network (Figure 2.3; Everytown, 2021). This organization is an example of a large and powerful coalition that grew from the idea of one suburban Indiana mom, Shannon Watts, who was horrified by the shootings at Sandy Hook Elementary in December 2012 and decided to do something about it. Her initial advocacy and fundraising efforts have grown into the issues and solutions–based organization that exists now, with mobilized volunteers in every state of the nation. They have become the experts in connecting with stakeholders at the local, state, and federal levels to speak out against policies that are not supported by scientific evidence as being likely to reduce gun violence. They also work diligently to help legislators propose and mobilize stakeholders to support policies based on evidence to reduce gun violence. Strategies advocates can utilize to build these types of important relationships with stakeholders are described more thoroughly in Chapter 10.

Advocacy at the international level seems so vast and broad it would be almost impossible to achieve success, yet much success has been achieved over the years. These efforts include international organizations and agencies, like the World Health Organization; foundations whose mission is to work on global health issues; different countries' investment in advocacy efforts abroad; and committed individuals to follow through with changes needed. For example, many organizations worked together on global advocacy efforts for immunizations to eradicate smallpox from Earth. Currently, the Bill and Melinda Gates Foundation is working to improve gender equity around the globe, as research shows when women are valued and supported, the health and welfare of every community increases. The Bill and Melinda Gates Foundation works with stakeholders

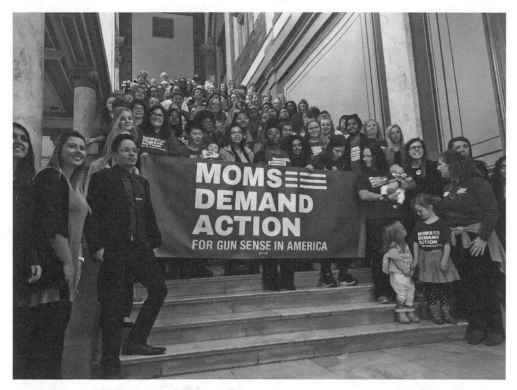

FIGURE 2.3 University of Indianapolis faculty and students join Moms Demand Action for their lobby day at the Indiana Statehouse in 2019.

from different continents and in local communities to make change happen and have demonstrated success (Gates, 2019).

Last, do not forget the most important stakeholder in any advocacy effort: the people or populations that it is intended to affect or help. These individuals should be central to all efforts and their advocacy ideas should be included to ensure efforts lead to empowerment, engagement, and ownership of the affected community. Also, keep in mind that advocacy does not happen in a vacuum or silo. When thinking about planning and implementation of advocacy efforts, other entities probably have advocated for a similar health issue in the past. Find out who their stakeholders were and how they went about engaging them, while answering any opponents along the way. Connecting with stakeholders for any advocacy effort requires thoughtful planning and engaging with each stakeholder about the advocacy effort. See Advocacy in Action Box 2.1 on tips for connecting and engaging with stakeholders.

ORGANIZATIONS THAT ENGAGE IN ADVOCACY

Advocacy is everywhere, but at the same time, it can be difficult to determine more formal avenues for advocacy efforts at the local, state, and national levels. Professional

BOX 2.1	Advocacy in Action Box 2.1

Tips for Connecting and Engaging With Stakeholders

- **Identify Stakeholders:** Remember these should include all agencies (community-based organizations; nongovernmental organizations); community champions (those who have influence, power, and/or money and those who will be working boots on the ground for the advocacy effort); the affected individuals and/or groups; and even opposition.
- **Build Relationships:** Advocacy efforts can take an enormous amount of time, and establishing trusting relationships with the individuals and agencies involved is important to keep them on target, motivated, and passionate about the cause.
- **Educate and Inform Stakeholders:** Make sure all individuals and groups involved are on the same page with the advocacy plan. Each should know the mission, goals, and activities of the advocacy effort and be involved in all steps of the process.

- **Set Expectations:** Each individual or group should know the overall plan for the advocacy effort and their individual contributions or tasks in order to achieve success.
- **Evaluate Advocacy Efforts:** Ensure that each stakeholder is meaningfully contributing to the advocacy effort; have honest conversations about progress and how efforts can be amplified. Also, be sure to publicize the advocacy's evaluation results to give credibility to the process and keep stakeholders aware of and invested in the effort.
- **Praise Successes:** To keep stakeholders passionate and motivated, praise the small wins toward bigger goals. Let people know that their work is moving the advocacy effort along and publicly share these successes.

Adapted from The INS Group. (n.d.). Engaging stakeholders as brand advocates (https://www.theinsgroup.com/engaging-stakeholders-as-brand-advocates/, retrieved February 12, 2021; and Centers for Disease Control and Prevention, Program Performance and Evaluation Office (2012), retrieved February 20, 2021.

organizations, nonprofit organizations, industry groups, and unions or worker groups are just some examples of organizations that engage in advocacy efforts. Finding organizations with similar advocacy goals to personal interests will help to better determine where to spend one's time and energy and even which organizations to support with membership and dues.

Public health education membership organizations regularly engage in advocacy efforts regarding issues that are important to their membership. National organizations, such as the Society for Public Health Education and American Public Health Association regularly advocate with policymakers on issues that membership has determined to be important through resolutions. These are often crafted in a smaller committee and then approved by an organization's board of directors. Resolutions give the organization's beliefs and stance on a health issue and give action steps about how the organization will better advocate for the issue. These are shared with membership and affiliates that exist on the state or local level. This way, advocacy can happen within and between all levels of public health education, and action steps can be enacted to affect the health issue of interest. As a separate, but related, organization, the National Commission on Health Education Credentialing also is interested in advocacy efforts at the local, state, and national levels as it is the credentialing party that formulates advocacy responsibilities and competencies for health education specialists. It is within the scope of this body to determine what individuals credentialed as a certified health education specialist or master certified health education specialist must be able to perform regarding advocacy in order to meet professional standards. In the same way, the National Board of Public Health Examiners is interested in advocacy for those credentialed as certified in public health. All of the above-mentioned organizations assist health education specialists with advocacy skills and training through continuing education, such as webinars, conference presentations, and experiential learning through meeting with policymakers.

Nonprofit organizations also advocate for issues within their purview and make excellent advocacy partners at the local, state, and national levels. Many of these agencies (community-based organizations, nongovernmental organizations) are designed around a singular health issue and can meet the demands of advocacy as part of their mission. Often, advocacy is central to their workload. Agencies such as the Michigan Association of Local Public Health, the Indiana Minority Health Coalition, Prevention Institute, and Advocates for Youth all advocate for health issues. Nonprofit agencies also exist in local communities, so it is important to know their structure and function and how they work to advance important health issues through advocacy efforts.

Industry groups, such as the American Hospital Association, American Lung Association, and American Cancer Society, all advocate for specific health issues that are important to reduce morbidity and mortality and increase the well-being of communities and the nation. They might also be involved in advocating at systemic levels, such as the quality, cost, and accessibility of healthcare; how to best distribute vaccines in a pandemic; or ensuring quality service during a hospital stay or clinic visit.

Many clubs are linked to chapters across the country. Groups like the Lions Club, Rotary Club, and others have members who work on local and larger health issues. For example, the Rotary Club made part of its mission to help eliminate polio from Earth. These organizations, and their passionate members, can be a home to those looking to localize their advocacy efforts outside of work and to connect with like-minded people in home communities. For example, a local Rotary Club in Mount Pleasant, Michigan, embraced the vision of its national organization to eradicate polio. Members who worked at the local university connected with the chapter sponsor of Eta Sigma Gamma to engage students in polio education during the club's events. Gammans also helped cohost events for students at the university that were designed to bring a heightened awareness about polio and how close world efforts were to eliminating its existence. These types of efforts across the country helped to make the United States a primary stakeholder in minimizing the spread of this horrific disease. Success would not have happened at the same level if members of Rotary Club did not buy into the vision and purpose and advocate with other public health professionals and organizations.

Unions and worker groups also advocate, usually on behalf of their members for their members' benefit. They bargain within work environments to advocate for worker health issues, such as safer working conditions and better healthcare coverage. One good example of this can be witnessed by the work of the United University Professions (UUP), which is the union representing the faculty and staff of the entire State University of New York (SUNY) system, also the largest higher education union in the United States (UUP, 2021b). During the COVID-19 global pandemic, the UUP worked with SUNY statewide leadership to ensure the health and safety of their workers through the offering of surveillance testing, new telecommuting options, and edits to their promotion expectations in order to alleviate some of the mental stress experienced by workers (Pittsley, 2020). As a result of their efforts, the SUNY Cortland campus reported as of December 2020 that not a single employee had been hospitalized or died as a result of COVID (Harms, 2020). In addition, the union posted recommendations for safe reengagement on their campuses in spring 2021, as outlined in their "United University Professions— Guidelines for Spring 2021 Return: Keeping Our Campuses Safe During the COVID-19 Pandemic" (UUP, 2021a). Documents such as this help ensure the concerns of employees are heard by administrators setting campus policies. The work of the UUP is a great example of how worker groups can successfully advocate for the health and safety of company employees.

Advocates also spring from their place of employment, often due to remarkable discoveries in their ordinary, everyday tasks. In these cases, they may be advocates as whistleblowers in a particular workplace or situation. Think of the Flint (Michigan) water crisis (Figure 2.4). This horrific tragedy, which affected mainly lower income and Black individuals and families within the city, was caused by changing the main water source from the Detroit to the Flint River. There were several occasions when this catastrophe could have been prevented or lessened by environmental health professionals and those appointed to the city's leadership by the governor at the time, but no one questioned the change in water supply. It took a courageous pediatrician, who noticed some developmental and other health concerns among her patients, to research more deeply into their causes and find that the lead-tainted water was the culprit. Dr. Mona Hanna-Attisha spent years investing her time and talents, often questioned by others and questioning herself, to determine the water supply was the cause and to this day advocates on behalf of Flint children to ensure they get the resources they need for their long-term health issues.

ADVOCACY PARTNERSHIPS

Like most endeavors in life, advocacy efforts will get further with partners. Collaborating with other agencies, organizations, and individuals through informal or formal partnerships, like coalitions, will help develop a unified message regarding the advocacy issue. There also will be strength in numbers, which is key in getting further reach for an advocacy message.

Connecting with local, regional, and national partners will help keep the advocacy effort at the forefront of multiple agendas and will keep key stakeholders engaged in the many efforts made to advocate for an issue. One good example of this in Indiana is the Top 10 Coalition. This coalition began in 2012 after representatives from a group of public health agencies, convened by the YMCA of Greater Indianapolis, originally got together to address poor health in central Indiana. After reviewing the Annual American Fitness Index produced by the American College of Sports Medicine, the group was distressed by the poor ranking of the metropolitan area surrounding Indianapolis and

Flint Water Crisis
Michigan – 2016

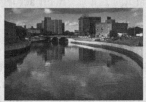

View of the Flint River in Flint, MI. Credit: U.S. Army Corps of Engineers

What was the need?

On April 25, 2014, the City of Flint, Michigan changed their municipal water supply source from the Detroit-supplied Lake Huron water to the Flint River. The switch caused water distribution pipes to corrode and leach lead and other contaminants into municipal drinking water. In October 2016, Flint residents were advised not to drink the municipal tap water unless it had been filtered through a NSF International approved filter certified to remove lead. Although the city reconnected to the original Detroit water system that same month, the potential damage was already done and a state of emergency was declared on January 16, 2016.

What were the objectives?

In addition to likely health effects from lead exposure, there were concerns about behavioral health of Flint residents, including feelings of anxiety or depression and substance abuse. To assess these concerns, we[1] conducted a Community Assessment for Public Health Emergency Response (CASPER) in May 2016 evaluating the following city-wide:

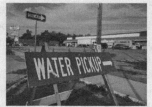

Water pickup sign in Flint, MI. Credit: USDA

- Behavioral and physical health concerns for adults (21+ years old) and children (less than 21 years old) in each household
- Household access to behavioral health services and barriers to access
- Resources used for water-related needs and barriers to access
- How community members were getting information about the crisis

KEY RESULTS

- 66% of households reported one or more adult members reported experiencing at least one behavioral health issue "more than usual"
- 54% of households reported that at least one child experienced at least one behavioral health issue "more than usual"
- 22.5% of households reporting difficulties getting access to behavioral health services
- 34% of individuals self-reported symptoms of anxiety and 29% self-reported symptoms of depression
- 51% of households felt that the physical health of at least one member had worsened due to Flint water crisis

What was the outcome?

Based on the results, federal, state, and local government and community health partners could guide their ongoing recovery efforts through focused behavioral health interventions and communication messages.

Data from the CASPER supported the need for continued mental health services along with five-year follow-up activities by the Substance Abuse and Mental Health Services Administration (SAMHSA) aimed to promote resilience in the Flint community.

These activities aim to support youth and their families, alleviate the impact of trauma, reduce behavioral health disparities, and increase opportunities and training for Flint's youth through strong community engagement[2].

Where can I find more information?

The CASPER report on the Flint Water Crisis is available online at https://www.cdc.gov/nceh/hsb/disaster/casper/docs/flint_mi_casper_report_508.pdf

[1] The Flint Community Resilience Group, Michigan Department of Health and Human Services, Genesee County Health Department, Genesee Health System, University of Michigan–Flint, and Centers for Disease Control and Prevention conducted the CASPER
[2] https://www.cityofflint.com/2016/10/11/flint-awarded-5-year-nearly-5-million-samhsa-grant-for-trauma-informed-care-in-flint/

National Center for Environmental Health
Division of Environmental Health Science and Practice

FIGURE 2.4 Overview of the 2016 water crisis in Flint, Michigan.

decided to do something about it. Over the next couple of years, leaders at the YMCA of Greater Indianapolis diligently worked to bring together experts from all across the region to discuss and begin tackling the most pertinent health issues facing the city. The original goal was to get Indianapolis into the top 10 healthiest cities on the rankings by 2020, thus the Top 10 name of the group. Though the goal has not yet been achieved, the group currently consists of 115 coalition partners and five work teams addressing the leading health indicators for the region in order to decrease the burden of chronic disease and develop a culture of health in Central Indiana by focusing on: "improving the built environment, increasing access to safe physical activity, increasing access to better nutrition, and promoting smoke free air and tobacco cessation" (Top 10 Coalition, n.d., para. 1). Realizing that establishing a *Health in All Policies* approach to policymaking is a key to changing the culture of health in the region, the group has a policy committee in charge of tracking bill proposals in the Indiana Statehouse and at the Indianapolis City Council, issuing resolutions on important health issues, sending action alerts to coalition members, providing policy updates to the entire coalition via the newsletter, and much more. This active committee is a great example of a way a large coalition can bring together the appropriate members to make sure advocacy actions are fulfilled.

Keep in mind that building partnerships and coalitions around advocacy goals will greatly increase the chances of success. When considering the best partners to bring to the table, critical thinking helps advocates consider how multiple agencies might work together in an advocacy effort; there might be an agency out there that is currently unknown that might be able to assist in creative ways!!! Using preestablished professional and personal networks can help advocates discover new and unique coalition partners. Don't forget to keep a running list of community agencies engaged in various types of advocacy related to health advocacy. This can be a great tool to draw on when considering partnership opportunities.

CONCLUSION

Advocacy efforts require many skills to be effective and efficient and eventually demonstrate success. These efforts, however, cannot be realized if those involved (you!) aren't fully aware of the lexicon involved in the process. In order to engage in effective advocacy, you will need to be able to "speak the language" of advocacy and be skilled in using that language to bring partners to the table. Knowing how to use the language of advocacy also helps ensure that there is a common language that's utilized by myriad diverse stakeholders when engaging in the advocacy efforts. This can help bring some consistency and professionalism to the process and keep advocacy efforts moving forward. Once these fundamental terms are understood, an advocate may feel more prepared to begin connecting with other individuals and organizations to further the advocacy process.

REFERENCES

Bolder Advocacy. (2021a). *Advocacy defined.* https://bolderadvocacy.org/advocacy-defined/

Bolder Advocacy. (2021b). *Terminology.* https://bolderadvocacy.org/resource-library/terminology/

Dorfman, L., & Krasnow, I. (2014). Public health and media advocacy. *Annual Review of Public Health, 35,* 293–306. https://www.annualreviews.org/doi/pdf/10.1146/annurev-publhealth-032013-182503

Everytown for Gun Safety. (2021). *Home page.* https://everytown.org/

Gates, M. (2019). *The moment of lift: How empowering women changes the world.* Flatiron Books.

Harms, D. (2020, December). Winter is coming: COVID-19 at Cortland. *Cortland Cause, 53*(1), 6.

Internal Revenue Service. (2020). *Lobbying.* https://www.irs.gov/charities-non-profits/lobbying

Lee, M., Smith, T., & Henry, R. (2013). Power politics: Advocacy to activism in social justice counseling. *Journal for Social Action in Counseling and Psychology, 5*(3), 70–94.

Musolino, C., Baum, F., Freeman, T., Labonté, R., Bodini, C., & Sanders, D. (2020). Global health activists' lessons on building social movements for Health for All. *International Journal for Equity in Health, 19,* 116. https://doi.org/10.1186/s12939-020-01232-1

Pittsley, J. (2020, December). What it is. *Cortland Cause, 53*(1), 1–3.

Tobacco Twenty-One. (n.d.). *Endorsements.* https://tobacco21.org/endorsements/

Top 10 Coalition. (n.d.). *Advocacy.* http://top10in.org/advocacy/

United University Professions. (2021a). *COVID-19 resources page.* https://uupinfo.org/resources/covid19/

United University Professions. (2021b). *Who are we? UUP!* https://uupinfo.org/history/whoweare.php

World Population Review. (2021). *State rankings: Infant mortality.* https://worldpopulationreview.com/state-rankings/infant-mortality-rate-by-state

CHAPTER 2: END-OF-CHAPTER ACTIVITIES

DISCUSSION QUESTIONS

1. How would you describe your own advocacy? Which organizations have you worked with to further advocacy efforts regarding a health issue? If you haven't yet been an advocate, how can you increase your skills to become involved?

2. What are the health advocacy agencies in your geographical area? How can you become involved with them?

3. If you were advocating for pandemic planning at the local level, which stakeholders would you include from your geographical area?

4. What is one nonprofit organization in your area that you could seek assistance from if planning advocacy efforts for gun violence prevention? How might you elicit help from national organizations?

5. What are four ways to advocate for change on a public health issue?

APPLICATION EXERCISES

1. Using the American Public Health Association website provided below under Additional Resources, find a public health issue for which there is an advocacy effort. Determine which local and state agencies you'd solicit to join the advocacy efforts for that health issue.

2. In a small group, brainstorm a list of public health issues that you could discuss with your local or state policymakers. Select one from the list and set up an advocacy plan for meeting with that legislator. What would you include? What would you say? Provide information backed with scientifically based research, facts, and literature.

3. This chapter discussed the Flint water crisis in Michigan and the importance of advocacy in bringing attention to this public health issue . However, Flint isn't the only city in the United States to experience drinking water problems. What other municipalities, towns, and cities in the United States can you find with drinking water problems? How are these areas advocating for improvements? Who are the stakeholders involved?

4. You are starting a coalition to address the infant mortality rate in your local and surrounding communities. List three agencies you'd want to include and explain why they would make appropriate allies or stakeholders.

5. List one public health issue that you are passionate about and discuss three ways you can advocate for that issue.

6. Find an example of an international public health issue that included advocacy efforts. Who were the stakeholders? Where were these stakeholders located? How did they work together for change?

ADDITIONAL RESOURCES

American Public Health Association. (n.d.). *Advocacy activities.* http://www.apha.org/policies-and-advocacy/advocacy-for-public-health/advocacy-activities

Community Guide. (n.d.). *Home page.* https://www.thecommunityguide.org/

County Health Rankings. (n.d.). *Home page.* https://www.countyhealthrankings.org

Federal government:

U.S. House of Representatives. (n.d.). *Home page.* https://www.house.gov

U.S. Senate. (n.d.). *Home page.* https://www.senate.gov

The White House. (n.d.). *Home page.* https://www.whitehouse.gov

Research America. (n.d.). *Home page.* http://www.researchamerica.org

Society for Public Health Education. (n.d.). *Advocating for public health.* https://www.sophe.org/advocacy

Trust for America's Health. (n.d.). *Home page.* https://www.tfah.org

Community Tool Box. (n.d.). *Home page.* University of Kansas. http://ctb.ku.edu/en

QUIZ QUESTIONS

1. When starting a local advocacy effort, which of the following is true?
   a. Find many state-level agencies to work on the local effort
   b. Determine which national agencies will give funding
   c. Include all local stakeholders who are interested in the issue
   d. Find international organizations that want to join

2. Which of the following is not true when advocating for change?
   a. Set the advocacy goals and objectives without input
   b. Find stakeholders in the community to champion the effort
   c. Determine the opposition and be prepared for their arguments
   d. Celebrate small successes with those involved

3. Which of the following is not true when distinguishing advocating from lobbying?
   a. Lobbying cannot be done by those in governmental positions.
   b. Advocating cannot be done by those in governmental positions.
   c. Lobbying includes the specifics of a piece of legislation to influence policymaker decisions.
   d. Advocating includes background information about public health issues.

4. Which of the following is NOT true if you work for a nonprofit organization and want to personally participate in a candidate's campaign for elected office?
   a. You can't work on a campaign if you work for a nonprofit organization.
   b. You must participate on your own time.
   c. You must use your own materials, including cell phone and computer.
   d. You need to ensure it doesn't conflict with any stated policies and procedures of your work organization.

5. Which of the following are true of advocacy?
   a. It is a process that uses a certain bill number to get change on a public health issue.
   b. It cannot be done by those who work for agencies with governmental funding.
   c. It is any action that speaks in favor of, recommends, argues for a cause, supports or defends, or pleads on behalf of others.
   d. All of the above are true about advocacy.

6. An advocate is someone who
   a. works for an agency to influence specific legislation.
   b. works toward change.
   c. is paid to work toward change on a public health issue.
   d. all of the above are true about advocacy.

7. Efforts to change policy through the legislative branch of government, such as Congress, local state houses, or city councils, is known as
   a. media advocacy
   b. lobbying
   c. politics
   d. legislative advocacy

8. Strategically using mass media to support community organizing and advance healthy public policy is known as
   a. media advocacy
   b. lobbying
   c. politics
   d. legislative advocacy

9. A group of two or more organizations that are working together jointly on a specific issue or cause is known as
   a. stakeholders
   b. a coalition
   c. advocacy
   d. lobbying

10. A person, group, organization, or system that affects or can be affected by an advocacy or organizing action is known as a(n)
    a. stakeholder
    b. coalition
    c. advocate
    d. lobbyist

ANSWER KEY
1. **C.** Include all local stakeholders who are interested in the issue
2. **A.** Set the advocacy goals and objectives without input
3. **B.** Advocating cannot be done by those in governmental positions.
4. **A.** You can't work on a campaign if you work for a nonprofit organization.

5. **C.** It is any action that speaks in favor of, recommends, argues for a cause, supports or defends, or pleads on behalf of others.
6. **B.** works toward change
7. **D.** legislative advocacy
8. **A.** media advocacy
9. **B.** a coalition
10. **A.** stakeholder

Everyday Opportunities for Advocacy

KEELY S. REES, AMY J. THOMPSON, AND EMILY WHITNEY

How wonderful it is that nobody need wait a single
moment to improve the world.

—ANNE FRANK

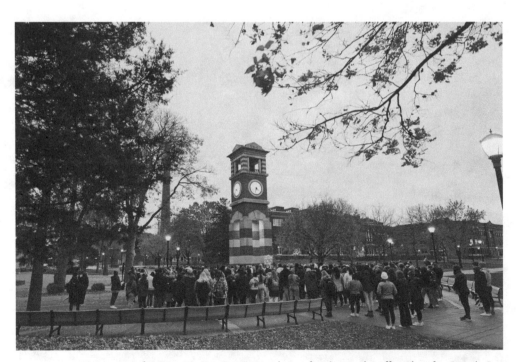

FIGURE 3.1 University of Wisconsin–La Crosse students, faculty, and staff gather for Speak Out
and Support Sexual Assault Survivors, fall 2021.

Source: University Communications, University of Wisconsin–La Crosse.

Keely S. Rees, Amy J. Thompson, and Emily Whitney, *Everyday Opportunities for Advocacy*. In: *Be the Change*. Edited by Keely S. Rees,
Jody Early, and Cicily Hampton, Oxford University Press. © Oxford University Press 2023. DOI: 10.1093/oso/9780197570890.003.0003

Objectives

1. Describe how health professionals engage in informal versus formal advocacy efforts.
2. Recognize the changing elements of public health advocacy skills.
3. Describe skills health advocates will need depending on the setting.
4. Identify local or national health advocates.
5. Develop your skills to become an emerging leader in the advocacy field.

INTRODUCTION

Advocacy works in tandem with policy development and implementation. While we fully address public health policy work in Chapter 6, it is important to see how policies affect our daily life through advocacy activities. We are often told that policy and advocacy initiatives take days and often decades to see the fruits of all the labor. While it can take time to see outcomes or results, it is the everyday actions and small decisions that have significant impacts. Advocacy ideally should become a part of our daily personal and professional identity. The policy and advocacy work that public health professionals engage in will vary depending on the setting, type of organization you work for, and the health issues in focus.

Historically, many health issues are siloed or even politicized and not viewed as an area deemed appropriate for health professionals to engage in policy work. In the last decade, issues such as climate change, gun violence, and fair housing are examples of complicated, multifaceted health concerns that public health organizations and individuals have shed much light on in the nation. Health-promoting organizations and professionals advocate for many different issues, and it takes us working together with many different groups and individuals to create positive change. You each have your own passion areas of health, personal health experiences, and corners of local, state, and global health work where you will make your mark. It is incumbent on health professionals to garner skill sets and practice everyday advocacy efforts that lead to the little p and big P policy changes in our communities (Box 3.1). While one-time or one-shot advocacy activities are certainly important, they need to become part of the day-to-day responsibilities of the profession, be performed on a regular basis (Hancher-Rauch et al., 2020), and build momentum for an issue or health area to really see the outcome necessary.

ENGAGING IN ADVOCACY

Engaging in advocacy may seem overwhelming to many health professionals, but the opportunities and topic areas are truly limitless. Advocacy work is where we make a difference on a daily basis. Advocacy work becomes part of the day-to-day responsibilities in the profession and performed on a regular basis (NCHEC & SOPHE, 2020). When first engaged in advocacy work, you will work hard to find your voice. It is important for you to have everyday opportunities to practice advocacy. Advocates need to learn how to identify current and emerging issues, how to access high-quality advocacy resources, and

| ADVOCACY IN ACTION BOX 3.1 | Everyday Advocate Exercise |

Title: Where Is the Advocate? (also known as Where Is Waldo?)

Description: Advocate scavenger hunt (can be completed with a partner or individually).

Objectives: To identify health advocates at the local, state, and national levels; to analyze where they are "doing" the advocacy work, who they are, and what impacts or outcomes you observe.

Use: Your institution's academic library, Google, Google Scholar, Twitter, Instagram, or Facebook.

Choose an area of health that interests you and your partner (i.e., clean water, distracted driving, depression, Tobacco 21, or teen pregnancy—you chose!).

Once you have chosen your health topic:

- Explore WHO are the advocates. If you are unsure who to research, look to your state or national professional organizations. Who are the leaders, board members, executive directors, and coordinators? What names keep showing up in your searches with that health topic?

- Determine WHERE they are conducting this advocacy work. For example, what are the different settings or levels (local, state, national) or what agency or professional organization is involved?

- Observe WHAT outcomes these advocates write about, share, and evaluate.

Hint: Here are some key advocates in our profession to look for on social media if you are stuck: Look up Dr. Amy Thompson's scholarly work around Tobacco 21. What are some of her key areas of advocacy? Or, examine Dr. Tyler James's work on accessibility or Morgan Drexler's advocacy relating to preventing impaired driving.

how to tailor messages for the intended audience. This type of informal advocacy occurs most often on local and interpersonal levels.

Informal advocacy may happen telephonically, be web based, include social media messaging, or sharing stories in various settings (e.g., face to face with family and those in your social networks). There are many examples of informal advocacy right in your community or campus. You might see get out the vote campaigns, tabling events or health fairs, visual advocacy in the form of ribbon campaigns, walks/runs, speaker events, and so many other opportunities. **Everyday** (informal) **advocacy** can also be described as "biting off small pieces" and can look like a lot of small advocacy acts you engage in daily or throughout your week. These small acts of advocacy lead to the bigger campaigns and planned strategies to initiate legislation, adopt a policy at city level, or create a national movement to stop human trafficking (Figure 3.1).

A person who engages in these smaller but important advocacy strategies is what we term an **everyday advocate**. An everyday advocate engages in acts of consistent interpersonal advocacy in their local or regional areas, which then can contribute to larger, systemic efforts. For example, everyday advocates might respond to a legislative alert and send an email to their local representative about a policy up for a vote. Or, they may help others around them better understand an issue and show them where to find credible information about that issue. An everyday advocate could cast a vote at the ballot box or help others get a ride to the polls. Everyday advocates who engage in these types of informal advocacy are all around us. Whom do you see as an everyday advocate in your group or community?

What have you noticed on your campus, community, or workplace in terms of informal advocacy?

Conversely, formal advocacy builds on these informal opportunities and may have an impact on a larger scale (Figure 3.2). Formal advocacy may involve your role as a professional within an organization, representing an initiative or legislation, and not just your personal, private efforts to do so. Formal advocacy leads to advocacy and policy at local or national levels, with the intent of making lasting change that impacts more people. Formal advocacy is further explored in more detail in Chapters 6 and 7.

CHANGING TIMES

The word *change* has been at the forefront of our nation in the past decade, and it is even more evident due to the recent pandemic. Our intention with this chapter is to provide a glimpse at some of the ways health professionals are advocating and adapting policies in these changing times. One needs to only turn on the news, read social media, or review public health data and periodicals to know the countless areas where health disparities exist, the need for social justice, and the call for dismantling systemic racism in ourselves, our policies, and our procedures. Your role as a public health practitioner in advocacy engagement has been well established (Caira, 2003; Cox, 2014; Galer-Unti et al., 2004; Galer-Unti, 2009; Garcia et al., 2015; HESPA II, 2020; Mahas et al., 2016; Rivera et al., 2016; Thompson et al., 2012). Previous research by Thompson et al. (2012) found that health educators were still only moderately engaged in advocacy activities. The need for more engagement and skilled advocates has been addressed in public health and health education preparation programs on campuses due to changing competency development within the last 10 years. You will learn about this more in Chapter 4 and understand how the areas of responsibilities for public health education educators have been updated to include an eighth responsibility, advocacy, as a stand-alone responsibility with subcompetencies (Knowlden et al., 2020; NCHEC & SOPHE, 2020). It is important to note that some of the biggest changes we have seen in public health advocacy take some significant effort and time to accomplish.

SETTINGS FOR EVERYDAY ADVOCACY

When we assess where health education specialists and other public health professionals are employed, this enables us to understand where and how they are engaging in policy and advocacy endeavors. The most common settings have been categorized and fall predominantly under community, school (K–12), healthcare organizations, for-profit business/industry, college/university, and government agencies at the local, state, or national settings. Each setting will require health professionals to acquire a unique understanding of their workplace policies regarding advocacy work. Next are various examples of informal and formal advocacy in various settings.

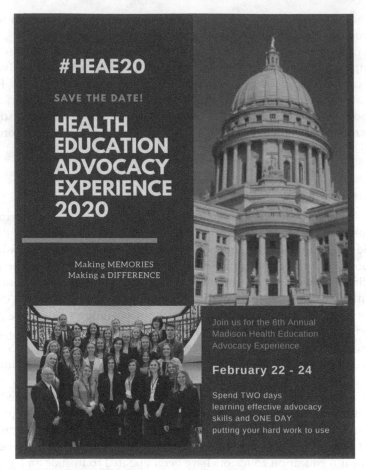

FIGURE 3.2 Everyday advocates head to more formal advocacy at the state capitol. University of Wisconsin–La Crosse faculty, staff, and students in Madison.
Source: Keely Rees.

Community Setting. In a community setting, health education specialists might act as lay health education specialists for an asthma program to reduce environmental triggers in the home. Health education specialists can also act as advocates for community health needs, such as lobbying the local government to use funds in ways that help promote the community's health or to create local laws or ordinances that promote community health.

School (K–12) Setting. When employed in a school setting, a health education specialist might be responsible for promoting the whole school, whole community, whole child (WSCC) approach by presenting curriculum information and student health information needs and concerns to groups of parents (Lewallen et al., 2015). Health education specialists can also advocate for student or faculty health in a school setting by creating school health councils or by suggesting ways to modify a curriculum.

Healthcare Setting. In this setting, the health education specialist might be responsible for a program to support patients' smoking cessation efforts. The health education specialist would need to communicate with providers the importance of the program, as well as the health education specialist's appropriateness for launching such an effort. The health education specialist could advocate for corporate responsibility to engage in health promotion and prevention efforts.

Business/Industry Setting. The health education specialist could communicate and advocate the need for a work site wellness program. Using their background in behavioral and biological sciences, the health education specialist would interpret the problem for management and articulate the possible ways of addressing the problem, such as offering a program or screening or changing organizational policy. Acknowledging concerns specific to management, the health education specialist could then advocate ways in which a health education program or policy might benefit management and the worker.

College/University Setting. A health education specialist in a college/university setting might be faced with the challenge of advocating for health education's "place" in the college curriculum. Recognizing multiple perspectives on expected student learning outcomes, the health education specialist would consider colleagues' professional backgrounds and use that information in formulating presentations on the importance of health education programs in the university environment. Communication might be handled through reports to curriculum committees, presentations to administrators, electronic communications, or small group discussions with students and faculty. University health education specialists may develop an advocacy plan in order to improve the health of current and future students.

University Health Services Setting. In a university health services setting, the health education specialist interfaces with students, healthcare providers, faculty, and other stakeholders. In this arena, the health education specialist might be charged with providing an educational program or social norm campaign to improve students' decision-making about use of drugs and alcohol. The health education specialist would communicate to healthcare providers the need for such a campaign and contribute to the program to ensure the providers' support and participation. The health education specialist would communicate the educational purpose of the program and/or relevant social norms data to students and interpret their value relative to their health education needs and concerns. This communication could be handled through electronic or print channels to individual students, posters placed around campus, and presentations before small groups within dormitories. The health education specialist might also work with select student organizations to encourage policy development regarding alcohol consumption on campus or alternatives to alcohol consumption and advocate for local laws or ordinances that stiffen alcohol or drug-related offenses for businesses.

Policies will be inherent within the organizations or settings; however, the types of advocating will need nuanced attention. Health professionals will implement advocacy projects and campaigns; teach about advocacy in schools, universities, and communities; and tirelessly strive to improve health status and quality of life for their communities. For instance, the contributing coauthors of this textbook represent a wide array of health professionals and experiences. These individuals represent many organizations, from universities to nonprofit healthcare systems, with all engaging in a wide array of advocacy activities. Importantly, you need to see, read about, and understand how individuals engage in everyday advocacy as well as helping you develop personal insights to learn about current best practices and recommendations for working with changing populations.

BASICS FOR EVERYDAY ADVOCACY

As you work to improve the health of a community or nation, it requires change in regulations and policy. To do this, public health professionals will engage in policy work using advocacy strategies. These strategies will vary based on the setting where you work and the health issue. The first step will be to understand the health issue. Health education professionals make excellent advocates for this reason; they know how to research the issue and find credible sources of information. They study the issue from all angles, are rooted in scholarly literature, and know where to access timely and accurate information. Many health professionals will spend a decade or more of their career dedicated to exploring a health issue or area as this type of investigation may be tied to their research agenda, the health association or agency they work for, or a personal or familial health experience (Box 3.2).

Next, do you understand this health issue from all angles? Advocates must research the issues from all perspectives. For example, do you know which organizations or groups might oppose the issue and may work against you or your organization to prevent a policy change? Understanding the health issue from the opposing side's values, principles, and beliefs will help you prepare and plan better. Knowing the opposition is almost more important than knowing your allies at first. When you reach out and connect with a stakeholder that might take a different stance on a health topic, set up a scheduled time to meet in person, virtually, or by phone. Be up front with what you want to talk about and your goal for the meeting and go in with an open mind; ask open-ended questions and be realistic as you will likely not change their mind or position on the policy or issue that day (or ever). Down the road, you will find this type of engagement helps build a foundation of cooperation and respect and often can lead to insights that move the policy forward. In creating these connections, you and your colleagues will have a better understanding of the opposition's values, narrative, and where they stand. These individuals might be school board members who have a child in the very school where you are trying to adopt a comprehensive sexuality education curriculum, a business owner worried about losing customers and money if you implement a Tobacco 21 policy, or a legislator rooted in their fiscal objectives versus family medical leave policies. At the core, the opposition is human. These are people with their own fears, values, and beliefs, and it is our role to inquire, engage, and find a way to either work toward a small policy win or know when to walk away.

Once you have identified your health issue, conducted your thorough research on the topic, and engaged with your allies and opponents, it is time to develop the **advocacy plan**. An advocacy plan is a comprehensive blueprint with your goals, objectives, and a clear idea of the outcome or changes you wish to see. An advocacy plan is a process

---

ADVOCACY IN ACTION BOX 3.2 | **What Will You Advocate For?**

What health area are you passionate about? What do you read about in your spare time? What topics can you listen to on podcasts or webinars? What topic do you turn to in a text or search endlessly online? What information do you love to share with your friends or social media? Pause again: Why did you become excited and passionate about this aspect of health?

tied to an expected outcome of what change you want to occur. When you create an advocacy plan, you pull from your vast tool-box of advocacy skills as each health issue or community will require tailored advocacy applications. Once your team or organization has a clear plan with a reasonable and feasible timeline—you start implementation. Knowing where to begin is often the hardest step in developing your plan. Many advocacy efforts begin with a brainstorm or conversation over lunch, and two months later it launches into your department's next media advocacy campaign to reduce distracted driving in your county. When designing your plan, it will include identifying resources (budget, personnel, and materials). Advocacy plans will utilize theoretical frameworks, grant-writing skills, and program planning and evaluation measures to fully engage in a strong advocacy endeavor that will withstand the time it takes to see an outcome occur.

As health professionals, we work alongside everyday advocates that include members from your communities, schools, and workplaces who also care about the health issue you are addressing. Being an effective advocate often requires the capacity to work with many stakeholders and those who work in grassroots settings. We need to assemble an advocacy planning group to include individuals from many facets of the health issue and settings in order to really create momentum, energy, and synergy toward an outcome that better serves the health and well-being of the most people. As a health education specialist, this is where your network of human connections, mentors, and leaders in your health-specific area or your geographical region becomes vital to your advocacy plan. For instance, Galer-Unti (2009) worked diligently to create advocacy momentum around "guerilla advocacy." This means taking assertive marketing tactics and skills from Jay Conrad Levison's work called *Guerilla Marketing* and applying them to our health educator advocacy toolboxes. Galer-Unti (2009) focused on how health professionals need strong skills in marketing. A few of these are crucial for health professionals to utilize. For example, assess your resource investment and time commitment as we have a finite amount of hours in a workday, and many of you will juggle numerous roles in your jobs. Galer-Unti emphasized using creativity and bringing energy and amazement to the issue. This method includes thinking of creative ways to capture your audience's attention and keep energy flowing to the issue over time. Another key guerilla tactic that is vital is keeping your focus. It is easy to divert and be pulled in another direction due to pressing issues or time constraints, and it will drain energy and momentum when you diversify too much.

SKILLS FUNDAMENTAL TO ADVOCATES

As mentioned throughout this chapter, advocacy requires some fundamental skills. We list some of the most common in Box 3.3 below. One of the most important skills of a public health advocate is adaptability. Advocates will need to adjust to changes in systems, setbacks, organizational structures, and overall political scenes that require adaptability. As you prepare to become a leader in the workforce, you will want to think about ways you can grow and learn to adapt as well as your strengths and skills. How will you lead in advocacy? For example, are you a strong technical writer and enjoy conducting research and fact finding, or do you have a passion for spoken word? Maybe you will lead through webinars, podcasts, and media outlets. Practice honing your skills and be concise and impactful. How can you convey your advocacy message and have it land with

ADVOCACY IN ACTION BOX 3.3	Fundamental Skills for Everyday Advocates
Strong communication skills	Trauma informed
Excellent interpersonal communications and networks	Dedicated and persistent
Strong writing abilities	Passionate and level headed
Savvy with technology	Strong leader, with ability to step back
Ability to listen	Capacity builder
Know when to lead versus follow	Strong empathy skills
Ability to adapt to different situations	Excellent facilitator
Good at conflict resolution and mediation	Creative and innovative
Debate with confidence	Problem-solver
Skilled at building trust	

Source: Keely Rees

your audience so that it "sticks"? It must be clear, concise, and compelling. Last, as an advocate, you can do something every day. Do something small. It can be a social media post, a response to an advocacy action alert, a conversation in the hallway, or a phone call to a policymaker. Your efforts will add up in an everyday way.

APPLYING YOUR STRENGTHS AND TALENTS TO ADVOCACY

Your work as an everyday advocate probably started before you entered the public health classroom, boardroom, department, or agency. Your skills may have begun in a sport, a debate team, or awareness of a personal or familial health concern. Many advocates find themselves here because of those very personal experiences and find ways to be heard in a healthcare setting, community, or school addressing the disparities around that issue. As you formalize your advocacy skills, you need to learn the process and impactful ways your voice becomes amplified. Over the course of two decades, working with young health advocates on legislative and more formal advocacy in state and federal offices, there are some characteristics and strengths (see Figure 3.3) that emerge from watching students and new professionals grow their advocacy muscles. Exercising these skills will enhance your informal and formal advocacy skills. A few of these are described below.

Listening Skills. Listening skills require the ability to hear the stories from the people and communities and bring their stories and experiences forward when thinking about ways to change policy or provide education. For example, working with teen advocates in a national program called Providers and Teens Communicating for Health (PATCH®; 2021), we learn the value of deep listening. The teens understand best what they and their peers are experiencing and share with health providers how to best listen and interact with teens, ultimately providing them the ability to provide the best healthcare and services to teens.

Engagement. An advocate must create a network of stakeholders, leaders, and other activists to help them move their issues forward locally or nationally. Engagement looks

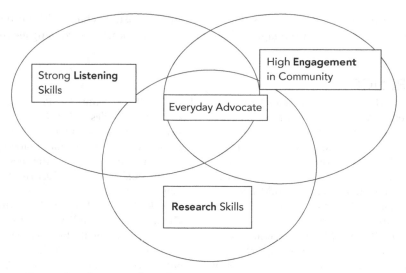

FIGURE 3.3 Strengths of an everyday advocate
Source: Keely Rees

like good old fashion networking: listening first, sharing stories, and talking with people; attending coalition meetings; or working with other agencies that have stakes in the health topic or issue. This is the work of connectors and relators, folks who have the ability to see relationships, find the connecting dots, and make things happen. You want this skill or have individuals on your advocacy team that seem to have a strong networking skill set.

Research. Strong everyday advocates have the ability to seek out valid and reliable sources of data, information, and resources that will further the understanding of the health issue and assist in their fight for the issue. This skill must be garnered early and practiced often and provide a discerning eye for good sources. This can be tricky because in the age of information, we know how many biases and different types of outlets for information we can go find when "googling" a topic. Advocates must have access to reliable and valid research to provide for their patients, students, communities, stakeholders, and policymakers.

CONCLUSION

Everyday acts of advocacy may lead to significant impacts in our communities, in our relationship with others, and in our personal lives. Engaging in informal advocacy can motivate us and help us to develop skills to further engage in advocacy efforts on a larger scale and level. Everyday advocacy can also motivate and persuade those you engage with. You have likely observed and experienced your own level of motivation, passion, and excitement to be a part of a profession that is so committed and dedicated to improving the human condition. Everyday advocates are in every corner of our world, promoting health and working to harness and mobilize the multitude of societal, cultural, medical, technological, and political forces that contribute to positive change. There has never been a more crucial time to engage in this work. What advocacy will you engage in today?

REFERENCES

Cox, C., Haidar, S., Brookins-Fisher, J., Thompson, A., Deakins, B., Bishop, C. (2014) Health Educator, *46*(2), 36–45.

Doyle, E. I., Caro, C. M., Lysoby, L., Auld, M. E., Smith, B. J., & Muenzen, P. M. (2012). The National Health Educator Job Analysis 2010: Process and outcomes. *Health Education & Behavior, 39*(6), 695–708. https://doi.org/10.1177/1090198112463393

Galer-Unti, R. A. (2009). Guerilla advocacy: Using aggressive marketing techniques for health policy change. *Health Promotion Practice, 10*(3), 325–327. https://doi.org/10.1177/1524839909334513

Galer-Unti, R. A., Tappe, M. K., & Lachenmayr, S. (2004). Advocacy 101: Getting Started in Health Education Advocacy. *Health Promotion Practice, 5*(3), 280–288. https://doi.org/10.1177/1524839903257697

Garcia, L. B., Hernandez, K. E., & Mata, H. (2015). Professional development through policy advocacy: Communicating and advocating for health and health equity. *Health Promotion Practice, 16*, 162–165.

Hancher-Rauch, H. L., Gebra, Y., & Carson, A. (2019). Health advocacy for busy professionals: Effective advocacy with little time. *Health Promotion Practice, 20*(4), 489–493. https://doi.org/10.1177/1524839919830927

Knowlden, A. P., Cottrell, R. R., Henderson, J., Allison, K., Auld, M. E., Kusorgbor-Narh, C. S., Lysoby, L., & McKenzie, J. F. (2020). Health Education Specialist Practice Analysis II 2020: Processes and outcomes. *Health Education & Behavior, 47*(4), 642–651.

Lewallen, T. C., Hunt, H., Potts-Datema, W., Zaza, S., & Giles, W. (2015). The whole school, whole community, whole child model: A new approach for improving educational attainment and healthy development for students. *Journal of School Health, 85*(11), 729–739. https://doi.org/10.1111/josh.12310

Mahas, R., Van Wasshenova, E., Everhart, F. J., Thompson, A., Boardley, D. (2016). Public Policy Involvement by Certified Health Education Specialists: Results of a National Study. *Health Promotion Practice, 17*(5), 668–674. doi:10.1177/1524839916658652

National Commission for Health Education Credentialing, Inc. (NCHEC), & Society for Public Health Education, Inc. (SOPHE). (2020). *A competency-based framework for health education specialists—2020.* Providers and Teens Communicating for Health (PATCH®). (2021). Home page. https://patchprogram.org/

Rivera, L., Starry, B., Gangi, C., Lube, L. M., Cedergren, A., Whitney, E., & Rees, K. (2016). From Classroom to Capitol: Building Advocacy Capacity Through State-Level Advocacy Experiences. *Health Promotion Practice, 17*(6), 771–774. https://doi.org/10.1177/1524839916669131

Thompson, A., Kerr, D., Dowling, J., & Wagner, L. (2012). Advocacy 201: Incorporating advocacy training in health education professional preparation programs. *Health Education Journal, 71*(3), 268–277. https://doi.org/10.1177/0017896911408814

CHAPTER 3: END-OF-CHAPTER ACTIVITIES
DISCUSSION QUESTIONS

1. Notice the *everyday advocacy* happening on your campus or community. Who are the key advocates and key organizations, and what role do they have in local public health efforts?

2. After reading about the *settings* in Chapter 3, describe in a small group (triad or dyad) the settings where health educators are in your community or even state. Do you know where some of your alumni are working and advocating for specific health issues?

3. You find yourself scrolling through social media (or running the social media accounts for your agency, organization) and notice inaccurate information being posted, discussed, and reshared around a health issue. Discuss your role as a health educator.

APPLICATION ACTIVITIES

1. Find the website for a public health or health education professional organization (national or state level) and find their advocacy and policy information in their menu. What are the top priorities? Do they have action alerts? Is there a way you can get involved?

2. Research and find podcasts related to a health issue you care about or want to learn more about. Are there advocacy groups, organizations that produce podcasts on your topic? For example, you are researching something on *water quality*, start with a Google search, Spotify, or podcast apps. Use your search terms related to your health topic. Share with your peers in a group discussion, a walk and talk, or in an online discussion forum.

3. Photovoice is a really powerful methodology we use in health education/public health. It helps us understand a population, a health issue, and a topic. Take a photo of some object, thing, you, person, an animal, or something else that expresses how you are coping, feeling, working, studying, or thinking this week/day. It does NOT have to have you in it, just something that represents your current feeling, ideas, advocacy, emotions, state, or thought process. Then add ONE (minimum) to FIVE (maximum) words to the photo, on the photo, or in the caption. You can share these in an online discussion board, share in a group sharing your phones or laptops, or create a class Padlet with these on them (https://padlet.com).

ADDITIONAL RESOURCES

Abroms, L. C., Gold, R. S., & Allegrante, J. P. (2019). Promoting health on social media: The way forward. *Health Education & Behavior*, 46(2, Suppl.), 9S–11S. https://doi.org/10.1177/1090198119879096

American Public Health Association. (n.d.) Advocacy for public health. https://www.apha.org/policies-and-advocacy/advocacy-for-public-health

Center for Rural Health. *Communication toolkit.* (n.d.) https://ruralhealth.und.edu/communication

Chapman, S. (2001). Advocacy in public health: Roles and challenges. *International Journal of Epidemiology, 30*(6), 1226–1232. https://doi.org/10.1093/ije/30.6.1226

Harris, D. (n.d.). *Active listening.* NAMI Palm Beach County. https://namipbc.org/keys-to-listening/

Rabinowitz, P. (n.d.). *Implementing Photovoice in your community.* Community Tool Box. https://ctb. ku.edu/en/table-of-contents/assessment/assessing-community-needs-and-resources/photovoice/main

Wang, C., & Burris, M.A. (1999). *Photovoice: A participatory action research strategy applied to women's health, Journal of Women's Health,* 8(2), 185–192.

QUIZ QUESTIONS

1. Which one of the following is an example of informal advocacy?
   a. People within the community gather to advocate for vulnerable people, such as the homeless.
   b. An established organization pays and trains its staff to advocate for a vulnerable population.
   c. A trained individual supports clients who struggle with housing issues.
   d. A paid lobbyist meets with legislators or their staff to discuss specific legislation regarding homelessness.

2. To truly hear and be engaged with experiences people share with their health providers is which of the following advocacy skills?
   a. engagement
   b. counseling
   c. listening
   d. research

3. In a university health services setting, health education specialists may engage and work closely with some student organizations to
   a. reconstruct all health promotion activities to decrease the number of strategies for self-awareness.
   b. re-create the business model in an academic setting.
   c. assist the university in lowering costs and reducing access to health services on and off-campus.
   d. create, implement, oversee, and analyze programs and strategies that promote health and well-being.

4. Which of the following skills would not be considered fundamental to advocates?
   a. adaptability
   b. listening
   c. dedication
   d. argumentative

5. When it comes to being engaged as an advocate networking with others, engagement will include which of the following?
   a. repairing, copying, looking, asserting, and bypassing
   b. listening, sharing, communicating, attending, and collaborating
   c. arguing, manipulating, selling, and dismissing
   d. encouraging, inspiring, uplifting, and demeaning

6. For advocates to provide research to their stakeholders, policymakers, and communities, advocates need to be able to access
   a. common surveys in everyday magazines
   b. only controversial research to prove their point
   c. valid and reliable research
   d. incongruent findings and financial resources

7. When working in a middle school setting, which one of the following is not what a health education specialist may be responsible for?
   a. whole child
   b. whole community
   c. whole school
   d. whole math curriculum

8. A health education specialist who may be communicating with providers about the importance of an obesity program, as well as the importance of developing and implementing such a program, would more than likely be in a _____.
   a. healthcare setting
   b. industry setting
   c. workforce reduction setting
   d. law enforcement setting

9. In the Advocacy Spotlight interview with Sara Finger, what advice did she provide?
   a. Seek out the support of others because you are not alone.
   b. Learn to appreciate the power of your voice, your experiences, and your insight.
   c. Know that there is no one way to be an advocate.
   d. All of the above.

10. _____ "is a comprehensive blueprint with your goals, objectives, and a clear idea of the outcome or changes you wish to see."
    a. a theoretical perspective
    b. an advocacy plan
    c. a lobbyist's responsibility
    d. a healthcare plan

ANSWER KEY
1. **A.** People within the community gather to advocate for vulnerable people, such as the homeless
2. **C.** Listening
3. **D.** Create, implement, oversee, and analyze programs and strategies that promote health and well-being

4. **D.** Argumentative
5. **B.** Listening, sharing, communicating, attending, and collaborating
6. **C.** Valid and reliable research
7. **D.** Whole math curriculum
8. **A.** Healthcare setting
9. **D.** All of the above
10. **B.** An advocacy plan

3.2 SARA FINGER

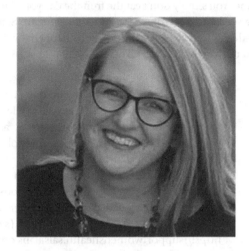

As the founder and executive director of the Wisconsin Alliance for Women's Health (WAWH), Sara Finger works to advance comprehensive women's health in Wisconsin by engaging, educating, empowering, and mobilizing individuals and organizations.

Q. What Led You to Establish the Wisconsin Alliance for Women's Health?

While seeking a political science undergraduate degree, I realized that I didn't want to just lobby on someone's behalf—I wanted to empower individuals to be their own advocates. I am motivated by the power of educating, equipping, and mobilizing the voices of many to speak as one in order to create change. In creating change, it's important to realize that some voices are quieter than others, but no less important. In an effort to make all voices heard in healthcare policy discussions, the WAWH is dedicated to empowering and activating a broad base of advocates, including healthcare professionals, clergy, legislators, other community leaders, and rural and urban women and families of all ages, races, faiths, education, orientation, and backgrounds. Through many successful coalitions, we have been able to help transform many ordinary citizens into potent forces for change as they raise their voice for policies that move Wisconsin toward a healthier future.

Q. What Are the Mission and Goals of the WAWH?

I'm incredibly proud of our organization's work to educate, engage, and empower women to be their own advocates in the healthcare reform debate. Healthcare reform is one of the most important women's health issues. Women everywhere are already winning with the Affordable Care Act with preexisting condition protections, covered preventive care, consumer protections, and affordable, accessible care. We continue to fight for meaningful implementation of the Affordable Care Act in our state to help women and their families access the affordable and quality healthcare they need and deserve.

Q. What Do You See as Some of the Biggest Accomplishments of the WAWH So Far?

Since our founding in 2004, one of our greatest overall accomplishments is helping more people find their way to and into the policymaking "kitchen." We estimate that less than 7% of eligible voters in Wisconsin can identify who their state elected leaders are—leaving 93% of eligible voters who are not familiar with who works for them in the state legislature. That's a lot of people who don't know who to reach out to and who to inform on key policy decisions impacting their lives. And if you don't know who your elected leaders are, you're likely not aware of their voting record. And if you're not aware of your legislators' voting record, how can you hold these individuals accountable? Helping more people be educated, engaged, and empowered around advocacy is an imperative if policy is going to happen WITH us rather than TO us!

Q. What Keeps You Engaged and Motivated as an Advocate?

The potential and promise of change keeps me engaged and motivated. By design, the level of civic engagement in our state and county is extremely low. Most people are sitting on the "sidelines" of democracy because they simply don't have the extra time, capacity, resources, or know-how to "get in the game" and be actively involved in advocacy on a regular basis. If we can help identify and remove the barriers that keep people from being informed, involved, and inspired to be effective advocates, there is such incredible potential to transform the way policy decisions and system changes are made.

Q. What Advice Do You Have for Current and Future Advocates?

Be gentle and kind to yourself. Advocacy is a long game: You simply don't eat the fruit the day you plant the seeds! Change does not happen overnight. Start by deciding that you want policy to happen "with" you rather than "to" you. Then take the next steps:

1. Learn to appreciate the power of your voice, your experiences, and your insight. You don't have to be a "sous chef" to enter that policymaking kitchen. Your reality and your stories are yours, and they are critical to informing policy decision-making at all levels.

2. Know that there is no one way to be an advocate. Do what feels right to you. Choose from a "menu" of ways to make a difference, such as finding out who represents you (see https://supportwomenshealth.salsalabs.org/whorepresentsme/index.html).

3. Remind yourself that you're not alone, and it's not up to you to single-handedly change things for the better. Lean on advocacy organizations like the WAWH, which are here to monitor policy threats and opportunities and alert you to when it makes the most sense to take action.

Advocacy

An Essential Skill for Health Education Specialists

KATHLEEN G. ALLISON, DIANNE KERR, AND AMY HEDMAN-ROBERTSON

Start where you are, use what you have, do what you can.

—ARTHUR ASHE

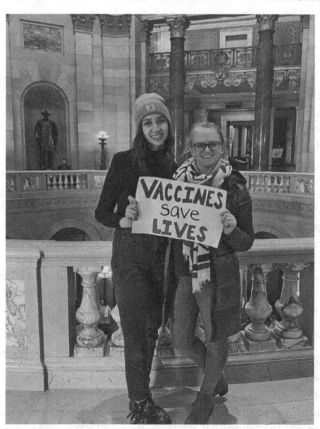

FIGURE 4.1 Vaccines save lives. Students Aniz and Marlee, majors in public health at the University of St. Thomas, do their part to promote vaccinations at Celebrate Immunization MN at the Minnesota State capitol, St. Paul.

Kathleen G. Allison, Dianne Kerr, and Amy Hedman-Robertson, *Advocacy*. In: *Be the Change*. Edited by Keely S. Rees, Jody Early, and Cicily Hampton, Oxford University Press. © Oxford University Press 2023. DOI: 10.1093/oso/9780197570890.003.0004

Objectives

1. Explain the importance of advocacy for the health education specialist (HES).
2. Describe the role of practice analyses for the health education and promotion profession.
3. Explain the role of credentialing in health education and its value for HESs.
4. Describe advocacy expectations related to entry- and advanced-level practice of HESs.
5. Create an action plan to enhance personal advocacy skills.

INTRODUCTION

In the first three chapters you learned about the importance of advocacy and some of the relevant terms related to advocacy. In this chapter, you will learn how these concepts relate to public health education. Before your studies in health education, you may have thought that the health education profession was almost exclusively about delivering health information. After all, the traditional definition of health education focuses on the acquisition of knowledge, attitudes, and skills for improving personal and community health (Green & Kreuter, 2005). And although health education includes teaching–learning processes, the profession of health education is so much more. Present-day health education practice incorporates health promotion activities (Figure 4.1), addressing social, organizational, environmental, policy, economic, and social factors that impact health (Cottrell et al., 2018). Health education as a strategy and as a discipline has been considered a key component of public health for decades. As such, health education specialists (HESs) are well versed in public health's core functions and essential services (Figure 4.2). The profession specializes in the skills found in the core function of policy development, most notably the essential health services of (a) communicating to inform and educate and (b) mobilizing communities and partnerships. The profession of health education is guided by "behavioral or organizational principles" for the improvement of health by individuals, groups, and communities (Videto et al., 2021). Advocacy is one of these principles, and it has become an increasingly valuable tool in the health education tool-box for improving health.

In this chapter, you will learn about the evolution of advocacy as a skill for the health education profession, how the skill is formalized in the credentialing processes of certification and accreditation, and why it is important for you to develop your advocacy skills for improving the health of individuals and communities.

THE HISTORY OF ADVOCACY IN HEALTH EDUCATION AND PROMOTION PRACTICE

Have you ever thought about how advocacy strategies have become part of health education and promotion practice? The current definition of the health education profession alludes to advocacy in stating that evidence-based practice and change principles are employed "to achieve personal, environmental, and social health" (Videto et al., 2021, p. 2). Additionally, the profession's code of ethics describes advocacy as a strategy to improve health, reduce health risks, and address health inequities (Coalition of National

THE 10 ESSENTIAL PUBLIC HEALTH SERVICES

To protect and promote the health of all people in all communities

The 10 Essential Public Health Services provide a framework for public health to protect and promote the health of all people in all communities. To achieve optimal health for all, the Essential Public Health Services actively promote policies, systems, and services that enable good health and seek to remove obstacles and systemic and structural barriers, such as poverty, racism, gender discrimination, and other forms of oppression, that have resulted in health inequities. Everyone should have a fair and just opportunity to achieve good health and well-being.

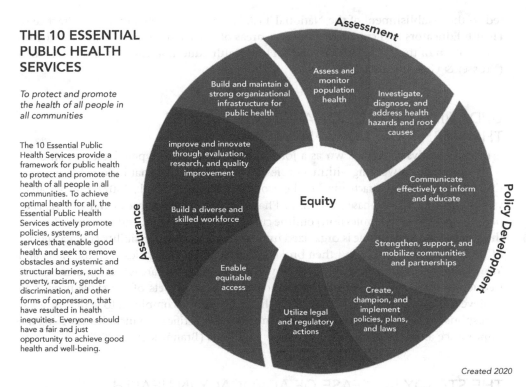

Created 2020

FIGURE 4.2 The 10 Essential Public Health Services.

Source: Centers for Disease Control and Prevention, Public Health Gateway. https://www.cdc.gov/publiche althgateway/publichealthservices/essentialhealthservices.html

Health Education Organizations, 2020). As obvious as it may seem that the profession's philosophical underpinning of improving health would involve advocacy, identifying it as a key element of the profession required verification from individuals working as HESs. The verification of the skills required for competence within a profession is accomplished through special research studies known as practice, or job, analyses.

A BRIEF HISTORY OF HEALTH EDUCATION

Individuals have been conducting health education for millennia—but health education, as a formalized profession, has a much more recent history. Professional health education organizations, preparation programs, and workforce positions have existed for nearly a century, with Sally Lucas Jean being credited with coining the term "health education" in 1922 (Henderson et al., 1980). However, health education as a profession was fragmented prior to the 1970s. There was no unified opinion about the purpose, duties, roles, or responsibilities of those calling themselves health educators (Prosser & Gautam, 2011). Helen Cleary (1995), president of the Society for Public Health Education (SOPHE) in 1974, stated that the profession urgently needed established professional standards. Her call to action set into motion a series of conferences that initially led to the establishment of the National Task Force on the Preparation and Practice of Health Educators and culminated in seven areas of entry-level responsibility and the incorporation of the National Commission for Health Education Credentialing (NCHEC) (Prosser & Gautam, 2011).

UPDATING PROFESSIONAL COMPETENCIES THROUGH PRACTICE ANALYSES

A practice analysis, also known as a job analysis, is a specific type of research study in which individuals working within a profession detail the work that is done by those actively engaged in, or "practicing," in the profession (Brannick et al., 2007). Practice analysis is typically a two-phase process. In Phase 1, a group of subject matter experts (i.e., people working in the profession) outline current job duties, tasks, and responsibilities of the profession. The outline is organized into larger areas of responsibility (i.e., categories of the profession's work) and then broken down into competencies (i.e., the skills and knowledge needed to conduct the work within the identified areas). Competencies are frequently broken down further into subcompetencies, subsets of the skills needed to achieve the competencies. In Phase 2, a validation study is completed to verify the areas of responsibility, competencies, and subcompetencies. Verification includes assessing the importance and frequency of competencies and skills (Brannick et al., 2007).

THE STEADY INCREASE OF ADVOCACY IN HEALTH EDUCATION PRACTICE ANALYSES

There have been five large-scale practice analyses in health education (Table 4.1). The first was the Role Delineation Project, spearheaded by Helen Cleary and a task force of health educators from the national organizations with health education constituencies. The project was funded by the Bureau of Health Manpower in the late 1970s (Henderson et al., 1980; Pollock & Carlyon, 1996). The Role Delineation Project and its successors, the Competencies Update Project (CUP) in 2004; Health Education Job Analysis (HEJA) in 2010; Health Education Specialist Practice Analysis (HESPA) in 2015; and Health Education Specialist Practice Analysis II–2020 (HESPA II-2020) reflected an evolving consensus of the contemporary practice of HESs (formerly called health educators). Competencies identifying the skills of those in graduate-level, advanced practice occurred in 1999 after the completion of the 1997 research project by the Joint Committee for Graduate Standards (American Association for Health Education [AAHE] et al., 1999).

ROLE DELINEATION PROJECT (1978–1981)

The Role Delineation Project established entry-level practice responsibilities and expectations of health educators, regardless of work setting (Henderson et al., 1980). Advocating health education in policy formulation was identified as a function in the initial specifications of the Responsibilities of entry-level health educators (Henderson et al., 1981), but was not overtly stated in the final Competencies of this original practice analysis, released as the Entry-level framework (NCHEC, 1985). The requisite skills

TABLE 4.1 Advocacy Highlights Found Within Practice Analyses for the Health Education Profession

Practice Analysis	Advocacy Highlights within Areas of Responsibility, Competencies, and Subcompetencies
Role Delineation Project (RDP) 1985	Requisite skills of communicating health and health education needs were identified (Henderson et al., 1981; NCHEC, 1985)
Graduate-level framework 1999	Graduate-level subcompetencies relating to persuasive communication were added (AAHE et al., 1999)
Competencies Update Project (CUP) 2004	Area of Responsibility VII was renamed to include the term advocacy; influence health policy was included as an advocacy competency (NCHEC & SOPHE, 2010)
Health Education Job Analysis (HEJA) 2010	Area of Responsibility VII was expanded to include more advocacy competencies (CUP competencies + 2 more) and more advocacy subcompetencies (addition of 12) were added (NCHEC & SOPHE, 2010)
Health Education Specialist Practice Analysis (HESPA) 2015	Media, political, and legislative advocacy were clearly noted; leading advocacy initiatives was verified as an entry-level subcompetency (NCHEC & SOPHE, 2015)
Health Education Specialist Practice Analysis II–2020 (HESPA II-2020) 2020	Advocacy is a stand-alone area of responsibility and new subcompetencies addressing advocacy at policy and systems levels and identifying coalitions as an advocacy strategy were added (NCHEC & SOPHE, 2020)

of advocacy, however, were included in the entry-level framework Area of Responsibility VII: Communicating Health and Health Education Needs, Concerns, and Resources for entry-level practice (NCHEC, 1985). These sub-competencies were found in Competency C: *Select a variety of community of communication methods and techniques in providing health information.* The associated sub-competencies 1) *Utilize a wide range of techniques for communicating health and health education information,* and 2) *Demonstrate proficiency in communicating health information and health education needs* imply the skills needed to engage in advocacy strategies.

GRADUATE-LEVEL FRAMEWORK (1999)
The first health education practice analysis (Role Delineation Project) focused on entry-level practice, however, many health educators practiced beyond the entry-level. In 1992, the AAHE and SOPHE established a Joint Committee for Graduate Standards (AAHE et al., 1999), leading to a graduate-level framework with additional areas of responsibility, competencies, and subcompetencies. The authors of the framework clarified the subcompetencies within the graduate-level framework with objectives. The

foundation of advocacy was clearly added with two Area VII subcompetencies. The first, Subcompetency VII.B.3, *Analyze Social, Cultural, Demographic, and Political Factors That Influence Decision-Makers*, overtly relates to advocacy efforts. The addition of another Area VII subcompetency, VII.C.3, *Demonstrate Both Proficiency and Accuracy in Oral and Written Presentations*, included as its objectives "prepare a written document that provides a convincing argument in support of a complex health issue" and "prepare and present a public address that provides a persuasive argument in support of a complex health issue" (AAHE et al., 1999, p. 43). The skill of persuasive communication for health was verified and adopted by the profession.

NATIONAL HEALTH EDUCATOR COMPETENCIES UPDATE PROJECT (2004)

The National Health Educator Competencies Update Project, known as the CUP, updated and refined the areas of responsibility, competencies, and subcompetencies from the Role Delineation Project and Graduate Framework study and combined them into one hierarchical framework. Two notable updates occurred with this reverification study, requiring the direct need for advocacy skills: (1) the renaming of Area of Responsibility VII to Communicate and Advocate for Health and Health Education and (2) the addition of the Competency VII.D *Influence Health Policy to Promote Health* (NCHEC et al., 2010).

The subcompetencies and competencies of the renamed area of competency in the CUP (NCHEC et al., 2010) convey skills needed for effective advocacy, such as Competency VII.D, *Influence Health Policy to Promote Health*, and the subcompetencies VII.B.5, *Use Appropriate Techniques When Communicating Health and Health Education Information*, and VII.D.1, *Identify the Significance and Implications of Health Care Providers' Messages to Consumers*, which require proficiency for conveying information on not only the individual level, but also the community and organization levels. They also relate the importance of understanding how messages and policies can potentially affect a population.

HEALTH EDUCATION JOB ANALYSIS (2010)

The next practice analysis was the Health Education Job Analysis (2010), also known as HEJA. HEJA expanded the advocacy competencies and subcompetencies initiated in the CUP model. Area VII Competencies 7.1, *Assess and Prioritize Health Information and Advocacy Needs*; 7.4, *Engage in Health Education Advocacy*; and 7.5, *Influence Policy to Promote Health*, were defined with twelve new Sub-competencies. The Sub-competencies address the use of technology (media advocacy), advocating for environmental changes such as policies and regulations, and including stakeholders in advocacy activities (NCHEC et al., 2010).

HEALTH EDUCATION SPECIALIST PRACTICE ANALYSIS (2015)

The Health Education Specialist Practice Analysis (2015), known as HESPA, reverified the competencies from HEJA. Area of Responsibility VII was renamed Communicate, Promote, and Advocate for Health Education/Promotion, and the Profession, emphasizing the importance of the changes external to the individual (e.g., cultural, community, and policy factors). The concept of health promotion was a thread throughout HESPA. Health promotion goes beyond health education and encompasses "educational, political, environmental, regulatory, or organizational mechanisms" to improve health (Videto et al., 2021, p. 5). This philosophy forwarded the advocacy competencies found within HEJA. Media advocacy, policy advocacy, and legislative advocacy became separate subcompetencies. The increased emphasis on a variety of advocacy methods demonstrated the differing skill subsets found within advocacy activities. Leading advocacy initiatives was verified as an entry-level subcompetency (NCHEC & SOPHE, 2015), relating to the increased expectations of advocacy skills for those new to health education and promotion.

HEALTH EDUCATION SPECIALIST PRACTICE ANALYSIS II–2020 (2020)

The most recent practice analysis, known as HESPA II-2020, reflects the distinct continuing evolution of advocacy and verifies advocacy as a separate Area of Responsibility (Area of Responsibility V). All aspects of advocacy in HESPA can be found within HESPA II-2020. A significant and clearly delineated addition to HESPA II-2020 is the use of coalitions as an advocacy strategy. Two new competencies were defined and verified: (1) 5.1, *Identify a Current or Emerging Health Issue Requiring Policy, Systems, or Environmental Change*, and (2) 5.2, *Engage Coalitions and Stakeholders in Addressing the Health Issue and Planning Advocacy Efforts*. Another notable aspect of the second competency is that HESs require the knowledge and skills to engage others in the advocacy efforts. Including stakeholders in assessment of needs and when planning strategies is not new in health education practice. What is new is the overt emphasis on applying those skills at policy and systems levels (NCHEC & SOPHE, 2020).

In addition to competencies, core knowledge items have been included in practice analyses beginning with HEJA. Although more content may be needed for some work settings, the 145 verified core knowledge items of HESPA II-2020 represent essential knowledge of HESs across work settings. Principles and methods of advocacy, civic responsibility, media advocacy, policy development, and understanding the bodies and structures of decision makers (e.g., administrative and judicial bodies) are considered to be essential knowledge for HESs (NCHEC & SOPHE, 2020).

FREQUENCY OF PRACTICE ANALYSES TO UPDATE COMPETENCIES AND INFORM PREPARATION

Practice analyses need to be conducted as professional practice changes. In a rapidly changing environment, a practice analysis may need to be conducted every few years. A typical time frame for a practice analysis is approximately every 5 years. This allows professionals to identify emerging areas of work while simultaneously allowing a profession to adapt preparation programs and continuing education programming (Brannick et al., 2007).

The results of the health education practice analysis research studies serve as a framework for professional preparation programs and the Certified Health Education Specialist (CHES®) and Master Certified Health Education Specialist (MCHES®) credentialing exams. They also inform continuing education providers regarding workforce expectations. Lastly, they allow individuals within the profession to self-assess their strengths and training needs. Each practice analysis allows for the monitoring of the profession and thus enables the profession to adapt its formal and informal educational offerings, enhancing health education professionals' abilities (skills and competence) to meet the established and emerging needs of the populations they serve.

ADVOCACY AS A STAND-ALONE AREA OF RESPONSIBILITY FOR HESs

Looking over the practice analyses from the early 1980s through the present, one can see a greater application of advocacy to improve health. This is directly related to our understanding of the social determinants of health and the strategies that are most effective in addressing those factors, external to individuals, that influence the health of individuals and communities. Social determinants of health (see Figure 4.3) are all of the contextual factors, such as economics, healthcare access and quality, education access, neighborhood, as well as social and community context, that influence the health and quality of life for people (Centers for Disease Control and Prevention, 2020). Effective strategies for improving the social determinants require policy and

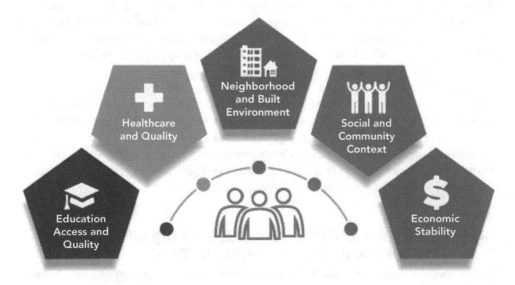

FIGURE 4.3 Social determinants of health.

systems changes, and advocacy is a key competency for affecting these upstream changes.

Thus far in the chapter you have learned about how advocacy has evolved in the health education profession and how it is identified by those working within the profession. To ensure that current and future professionals are up to date with the skills needed to effectively function in the public health education profession, the results of the practice analyses serve as the framework for the credentialing of individuals and programs.

OVERVIEW OF CREDENTIALING AND ACCREDITING BODIES

How can a person convey that they have a working knowledge of advocacy methods? One way is through a credential that includes advocacy competencies. According to Dictionary.com, a credential is "evidence of authority, status, rights, entitlement to privileges or the like, usually in written form" (Dictionary.com, n.d.). Credentials may be earned by individuals in health education and public health. In these disciplines, the credentialing process is a certification conducted by two agencies, the NCHEC and the National Board of Public Health Examiners (NBPHE), respectively.

Why You Might Consider Certification

A certification is more than a résumé builder and much more than a certificate you would get from completing a course or training. It shows you have met a national professional standard, which gives you more credibility. This may be advantageous in getting a job as some workplaces "require" or "prefer" to hire certified individuals and include that credential in their job postings. So, being certified may give you an advantage in getting hired. Getting certified also demonstrates a level of competence and validation of your skills by a national organization as well as a commitment to your profession.

EXAMPLES OF CREDENTIALS FOR THOSE IN PUBLIC HEALTH EDUCATION

According to Videto et al. (2021), the Joint Committee on Health Education and Promotion Terminology (2020) defined an HES as "an individual who has met, at a minimum, baccalaureate-level health education academic preparation. This individual must be competent to use appropriate educational strategies and methods to facilitate the development of policies, procedures, interventions, and systems conducive to the health and well-being of individuals, groups, and communities. Specialists may serve in a variety of settings" (Videto et al., 2021, p. 11). There are three primary certifications in health education and public health, the CHES®, MCHES®, and Certified in Public Health (CPH) credentials (see Table 4.2).

TABLE 4.2 CHES®, MCHES®, and CPH Certification Requirements

Certification	CHES®	MCHES®	CPH
Eligibility	Bachelor's degree or above in health education or a related degree with at least 25 semester credits (or 37 quarter hours) of coursework specific to the areas of responsibility for health education specialists	For non-CHES or CHES with fewer than 5 years active status: a master's degree or higher in health education, public health education, community health education, or the like OR a master's degree or higher with academic transcript reflecting the same credits as required for CHES; 5 years documented experience as a CHES	Bachelor's degree and above and 5+ years of work experience in public health OR student/graduate of CEPH-accredited school or program
Exam	Pass the CHES exam based on the NCHEC areas of responsibility at entry level	Pass the MCHES exam based on the NCHEC areas of responsibility at entry and advanced levels	Pass the CPH exam based on the CPH 10 domains
Work experience	Not required	5 years as a health education specialist	Those with a bachelor's degree must have at least 5 years of continuous public health practice experience Those with graduate degrees in public health not required to have work experience
Maintenance	75 Continuing Education Contact Hours (CECH) within 5 years to maintain certification	75 CECH within 5 years to maintain certification	50 credits every 2 years to maintain certification

Adapted from Kerr, D. L., Blavos, A., Hancher-Rauch, H., Brookins-Fisher, J., & Thompson, A. (2019). CHES, MCHES, and/or CPH? Selecting the best credential for you. *Health Promotion Practice, 20*(2), 167–172. https://doi.org/10.1177/152483991 8825132

NCHEC CERTIFICATIONS

The credentials awarded by NCHEC are the CHES® and the MCHES®. If you are just starting out with a bachelor's degree, CHES® is the NCHEC certification for you (Kerr et al., 2019). If you are further along in your career, the MCHES® is an advanced-level certification. If you are a college student, you may notice some of your professors have these credentials.

BECOMING CHES® CERTIFIED

According to NCHEC, to become CHES® certified you must submit the following:

- "an official transcript (including course titles) that clearly shows a major in health education, e.g., Health Education, Community Health Education, Public Health Education, School Health Education, etc. Degree/major must explicitly be in a discipline of 'Health Education'" OR
- "an official transcript that reflects at least 25 semester credits or 37 quarter hours of course work (with a grade "c" or better) with specific preparation addressing the Eight Areas of Responsibility and Competency for Health Education Specialists" (NCHEC, n.d.).

If you are unsure if some of your course credits count, NCHEC office staff can assist you with a review of your transcript. Next, you need to study and register to take the CHES® exam. This is a competency-based exam on the field of practice that includes the following eight areas of responsibility: (1) assessing needs and capacity; (2) planning; (3) implementation; (4) evaluation and research; (5) advocacy; (6) communication; (7) leadership and management; and (8) ethics and professionalism. The advocacy area, in particular, is the focus of this textbook.

The CHES® and MCHES® exams are computer based and can be taken at national testing centers during the months of October and April. In 2020, NCHEC added an option to take the exam at home with Live Remote Proctoring (LRP) during the same time frames. During the LRP the proctor can view you taking the exam through your computer camera to ensure the security of the exam process. Once you pass the exam, you have your credential! You need to recertify every 5 years by earning a total of 75 Continuing Education Credit Hours (CECH) to maintain your CHES® or MCHES® certification.

The MCHES® is a higher level of certification than the CHES®. You can apply to be MCHES® certified after 5 years of experience practicing as a CHES®. You do not have to be CHES® prior to becoming MCHES® as long as you meet other eligibility requirements. More about MCHES® eligibility can be found on the NCHEC website (https://www.nchec.org/mches-exam-eligibility).

CPH CERTIFICATION

Another certification more specific to public health is the CPH credential, sponsored by the NBPHE. This certification primarily demonstrates expertise in the following 10 domains of public health: (1) evidence-based approaches to public health; (2) communication; (3) leadership; (4) law and ethics; (5) public health biology and human disease risk; (6) collaboration and partnership; (7) program planning and evaluation; (8) program management; (9) policy and public health; and (10) health equity and social justice. Each domain represents 10% of the CPH exam (NBPHE, 2016).

Within the CPH certification, you will find elements of advocacy emphasized. The CPH certification refers to "policy" rather than "advocacy" in its domain areas. The terms "policy" and "policies" are referred to in several CPH domain areas beyond the domain area of the policy in public health. For example, "evaluating policy" is found under the program planning and evaluation domain and "engaging stakeholders in the process of policy development" is listed beneath the collaboration and partnership domain (NBPHE, 2019). The terms "policy," "policies," and "political" are referred to over 30 times in the CPH domain areas, clearly emphasizing their importance (NBPHE, 2019).

To obtain the CPH credential, you must attend a graduate school or program accredited by the Council on Education for Public Health (CEPH) or be an alumnus of a CEPH-accredited school and have completed all requirements for a master's or doctoral degree. Also, if you have at least a bachelor's degree and at least 5 years of public health work experience or a least a master's degree and 3 years of public health work experience, you are eligible to take the CPH exam (NBPHE, 2020). You can confirm your eligibility with the certification program manager at NBPHE. If, as a public health student, you have not yet graduated and pass the exam, you receive a provisional CPH certification until you graduate. Once your university verifies you have graduated, you are officially included on the CPH registry (NBPHE, 2021).

ACCREDITATION

While individuals can be certified in health education or public health, certification programs and college and university programs can be accredited. In this chapter, we define accreditation as an official certification that a school or course has met standards set by external regulators (Cottrell et al., 2018).

For example, the CHES® certification program was accredited by the National Commission for Certifying Agencies in 2008 and the MCHES® in 2013 (NCHEC & SOPHE, 2020). In addition, NCHEC earned the International Organization for Standardization 17024 accreditation from the International Accreditation Service as a Personnel Certification Body. This accreditation confirms that NCHEC's processes and systems align with acceptable program standards for personnel certifying organizations (NCHEC & SOPHE, 2020). Many universities offering health education programs base their curricula on the CHES® and MCHES® eight areas of responsibility, competencies, and subcompetencies.

The CEPH accredits graduate programs in public health as well as undergraduate programs. These include programs at schools or colleges of public health and public health programs that must include a master's degree. CEPH has accredited schools and colleges of public health since 2013, when the American Public Health Association (APHA) and the Association of School and Programs of Public Health transferred the evaluation of schools of public health to them (CEPH, 2018). In 2013, CEPH adopted accreditation criteria available to all baccalaureate public health programs, including undergraduate health education programs. Currently CEPH is the independent agency recognized by the U.S. Department of Education (DOE) to accredit schools of public health and public health programs outside of schools of public health. In July 2019 CEPH was recognized again by the DOE as the accreditation agency for public health programs (CEPH, 2021). Public health programs must meet criteria and pay fees for CEPH accreditation. To assist applicants to prepare for possible accreditation, CEPH offers several workshops and consultation experiences. Ultimately the CEPH Board of Councilors is the independent body that makes accreditation decisions (CEPH, 2018).

Health advocacy also plays an important role for those working in school health education. This can be found in the accreditation of school health teacher preparation programs. The accreditation agency available for teacher preparation programs (including school health), called the Council for the Accreditation of Educator Preparation (CAEP), originally founded in 1954 as the National Council for the Accreditation of Teacher Education (CAEP, 2015). This accreditation provides an "opportunity to create a unified accreditation system that strengthens the performance standards of teacher education candidates, raises the stature of the teaching profession, and improves the standards for the evidence that supports claims of quality" (NCHEC & SOPHE, 2020, p. 9). CAEP uses a specialized professional association (SPA) to determine quality in a variety of topical areas, including health education. In fall 2019, SOPHE was identified by CAEP as a SPA in health education teacher preparation (NCHEC & SOPHE, 2020). The practice analysis results, including those related to advocacy, are used for the credentialing of school health preparation programs.

There is even an accreditation for public health departments. This accreditation is performed by the Public Health Accreditation Board (PHAB). In order to be accredited, health departments must meet certain standards and measures. They must submit a detailed report as well as engage in a site visit from PHAB representatives to be assessed. After the visit, the health department receives a rating of accredited, reaccredited, or not accredited. After a health department is initially accredited, they have 5 years to apply for reaccreditation. This process helps health departments determine their strengths and weaknesses. In addition, going through the certification process may help them improve the quality of their work to better serve their communities (PHAB, n.d.). So, if you are searching for a job in a health department, you may want to check to see if they are accredited by PHAB (see Advocacy in Action Box 4.1). Just like a certification, it indicates certain standards have been achieved.

WHY ADVOCACY IS IMPORTANT TO HEALTH EDUCATION AND PROMOTION

It may surprise you to learn that law and policy are said to involve one of the most effective strategies to improve population health (Office of Disease Prevention and Health Promotion, n.d.). Many health education professionals work in the areas of policy development and implementation as well as advocacy, acting to influence the opinions of the public and policymakers to support public health policies and programs (APHA, n.d.). "Much of the work of today's health education specialist involves advocating for changes in policies or systems that affect the health of vulnerable and priority populations. Health education specialists must use their expertise and experience to promote national, state, or local, regulations, and other policy decisions to support the public's health" (Auld et al., 2019, p. 26).

As you have already learned, within the HES profession, the emphasis on advocacy has increased over the years. No matter your work setting, you will likely find advocacy to be a skill in demand. To learn what advocacy currently looks like in the health education profession, we can look to the organizations that sponsor certifications in the health education field: the National Commission for Health Education Credentialing (CHES® and MCHES® certifications) and the National Board of Public Health Examiners (CPH certification).

| ADVOCACY IN ACTION BOX 4.1 | Public Health Accreditation Board |

Search your county health department's website to determine if they are accredited by the Public Health Accreditation Board. If they are, you will probably see a round symbol denoting PHAB accreditation like the example below.

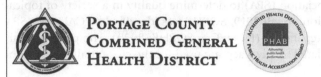

Look around the website to see what type of programs the health department is offering. Do they have a special section on health education? Are they promoting vaccines? If they are a larger county, they may even have a link to health careers or job openings that may be of interest to you. Report your findings in a class discussion about health department work, accreditation and any evidence of how they are advocating to improve community health.

THE IMPORTANCE OF ADVOCACY TO CHES® AND MCHES®

As discussed previously, advocacy's role in the profession has steadily increased in scope and significance. "Health education specialists are expected to advocate for and support initiatives that promote the health of priority populations. This means they should initiate and promote legislation, laws, rules, policies and procedures that are designed to enhance health" (NCHEC & SOPHE, 2020, p. 49). Advocacy takes many forms and takes place in a variety of health education practice settings, including community, school, health care, college/university, and worksite/business (NCHEC & SOPHE, 2020).

REFLECTING ON YOUR ADVOCACY SKILLS

The role of an HES is associated with 4 advocacy competencies and 18 subcompetencies. Use Table 4.3 to assess your interests and skills in the various sub-competencies falling under Area V Advocacy. Place a check mark (√) in the column that best describes your response to each subcompetency.

OTHER COMPETENCIES, SUBCOMPETENCIES, AND KNOWLEDGE RELATED TO ADVOCACY

In addition to the advocacy responsibility (Area V), advocacy is referred to in two other responsibilities (Area I, Assessment of Needs and Capacity; and Area VIII, Ethics and Professionalism). Within Area VIII, focus is on complying with legal standards and regulatory guidelines when engaged in advocacy processes (NCHEC & SOPHE, 2020, p. 66). Additionally, HESs are expected to advocate for their profession (NCHEC & SOPHE, 2020). You can learn more about all the areas of responsibility, competencies, and

TABLE 4.3 Rate Your Advocacy Skills (NCHEC & SOPHE, 2020)

Competency Subcompetency	I Can Do This	I Would Like to Develop in This	I Am Not Interested in This
Identify a current or emerging health issue requiring policy, systems, or environmental change.			
Examine the determinants of health and their underlying causes (e.g., poverty, trauma, and population-based discrimination) related to identified health issues.			
Examine evidence-based informed findings related to identified health issues and desired changes.			
Identify factors that facilitate and/or hinder advocacy efforts (e.g., amount of evidence to prove the issue, potential for partnerships, political readiness, organizational experience or risk, and feasibility of success).			
Write specific, measurable, achievable, realistic, and time-bound (SMART) advocacy objective(s).			
Identify existing coalition(s) or stakeholders that can be engaged in advocacy efforts.			
Engage coalitions and stakeholders in addressing the health issue and planning advocacy efforts.			
Identify existing coalitions and stakeholders that favor and oppose the proposed policy, system, or environmental change and their reasons.			
Identify factors that influence decision makers (e.g., societal and cultural norms, financial considerations, upcoming elections, and voting record).			
ª Create formal and/or informal alliances, task forces, and coalitions to address the proposed change.			
Educate stakeholders on the health issue and the proposed policy, system, or environmental change.			
Identify available resources and gaps (e.g., financial, personnel, information, and data).			
Identify organizational policies and procedures and federal, state, and local laws that pertain to the advocacy efforts.			
Develop persuasive messages and materials (e.g., briefs, resolutions, and fact sheets) to communicate the policy, system, or environmental change.			
Specify strategies, a timeline, and roles and responsibilities to address the proposed policy, system, or environmental change (e.g., develop ongoing relationships with decision makers and stakeholders, use social media, register others to vote, and seek political appointment).			
Engage in advocacy.			
Use media to conduct advocacy (e.g., social media, press releases, public service announcements, and op-eds).			
Use traditional, social, and emerging technologies and methods to mobilize support for policy, system, or environmental change.			
ª Sustain coalitions and stakeholder relationships to achieve and maintain policy, system, or environmental change.			

(continued)

TABLE 4.3 (Continued)

Competency Subcompetency	I Can Do This	I Would Like to Develop in This	I Am Not Interested in This
Evaluate advocacy.			
Conduct process, impact, and outcome evaluation of advocacy efforts.			
Use the results of the evaluation to inform next steps.			

[a] Advanced subcompetency (NCHEC & SOPHE, 2020, pp. 51–53).

Adapted from the "My Skills Checklist" by the Department of Education, Victoria, Australia. https://www.education.vic.gov.au/Documents/school/teachers/teachingresources/careers/personalskills.pdf

National Commission for Health Education Credentialing, Inc. (NCHEC), & Society for Public Health Education, Inc. (SOPHE). (2020). *A competency-based framework for health education specialists—2020.*

subcompetencies associated with CHES® and MCHES® by visiting the NCHEC website (https://www.nchec.org).

Being knowledgeable about advocacy will make your advocacy efforts more effective. For CHES® and MCHES®, advocacy-related knowledge includes that for administrative, legislative, regulatory, and judicial bodies and structure; civic responsibility (e.g., voter registration, run and/or hold political office, attend community meetings); organizational policy development and governance; advocacy terminology, principles, and methods; and media advocacy (NCHEC & SOPHE, 2020, p. 93). There is a lot of knowledge you will learn and skills you will master as you increase your proficiency in advocating for health. Look over Table 4.4 and think about how you may want to get started on your advocacy journey.

CONCLUSION

You learned a lot in this chapter about health education as a strategy and as a profession within public health. Advocacy has become a key component in health education practice; HESs engage stakeholders, plan and evaluate advocacy efforts, and advance policies that improve the health of individuals and communities. Advocacy-related skill expectations have been validated through practice analyses and have evolved to an Area of Responsibility for Health Education Specialists in HESPA II–2020. You also learned that the practice analyses influence professional preparation and continuing education as well as serve as the framework for credentialing, the certification of individuals, and the accreditation of programs. Gaining knowledge about planning, implementing, and evaluating advocacy efforts as well as assessing your personal interests in advocacy work will help you in your advocacy journey and learning the skills for becoming a CHES®, CPH, or other type of credentialed professional in public health.

TABLE 4.4 Steps to Get Started in Advocacy

Strategies to Get Involved With Advocacy Effort	I Am Going to Try This in the Next 3 Months (√)	I Am Going to Try This in the Next 6 Months (√)
Identify a passion/cause focus for my advocacy		
Join a health advocacy organization		
Get to know my policy leaders and other decision makers (e.g., local, state, and national legislators; school board members)		
Learn and engage in the legislative process		
Become familiar with legislative timelines		
Follow advocacy blogs, podcasts, listservs, etc.		
Join a national and/or state professional association (e.g., SOPHE, APHA)		
Volunteer with local nonprofit agency or organization		
Take advantage of advocacy educational trainings		
Join a social media action group		
Create a category for "Advocacy Activities" on my réesumé		

REFERENCES

American Association for Health Education (AAHE), National Commission for Health Education Credentialing, Inc. (NCHEC), & Society for Public Health Education (SOPHE). (1999). *A competency-based framework for graduate-level health educators*. National Commission for Health Education Credentialing.

American Public Health Association (APHA). (n.d.). *APHA legislative advocacy handbook: A guide for effective public health advocacy*.

Auld, M. E., Young, K. J., & Perko, M. (2019). Becoming a health education professional. In R. J. Bensley & J. Brookins-Fisher (Eds.), *Community and public health education methods* (4th ed., pp. 15–31). Jones & Bartlett Learning.

Brannick, M. T., Levine, E. L., & Morgeston, R. P. (2007). *Job and work analysis: Methods, research, and applications in human resource management* (2nd ed.). Sage.

Centers for Disease Control and Prevention (CDC). (2020, August 19). About social determinants of health. https://www.cdc.gov/socialdeterminants/about.html

Cleary, H. (1995). *The credentialing of health educators: An historical account*. National Commission for Health Education Credentialing.

Coalition of National Health Education Organizations (CNHEO). (2020). *Code of ethics for the Health Education Profession®*. http://www.cnheo.org/code-of-ethics.html

Cottrell, R. R., Girvan, J. T., Seabert, D. M., Spear, C., & McKenzie, J. F. (2018). *Principles and foundations of health promotion and education* (7th ed.). Pearson.

Council for the Accreditation of Educator Preparation (CAEP). (2015). History of CAEP. http://caepnet.org/about/history/

Council on Education for Public Health (CEPH). (2018). *Accreditation procedures schools of public health, public health programs, standalone baccalaureate programs*. https://ceph.org/about/org-info/criteria-procedures-documents/criteria-procedures/#

Council on Education for Public Health (CEPH). (2021). CEPH recognized by U.S. Department of Education. https://ceph.org/about/org-info/join-mailing-list/journal/ceph-recognized-us-department-education/

Dictionary.com. (n.d.). Definition of credentialing. https://www.dictionary.com/browse/credentialing

Green, L. W., & Kreuter, M. W. (2005). *Health program planning: An educational and ecological approach* (4th ed.). McGraw-Hill.

Henderson, A. C., McIntosh, D. V., & Carlyon, W. H. (1980). The initial phase of role delineation for health education: A summary report. *Journal of the American College Health Association, 29*, 119–123.

Henderson, A. C., McIntosh, D. V., & Schaller, W. E. (1981). Progress report of the Role Delineation Project. *Journal of School Health, 51*, 373–376.

Kerr, D., Blavos, A., Rauch, H., Brookins-Fisher, J., & Thompson, A. (2019). CHES, MCHES, and/or CPH? Selecting the best credential for you. *Health Promotion Practice, 20*(2), 167–172. https://doi.org/10.1177/1524839918825132

National Board of Public Health Examiners (NBPHE). (2019). *CPH content outline 2019.* https://nbphe-wp-production.s3.us-east-1.amazonaws.com/app/uploads/2017/05/ContentOutlineMay-21-2019.pd

National Board of Public Health Examiners (NBPHE). (2016). *A job analysis of the Certified in Public Health.* http://s3.amazonaws.com/nbphe-wp-production/app/uploads/2017/09/2016jta_report.pdf

National Board of Public Health Examiners (NBPHE). (2019). CPH content outline 2019. https://nbphe-wp-production.s3.us-east-1.amazonaws.com/app/uploads/2017/05/ContentOutlineMay-21-2019.pdf

National Board of Public Health Examiners (NBPHE). (2020). Candidate handbook. Certified in Public Health. https://nbphe-wp-production.s3.amazonaws.com/app/uploads/2017/05/CPH-Candidate-Handbook.pdf

National Board of Public Health Examiners (NBPHE), CPH Certified in Public Health. (2021). CPH FAQs. https://www.nbphe.org/cph-exam-faqs/

National Commission for Health Education Credentialing, Inc. (NCHEC). (n.d.). CHES exam eligibility. https://www.nchec.org/exam-eligibility-guide

National Commission for Health Education Credentialing, Inc. (NCHEC). (1985). *A framework for the development of competency-based curricula for entry-level health educators.*

National Commission for Health Education Credentialing, Inc. (NCHEC), & Society for Public Health Education, Inc. (SOPHE). (2015). *A competency-based framework for health education specialists—2015.*

National Commission for Health Education Credentialing, Inc. (NCHEC), & Society for Public Health Education, Inc. (SOPHE). (2020). *A competency-based framework for health education specialists—2020.*

National Commission for Health Education Credentialing, Inc. (NCHEC), Society for Public Health Education (SOPHE), & American Association for Health Education (AAHE). (2010). *A competency-based framework for health education specialists—2010.*

Office of Disease Prevention and Health Promotion. (n.d.). Law and health policy. https://www.healthypeople.gov/2020/law-and-health-policy

Pollock, M. B., & Carlyon, W. (1996). Seven responsibilities and how they grew: The story of a curriculum framework. *Journal of Health Education, 27*, 81–87.

Prosser, T. L., & Gautam, Y. R. (2011). Role delineation in health education. *Health Education Monograph Series, 28*(3), 60–65.

Public Health Accreditation Board. (n.d.). *The mission of the public health accreditation board.* https://phaboard.org/accreditation-background/

Videto, D. M., Dennis, D. L., & Joint Committee on Health Education and Promotion Terminology. (2021). Report of the 2020 Joint Committee on Health Education and Promotion Terminology. *Health Educator, 53*(1), 4–21.

CHAPTER 4: END-OF-CHAPTER ACTIVITIES

DISCUSSION QUESTIONS

1. Why is advocacy an important professional competency for health education specialists and other allied professions?

2. In what ways is advocacy considered a "skill"? What suggestions would you have for a public health professional seeking to gain and improve advocacy-related skills and abilities?

3. Look over the competencies and subcompetencies expected of entry-level health education specialists (Table 4.3). Were there any that surprised you? Which do you believe will be the most difficult to learn or conduct? Why? Are there any that you believe should be added?

APPLICATION ACTIVITIES

1. On completing Table 4.3, reflect on your responses. Write a reflection paper answering these questions: (a) Which of the subcompetencies do you feel most confident about? (b) Which of the subcompetencies interests you the most? (c) Which of the subcompetencies would you like to improve upon? What ideas do you have for opportunities to improve in these areas?

2. Find an individual with a health certification (CHES®, MCHES®, or CPH) and interview them. Here are some possible interview questions: Do you think it is important to get certified? Why did you get certified? Would you advise eligible young professionals to obtain a CHES® or CPH certification? Why or why not? Do you think certification of individuals and accreditation of programs in health education and public health is beneficial or unnecessary? Why or why not?

3. Work in small groups to create Venn diagrams comparing the emphases of CHES®/MCHES® and CPH on advocacy and policy; identify and discuss similarities and differences.

4. Consider how you can demonstrate your advocacy work using the checklist below:

    _____Media samples, such as letters to the editor, op-ed pieces, public service announcements, media kits, press releases

    _____Fact sheets for legislators on advocacy topics

    _____ Social media postings (of advocacy efforts)

    _____Photos from the advocacy activities, such as a health advocacy summit, meetings with legislators, town halls, and the like

    _____Infographic used in advocacy effort

ADDITIONAL RESOURCES

American Public Health Association Advocacy for Public Health. (n.d.). *Advocacy for public health*. https://www.apha.org/Policies-and-Advocacy/Advocacy-for-Public-Health

National Board of Public Health Examiners. (n.d.). CPH certification handbook. https://nbphe-wp-production.s3.amazonaws.com/app/uploads/2017/05/CPH-Candidate-Handbook.pdf

National Commission for Health Education Credentialing (NCHEC). (n.d.). CHES® exam eligibility questions. https://www.nchec.org/ches-exam-eligibility

National Commission for Health Education Credentialing. (n.d.). *Home page.* https://www.nchec.org

Society for Public Health Association Advocating for Public Health. (n.d.). *Advocating for public health.* https://www.sophe.org/advocacy/

QUIZ QUESTIONS

1. What is the primary purpose of a practice analysis?
   a. To verify current skills and knowledge needed for a given profession
   b. To develop credentialing examinations for individuals within a profession
   c. To design curricula for preparing individuals to enter a profession
   d. To ensure that determinants of health are addressed

2. How frequently are practice analyses in the health education profession typically conducted?
   a. Every year
   b. Every 2 years
   c. Every 5 years
   d. Every 10 years

3. What is the name of the most recent practice analysis in health education?
   a. HESPA
   b. HESPA II
   c. HEJA
   d. CUP

4. Which of the following is a program or school-level accreditation?
   a. MCHES®
   b. CHES®
   c. CPH
   d. CEPH

5. When comparing CPH and CHES® and MCHES®, advocacy is
   a. emphasized equally in both certifications.
   b. emphasized more in the CPH than the CHES® and MCHES®.
   c. emphasized more in the CHES® and MCHES® than CPH.
   d. emphasized only in CPH when policy is referred to.

6. Which of the following is an advocacy-related expectation for entry-level health education specialists?
   a. joining local protests that address health inequities
   b. developing policy proposals for legislators
   c. identifying stakeholders who oppose a proposed policy
   d. lobbying legislators to support a specific bill

7. CHES® and MCHES® advocacy-related knowledge includes which of the following?
    a. Knowledge about government structure and legislative process
    b. Understanding basics of the judicial system
    c. Advocacy terminology and strategies
    d. All of the above

8. The CHES® and CPH exams allow individuals to earn what?
    a. a license
    b. accreditation
    c. certification
    d. a degree

9. Which of the following of the eight areas of responsibility for health educators was created after a 2020 Health Education Specialist Practice Analysis (HESPA)?
    a. program planning
    b. health communication
    c. ethics and research
    d. advocacy

10. Steps you can take to get started in advocacy include
    a. learn and engage in the legislative process
    b. subscribe to action alerts from organizations in your field
    c. follow advocacy blogs, podcasts, listservs, and so on
    d. all of the above

ANSWER KEY

1. **A.** To verify current skills and knowledge needed for a given profession
2. **C.** Every 5 years
3. **B.** HESPA II
4. **D.** CEPH
5. **C.** Emphasized more in the CHES® and MCHES® than CPH
6. **C.** Identifying stakeholders who oppose a proposed policy
7. **D.** All of the above
8. **C.** Certification
9. **D.** Advocacy
10. **D.** All of the above

4.3 TYLER G. JAMES

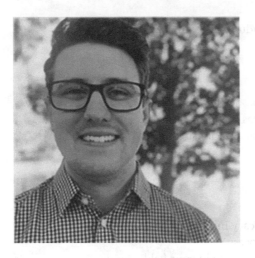

Q. What Led or Inspired You to Become Engaged in Advocacy—Specifically as It Relates to Policy Change and Public Health?

My advocacy work with people with disabilities and, more specifically, Deaf communities who use American Sign Language (ASL), started in the early years of my PhD program. As a non-Deaf undergraduate student attending Deaf community events, I heard stories of a lack of equal access to K–12 education environments, a lack of employment opportunities, and a lack of patient-centered care in healthcare settings. Collectively, these inequities are connected to a fundamental cause, audism: a system of advantage based on hearing ability (Bauman, 2004, p. 245). In 2017, I witnessed a Deaf friend and mentor be denied effective communication in the emergency room for over 8 hours: What happened to the Americans With Disabilities Act, passed 27 years prior? At that point, I gained clarity on the oppressive nature of healthcare environments for people with disabilities, began to recognize the significant limitations of existing policy and the implementation of those policies, and decided to dedicate my work to improving outcomes for people with disabilities in healthcare settings.

Q. Describe the Deaf and Disability Advocacy Work You Have Done Around Policy, Education at a Local, State, or National Level

The bulk of my experience to date has focused on local, individual-level issues. In the local Deaf community, I gained the reputation for "knowing the words to say" to advocate for effective communication access. My patient-level advocacy has taken me from the emergency department, to the intensive care unit, and to a mental health hospital. I have similar experience working with students with disabilities in higher education, fighting for equal communication access to graduate and professional coursework. I am deeply honored to be trusted to serve in this capacity in inherently private and vulnerable times. I also recognize that my existence in these situations is a demonstration of the systems of oppression: In a just world, I would not need to be present.

The focus on individual-level advocacy has been multifaceted. The people I have worked with have been empowered and enabled to be strong self-advocates, and, in most cases, their issues have been resolved. However, the system-level change rarely occurs—the same systems I have advocated in continue to oppress Deaf and disabled people.

In recognizing the limitations of individual-level advocacy, my work has started to transform to more state- and federal-level advocacy. I have worked as a fact witness in a lawsuit where people with disabilities are suing state agencies denying them equal access; I have started working with Deaf-led state coalitions, in Florida and in Michigan, dedicated to improving the health of people with disabilities through policy change; and my research with Deaf collaborators has started focusing on state and national policy issues.

Q. What Are Some of the Biggest Challenges You Have Faced as an Advocate?

Working against systems of oppression that are operating as designed can be frustrating. My historic focus on individual-level advocacy had more immediate reinforcement—either the Deaf patients were provided communication access or they were not. There is a lack of short-term reinforcement when working at higher levels of advocacy; this, paired with the frustration, may create conditions of burnout.

Q. What's One Piece of Advice You Would Like to Offer Emerging Advocates in Public Health?

Work with community partners; recognize that they are the experts of how policy affects them locally. Be comfortable with them challenging the way you think.

Ethics of Public Policy Frameworks

Systems and Environmental Change

SARA FINGER AND E. LISAKO J. MCKYER

Those closest to the problem are closest to the solution.

—**GLENN E. MARTIN**

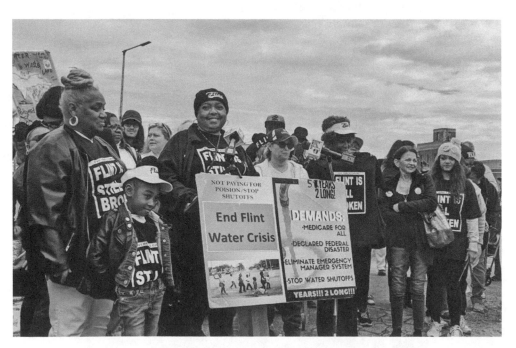

FIGURE 5.1 Protesters in Flint, Michigan, call for action and accountability over water contamination.

Photo by Pexels.com.

Sara Finger and E. Lisako J. McKyer, *Ethics of Public Policy Frameworks: Systems and Environmental Change.* In: *Be the Change.* Edited by Keely S. Rees, Jody Early, and Cicily Hampton, Oxford University Press. © Oxford University Press 2023. DOI: 10.1093/oso/9780197570890.003.0005

Objectives

1. Identify ethical frameworks used in public health.
2. Review examples of codes of ethics.
3. Critique the frameworks for ethical decision-making.
4. Review common sources of ethical standards.
5. Demonstrate how to apply an ethical lens to public health policies.
6. Analyze ethical scenarios related to public health and advocacy.

INTRODUCTION

We constantly face choices that have consequences, for ourselves and others. For those working to improve the health of individuals, communities, and populations, attempts to improve the public's health through policy change are a means to affect and alter systems and environments. In other words, the contexts in which people live. Yet, the most well-intentioned public policies can have unintended adverse effects. Thus, it is critical for public health professionals to consider the ethical implications of policies we seek to enact and/or evaluate.

Public health is an evidence-informed practice. The principles of ethics are not based on feelings, religion, law, accepted social practice, or science. In public health, ethics are about making decisions and upholding standards of behavior based on a common "code." According to the American Public Health Association's Code of Ethics (2019): "A code is not the only lens that society uses to evaluate the performance of its professions, but it is a visible statement of the collective conscience of a profession, and it is one benchmark against which specific professional practices can be measured" (p.1). The Coalition for Health Education Organizations (CNHEO) revised their Code of Ethics in 2020 and states its framework is for health education professionals and "is grounded in fundamental ethical principles, including: value of life, promoting justice, ensuring beneficence, and avoiding harm." (CNHEO, 2020, p. 1).

The concept of what is "ethical" relies heavily on culture and philosophical perspectives. Indeed, there is an entire field of scholarly endeavors focused on the various philosophies of ethics. Many of the philosophical approaches to ethics subscribed to in Western cultures like that of the United States are based on the works of ancient Greek philosophers. Some of the more contemporary and emerging ethical philosophies are hybrids of Western, Eastern, and everything in between. Thus, what is ethical is relative and depends on a person's perspectives and values. The Centers for Disease Control and Prevention (CDC; 2017) defined public health ethics as a "a systematic process to clarify, prioritize and justify possible courses of public health action based on ethical principles, values and beliefs of stakeholders, and scientific and other information."(https://www.cdc.gov/os/integrity/phethics/index.htm)

In this chapter, we provide a brief overview of common philosophies, share examples of ethical codes and guidelines, and explore scenarios in order to ensure public health professionals are grounded in the foundation of Western ethics. This is simply a first step in understanding ethics and its implications for public policy and advocacy.

SOCIOECOLOGY OF HEALTH

For the past 20 years, much of our focus in public health has been on individual behaviors and lifestyles. Unfortunately, this emphasis on the person versus the social influences impacting an individual's health has built a culture of victim blaming. In relation to individual-level changes, we must recognize their limitations and characteristics:

- they take place one time and are often short term;
- they often result in temporary changes;
- they are not a part of an ongoing plan; and
- they are nonsustaining.

The socioecological framework to health promotion (McLeroy et al., 1988) emphasizes that health promotion should not focus solely on intrapersonal behavioral factors, but must consider factors at multiple socioecological levels that influence health. Specific to system and environmental changes, this framework addresses the importance of interventions directed at changing interpersonal, organizational, community, and public policy factors that support and maintain unhealthy behaviors (Golden, et al., 2015). This perspective assumes that appropriate changes in the social environment will produce changes in individuals and, in turn, populations. Finally, the support of individuals in the population is essential for implementing environmental changes.

In contrast to individual-level change, systems and environmental changes are characterized as

- part of an ongoing, long-term strategy;
- influencing behavior changes over time;
- taking place at the population level; and
- sustainable.

MOVING FROM THE INDIVIDUAL TO FOCUSING ON SYSTEMS AND ENVIRONMENTAL CHANGE

If we only focus on the individual, we not only enable and perpetuate the victim-blaming culture, but also miss the enormous opportunities to have longer lasting, deeper, and broader impacts. In public health, we have the opportunity and obligation to go beyond programming and practice by focusing on changing the systems and environments that create the structures in which we work, live, and play.

Systems change focuses on modifying large-scale, complex systems serving as determinants of health, including how a place operates (Leischow, et al, 2008). This may include social environmental systems (e.g., schools, workplaces) and systems with less-than-obvious linkages to public health outcomes (Figure 5.1). Examples include the penal system and mortgage approval processes (banking systems). Changing systems requires coming to terms with the complexity (Leischow et al., 2008).

A system may be environmental, such as an ecosystem; biological, such as our own digestive system; or processes. In public health, the systems we refer to are often social in nature, such as our food distribution systems, educational systems, economic systems, and healthcare systems.

An example of a systems *change* may be a hospital adopting a baby-friendly hospital initiative as part of their required operations. In this case, the standard way of doing business is changed. Another example of system-level change is a county commission modifying their bylaws to require the inclusion of youth (or other marginalized populations) as voting members with full privileges on all issues brought to the council.

If your goal was to ensure access to healthy food in your community, some systems change approaches may include the following:

- *implementing a system of local farm-to-school programs*
- *connecting emergency food providers with local growers in a sustainable way*
- *implementing the national school lunch program across the state's school systems*
- *creating a certification process for school bake sales to ensure they are in line with school wellness policies*

These approaches should be designed and implemented such that they become part of the regular and institutionalized (i.e., permanent) way of doing business.

Environmental change focuses on modifications to the physical environment—"places" such as a school, park, workplace, or clinic (Bracht, 1999). Importantly, environmental changes are designed such that the environment as a context for behavior supports and even makes easy the desired behavior (Engbers et al., 2005).

An example of an environmental change may be a university campus that changes all on-campus streets to bicycle- and pedestrian-only roadways. Driving then becomes an inconvenience compared to biking or walking.

Other examples of changes to the environment might include:

- *designing buildings such that stairs are more easily accessible than elevators for the majority of people*
- *a municipality planning process ensures easy access and safe pedestrian and bicycle access to main roads and parks*
- *zoning changes to facilitate neighborhood corner markets featuring fresh fruits and vegetables and other healthy foods*

Similar to systems changes, environmental changes should be implemented such that they become part of people's everyday landscape. For example, all workplaces are designed and built with nursing mothers in mind, all neighborhoods are pedestrian friendly, or low-sugar/sugar-free beverages cost substantially less than sugar-laden drinks.

Unlike clinical health fields such as medicine or nursing where the individual patient knowingly subjects themselves to care, public health efforts often occur without people's knowledge or explicit consent. For example, physicians inform patients of treatment choices so they can jointly determine which approach to take. Environmental public health practitioners may modify drinking water treatment approaches without citizens ever knowing. A community health practitioner may advocate for legislative changes on behalf of a community, even if several community members are unaware.

Therein lies an ethical dilemma for public health professionals: Can we implement public health interventions among people who are unaware of, or even disagree with, our advocacy efforts, which are ostensibly on their behalf? How do we determine what is the right thing to do?

WHAT IT LOOKS LIKE TO BE ETHICAL

When we use the term "ethical," it means more than simply being good or bad, right or wrong, just or unjust. Often, we believe that we can discern the difference between these things. Indeed, from movies, books, and stories, it seems readily apparent there are two sides, making it easy to decipher the "good people" from the bad, the "righteous side" from the wrong. Yet when it comes to advocacy, the lines between "sides" are often blurred and relative to one's perspective. The validity of arguments are in the eye of the beholder.

For those of us in public health, it is critical that we set our own lodestar. We must establish the principles and beliefs that will guide our actions. More importantly, we must be aware of the sources of our own values and beliefs, as they heavily influence our decisions, actions, and ethical perspectives. We do not have to share the same ethical philosophies and we are not required to agree on the various approaches to achieving systemic and environmental change. We must, however, learn to recognize the source of our ethical beliefs and perspectives—the lens by which we view actions—in order for us to adequately evaluate the impact of public policies on systems and environments (Figure 5.2). In other words, we must train ourselves to recognize and understand our own implicit beliefs so that we may be accountable for our chosen actions based on what we believe to be just and inherently good.

As referenced in Chapter 2, public health involves promoting and protecting the health of people and communities where they live, learn, work, and play. So, at the heart of our profession, our aim is to proactively help people reach their optimal health. In that frame, for a public health professional to be ethical, they must champion the policies and systems that help people be their healthiest. Equally, we must fight against those policies and systems that create barriers to good health and lead to wide health disparities and inequities.

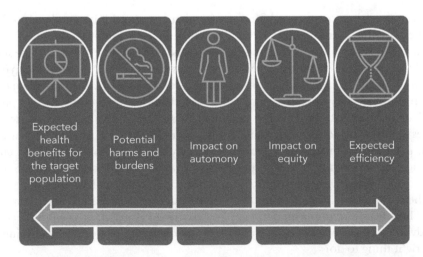

FIGURE 5.2 Substantive normative criteria that should guide ethical analysis in public health.

FRAMEWORKS FOR ETHICS

In the simplest of terms, ethical theories can be categorized broadly into two groups: consequentialist and nonconsequentialist (Gustafson, 2018).

Consequentialism

Within the consequentialist framework (Gustafson, 2018), a person acts in a way to produce the most good. It is all about achieving the best outcomes in each situation. In other words, "the end justifies the means."

For example, if someone believes that it could be right to kill one person to prevent the deaths of many others, they are, at least partially, a **consequentialist**.

Nonconsequentialism

In the nonconsequentialist framework (Gustafson, 2018), a person judges the rightness or wrongness of an action based on properties intrinsic to the action, not on its consequences.

A **nonconsequentialist** would believe it is inherently wrong to murder people and refuse to kill even one person, even if not killing that one person would lead to the death of many others.

Ethical Codes and Guidelines

Each human being is embedded in their own systems and environments, such as communities, families, and cultures, each with their respective ethical standards, rights, obligations. How that is defined and implemented can vary, of course. Similarly, most major health disciplines and respective professional organizations have rules, codes, or guidelines that outline the behavioral expectations of its professionals.

Many people are familiar with the paraphrase of the Hippocratic oath (2021), commonly translated as "first do no harm." In the mid-1800s, the American Medical Association (AMA) prepared (1848) and adopted a code of ethics based on the work of Hippocrates. Subsequently, other allied health professions developed and adopted their own codes with the intention of guiding their respective members to uphold a standard of practice.

Here are examples of two public health–related codes: shared principles health ethics and public health ethics.

Shared Principles Health Ethics

Principles are defined as a comprehensive and fundamental law, doctrine, or assumption. They are often seen as a rule or code of conduct. Given the common AMA-based ethical principle pedigree shared by public health and other allied health, there are several cross-cutting themes in common. Three of these major principles are reflected in the *Belmont Report* (U.S. Department of Health, Education, and Welfare, 1979). This report is a landmark document prepared in response to the horrific human rights violations committed during the Tuskegee Syphilis Study (National Commission for the Protection of Human Subjects of Biomedical and Behavioral Research, 1979). The three major ethical principles are as follows:

1. **Respect for Persons.** This is exemplified by ensuring individuals have autonomy and their desires and rights are respected. Further, individuals who are unable to exert their autonomy are to be afforded special protection.

2. **Beneficence.** This is the obligation to go beyond simple nonmaleficence (do no harm). Rather, this principle requires benefit to individuals AND collectives in the conduct of health-related research.
3. **Principle of justice.** This principle demands equitable opportunities (which is not the same as equal opportunities) as well as risk. In the context of health, Norman Daniels (2007) considered health equity a matter of fairness and justice.

PUBLIC HEALTH ETHICS: NOT THE SAME AS BIOETHICS

Public health's focus on populations takes on a macro-level perspective in determining what is beneficial and just. Indeed, one could argue that our obligation to maximizing populations' health may conflict with individual-level application of the principles of beneficence and nonmaleficence. Ron Bayer and Amy Fairchild (public health ethicists) wrote a thought-provoking article (2004) outlining how public health ethics should not be based in bioethics given the individual-centric foundations of the latter. Then, what should public health professionals use to guide our decision-making (Figure 5.3)? How do we hold ourselves accountable to ethical decision-making?

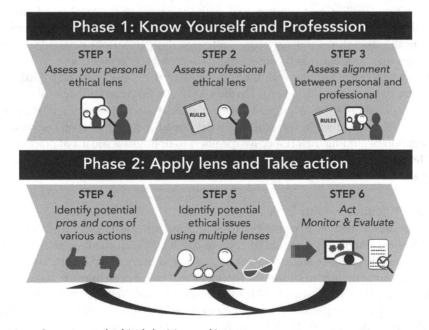

FIGURE 5.3 Steps toward ethical decision-making.

TABLE 5.1 Guiding Questions to Identify an Ethical Lens

Outcomes	Virtue	Rule	Justice
When faced with a difficult decision, the most important consideration for me is . . .			
The greater good	How it reflects my character	Fulfilling my responsibilities	Ensuring fairness
If I have to do something others might consider to be bad, I believe it is ethical . . .			
If the benefits to most people outweigh the bad to some	If it builds or maintains good character	If I adhere to preestablished rules about what is ethical	If it reduces inequities in the world
I am most comfortable with making decisions when the ethical guidelines . . .			
Gives me some latitude to evaluate costs and benefits	Are established by people of good character	Are not wishy-washy, but are clear-cut	Encompass a fair and equitable process
If I have to decide between helping 1 person versus 100, I will probably . . .			
Do what will help 100 people	Be guided by morals about what to do	Do whatever I am required to do, even if I disagree	Help the side that results in an equitable outcome

FRAMEWORKS FOR ETHICAL DECISION-MAKING

Ethics comes down to the decision-making process and the beliefs by which that process is informed. Having a method for ethical decision-making is critical (Table 5.1). Only by careful exploration of the problem, aided by the insights and different perspectives of others, can we make good ethical decisions. The *three broad frameworks to guide ethical decision making* are consequentialism, duty, and virtue.

- The *consequentialism framework* focuses on the future effects of possible courses of action, considering the people who will be directly or indirectly affected. We consider what outcomes are desirable in a given situation and believe ethical conduct to be whatever will achieve the best consequences. A person using the consequentialism framework desires to produce the most good.
- The *duty framework* focuses on the duties and obligations that we have in a given situation and considers what ethical obligations we have and what things we should never do. Ethical conduct is defined by doing one's duties and doing the right thing, and the goal is performing the correct action. Doing what is right is not about the consequences of our actions (something over which we ultimately have no control) but about having the proper intention in performing the action (Afghanistan).
- The *virtue framework* focuses on what kind of person we should be and what our actions say about our character. We define ethical behavior as whatever a virtuous person would do in a given situation, and we seek to develop similar virtues.

Table 5.2 from Brown University researchers Bonde and Firenze is designed to highlight the main contrasts between these three frameworks.

TABLE 5.2 Contrasting Frameworks for Ethical Decision-Making

	Consequentialism	Duty	Virtue
Deliberative process	What kind of outcomes should I produce or try to produce?	What are my obligations in this situation, and what are the things I should never do?	What kind of person should I be (or try to be), and what will my actions show about my character?
Focus	Focuses on future events of an action or the people who will be directly or indirectly affected by the action.	Focuses on the duties that exist prior to the situation and determines obligations.	Tries to discern character traits that are, or could be, motivating the people involved in the situation.
Definition of ethical conduct	Action that will achieve the best consequences.	Action that prioritizes individual will and intention over the consequences; never failing to do one's duty.	Action that a fully virtuous person would do under the circumstances.
Motivation	Produce the most good.	Perform the right action.	Develop one's character.

COMMON SOURCES FOR ETHICAL STANDARDS

Since the field of public health is complex and multifaceted, the guidelines and history of public health ethics also are. With the evolution of public health, numerous people have been involved with outlining ethical principles and frameworks over the years, including Kass in 2001; Childress et al. (2002); Roberts and Reich (2002); Upshur (2002); Power and Faden (2006); the Nuffield Bioethics Council (2007); Daniels (2007); and Arras and Fenton (2009). Common assumptions and beliefs carry through most of their frameworks, including the need to balance a moral obligation to prevent harm and health promotion with respect to individual autonomy in public health.

These many philosophers and ethicists have helped us determine what ethics are based on. They have suggested at least five different sources of ethical standards to use:

- **Rights Approach**—protects and respects the moral rights of those affected, including the right to make one's own choices about what kind of life to lead, to be told the truth, to not be injured, and to receive a degree of privacy.
- **Utilitarian Approach**—emphasizes actions that provide the most good and deals with consequences; it tries both to increase the good done and to reduce the harm done.
- **Fairness and Justice Approach**—promotes that all those involved should be treated equally.
- **Common Good Approach**—suggests that the interlocking relationships of society are the basis of ethical reasoning and that respect and compassion for all others—especially the vulnerable—are requirements of such reasoning. This approach also calls attention to the common conditions that are important to the welfare of everyone. It may be a system of laws, police and fire departments, healthcare, a public educational system, or even public recreational areas.

- **Virtue Approach**—emphasizes that ethical actions ought to be consistent with certain idealistic virtues like honesty, courage, compassion, generosity, tolerance, love, fidelity, integrity, fairness, self-control, and prudence. Virtue ethicists ask of any action: "What kind of person will I become if I do this?" or "Is this action consistent with acting at my best?"

APPLYING AN ETHICAL LENS TO PUBLIC HEALTH POLICIES

There are several tools available to help public health practitioners evaluate the ethics of healthcare and health policies. A review published in 2021 found 13 different tools available; the authors evaluated each tool for its ethical bent and its application to the various socioecological levels (e.g., local-level policy, national policy). The following is based on an example outlined in *A Framework for Making Ethical Decisions*, a product of dialogue and debate in the seminar Making Choices: Ethical Decisions at the Frontier of Global Science held at Brown University in the spring semester 201 (Brown, 2011).

Step 2: WHAT–Recognize an ethical issue.

Step 2: WHO–Consider who is involved. Consider all individuals and groups who may be impacted negatively and positively by your decision.

Step 3: WHY–Collect data and understand the situation. Identify information needed to make a decision, including where and from whom the input should come.

Step 4: HOW–Evaluate your decision-making options.
- Which action will produce the most good and do the least harm? (the utilitarian approach)
- Which action respects the rights of all who have a stake in the decision? (the rights approach)
- Which action treats people equally or proportionally? (the justice approach)
- Which action serves the community as a whole, not just some members? (the common good approach)
- Which action leads me to act as the sort of person I believe I should be? (the virtue approach)

Step 5: DECIDE–Evaluate which approach leads you to the decision you feel best about.

Step 6: ACT and REFLECT–Move forward with a decision and reflect on the consequences of your actions. Ask yourself if you would change anything on seeing the impact of your decision.

To help demonstrate what it looks like to be an ethical public health professional, the below narrative describes a real-life public health systems change approach by which Sara Finger's (executive director and founder of the Wisconsin Alliance for Women's Health [WAWH]) experience with the WAWH exposed an ethical shortcoming.

After reading the case scenario from WAWH above, consider the following questions:

- What theory of ethics drove WAWH's decision-making in their quest to "do good"?
- Knowing what happened and understanding the missteps they took, what ethical framework approach would you recommend for increasing access to LARCs? Explain your rationale.

ADVOCACY IN ACTION BOX 5.1	Increasing the Use of Long-Acting Reversible Contraception in Wisconsin

In the last decade, public health has lifted up long-acting reversible contraception (LARC) as a powerful tool to help plan, prevent, and space pregnancies. Around 2008, there were large investments, a great deal of attention paid, and a lot of energy expended to determine how to increase the usage of LARC among those of reproductive age in Wisconsin. Often, those who gathered to discuss how to increase LARC usage included mostly academic professionals and healthcare providers. While not unique to this situation, this table of decision makers was predominantly White and privileged. The public health experts who were expected and compensated to sit at that table had incredible ideas and were successful to the extent in which they accessed and held up best practices and evidence when making changes inside the healthcare system. They determined that more labor and delivery departments should stock and offer immediate postpartum insertion of LARC, and they aimed to train more pediatricians and family practice physicians on how to perform same-day insertion for patients. This group of decision makers mapped out exactly how to prime the healthcare system to make it easier for patients to get LARC. Yet, they made one major ethical misstep. They failed to incorporate the voices and experiences of patients and neglected to acknowledge the valid and deeply rooted distrust that many patients—especially patients of color—feel toward the healthcare system.

Nothing About Us, Without Us

While it was noble for these experts to gather, assess, and make plans to increase LARC usage to advance people's health, this wasn't the "field of dreams," and if they built it, people were not guaranteed to come. What surfaced as unjust about this public health work was that it failed to examine both sides of the healthcare "coin." The table they set did not include or incorporate community voices and largely ignored the perspectives of those most impacted by the issue. In fact, they directly contradicted the voices and experiences of patients who had for generations experienced reproductive coercion and oppression (reference Undivided Rights).

Still, with full frankness, this is how public health has traditionally been practiced. The experts who are typically White and privileged are paid to make decisions that affect the health and well-being of others. Those closest to the public health problems—the community—rarely are compensated for their time or sought for their opinions and engagement. Rather, they are often forced to settle with a quick survey, focus group, or listening session for the sake of checking the "community input" box on a list. It is a patronizing approach to problem-solving.

Until our nonprofits, academics, and healthcare workforces are more diverse and genuinely include voices and authentic involvement from a variety of perspectives, the ethical approach for us all to take is to intentionally evaluate who is missing from any given policy or system change conversation and to find ways not only to incorporate, but also to invest in and compensate community members for their valuable insight and contributions.

CONCLUSION

On the front lines of public health, you will be called on to think before you act, even in urgent situations. You will be called to navigate a complex menu of options and analyze the potential consequences of your decisions. Your imperative should be to preempt the negative consequences of an action by thoughtfully engaging with ethical frameworks and standards as outlined in this chapter.

Remember that the principles of ethics are not based on feelings, religion, law, accepted social practice, or science. Ethics is about making decisions and upholding a standard of behavior. Setting a consistent standard can set your own professional compass.

While your personal values have certainly guided you to the field of public health, it is your responsibility to allow your profession's code of ethics, not your personal beliefs, to guide your best decision-making as you aim to promote and protect the health of people and communities where they live, learn, work, and play.

REFERENCES

American Medical Association & New York Academy of Medicine. (1848). *Code of medical ethics.* Academy of Medicine.

American Public Health Association. (2019) Public health code of ethics. https://www.apha.org/-/media/files/pdf/membergroups/ethics/code_of_ethics.ashx

Fenton, E., & Arras, J.D. (2009). Bioethics and Human Rights: Curb Your Enthusiasm. *Cambridge Quarterly of Healthcare Ethics, 19,* 127–133.

Bayer, R., & Fairchild, A. L. (2004). The genesis of public health ethics. *Bioethics, 18*(6), 473–492. https://doi.org/10.1111/j.1467-8519.2004.00412.x

Brown University. A Framework for Making Ethical Decisions | Science and Technology Studies. (n.d.). https://www.brown.edu/academics/science-and-technology-studies/framework-making-ethical-decisions.

Bracht, N. F. (1999). *Health promotion at the community level: new advances* (Vol. 15). Sage Publications.

Centers for Disease Control & Prevention. (2017, October 11). *Public health ethics.* https://www.cdc.gov/os/integrity/phethics/index.htm

Childress, J., Faden, R., Gaare, R., Gostin, L., Kahn, J., Bonnie, R., Kass, N., Mastroianni, A., Moreno, J., & Nieburg, P. (2002). Public Health Ethics: Mapping the Terrain. *Journal of Law, Medicine & Ethics, 30*(2), 170–178. doi:10.1111/j.1748-720X.2002.tb00384.x

Coalition for National Health Education Organizations (CNHEO). (2020). *Code of Ethics for the Health Education Profession®.* http://cnheo.org/ethics-of-the-profession.html

Daniels, N. (2007). *Just health: Meeting health needs fairly.* Cambridge University Press.

Engbers, L. H., van Poppel, M. N., Paw, M. J. C. A., & van Mechelen, W. (2005). Worksite health promotion programs with environmental changes: A systematic review. *American Journal of Preventive Medicine, 29*(1), 61–70. https://doi.org/10.1016/j.amepre.2005.03.001

Golden, S. D., McLeroy, K. R., Green, L. W., Earp, J. A. L., & Lieberman, L. D. (2015). Upending the social ecological model to guide health promotion efforts toward policy and environmental change. *Health Education & Behavior, 42*(1, Suppl.), 8S–14S. https://doi.org/10.1177/1090198115575098

Gustafson, A. (2018). Consequentialism and non-consequentialism. In E. Heath, B. Kaldis, & A Marcoux (Eds.), *The Routledge companion to business ethics* (pp. 79–95). Routledge.

Hippocratic Oath. (2021, July 30). In *Wikipedia.* https://en.wikipedia.org/wiki/Hippocratic_Oath

Leischow, S. J., Best, A., Trochim, W. M., Clark, P. I., Gallagher, R. S., Marcus, S. E., & Matthews, E. (2008). Systems thinking to improve the public's health. *American Journal of Preventive Medicine, 35*(2), S196–S203. https://doi.org/10.1016/j.amepre.2008.05.014

McLeroy, K. R., Bibeau, D., Steckler, A., & Glanz, K. (1988). An ecological perspective on health promotion programs. *Health Education Quarterly, 15*(4), 351–377. https://doi.org/10.1177/109019818801500401

Merriam-Webster. (n.d.) *Principle.* https://www.merriam-webster.com/dictionary/principle

Roberts, M. J., & Reich, M. R. (2002). Ethical analysis in public health. *Lancet, 359,* 1055–1059.

Upshur R. E. (2002). Principles for the justification of public health intervention. *Canadian journal of public health = Revue canadienne de sante publique*, 93(2), 101–103. https://doi.org/10.1007/BF03404547

U.S. Department of Health Education and Welfare. (1979). *The Belmont report: Ethical principles and guidelines for the protection of human subjects of research.* National Commission for the Protection of Human Subjects of Biomedical and Behavioral Research.

CHAPTER 5: END-OF-CHAPTER ACTIVITIES

DISCUSSION QUESTIONS

1. What are the four general ethical frameworks that serve as the source of the public health ethics lens?

2. What are the three responsibilities that public health ethics practice are charged with?

3. What are some systems change approaches you could take to
    a. eliminate childhood hunger in your county?
    b. help more people get the COVID-19 vaccine?
    c. reduce injuries to bicyclists (improve bicycle safety) in your city/town?

4. What are some environmental changes you could make to
    a. eliminate childhood hunger in your county?
    b. help more people get the COVID-19 vaccine?
    c. reduce injuries to bicyclists (improve bicycle safety) in your city/town?

APPLICATION ACTIVITIES

1. Group Activity: Get into small groups and have members wear the "lens" of different ethical frameworks as you discuss the following scenario: You live in the nation of Autonomia, a country similar to the United States in terms of its culture, government, and social structures. Autonomia is experiencing a very contagious epidemic of the *Corpus animatum* virus—also known as the zombie flu. Your goal as a public health professional working for the Institute for Disease Eradication in Autonomia (IDEA) is to help the population become vaccinated.
    a. You encounter a family who insists it is their right not to be vaccinated. What is your response according to the lens you are using?
    b. Based on your assigned ethical lens, what are the benefits of requiring the antizombie vaccine? What are the negatives?

2. Select two professional organizations you are most likely to join (if you are not already a member). Evaluate their code of ethics or professional ethical guidelines to answer the following:
    a. Are there explicit guidelines detailing what is considered ethical or not? Provide examples.
    b. What are the consequences to members who violate their respective codes of conduct or ethical codes?

3. You live in the nation of Autonomia, a country similar to the United States in terms of its culture, government, and social structures. Autonomia is experiencing a highly contagious epidemic of the *Corpus animatum* virus–also known as the zombie flu. Your goal as a public health professional working for the Institute

for Disease Eradication in Autonomia (IDEA) is to help the population become vaccinated.

   a. What are some **systems change** approaches you could take?

   b. List **environmental changes** you could make to help more people get the antizombie vaccine.

ADDITIONAL RESOURCES

Brown University. (n.d.). *A framework for making ethical decisions.* https://www.brown.edu/academics/science-and-technology-studies/framework-making-ethical-decisions

Coalition for National Health Education Organizations (CNHEO). (2020). *Code of ethics for the health education profession.* www.cnheo.org/code-of-ethics.html

Coughlin, S. S. (2008, January 1). *How many principles for public health ethics? Open Public Health Journal, 1,* 8–16. https://www.ncbi.nlm.nih.gov/pmc/articles/PMC2804997/

Jennings, B. (2020). Ethics codes and reflective practice in public health. *Journal of Public Health, 42,* 188–193. https://academic.oup.com/jpubhealth/article-abstract/42/1/188/5077245?redirectedFrom=fulltext

Lorenzetti, J. P. (2010, March 12). Ethical frameworks for academic decision-making. Faculty focus. https://www.facultyfocus.com/articles/faculty-development/ethical-frameworks-for-academic-decision-making/

Marckmann, G., Schmidt, H., Sofaer, N., & Strech, D. (2015, February 6). Putting public health ethics into practice: A systematic framework. *Frontiers in Public Health, 3.* https://www.frontiersin.org/articles/10.3389/fpubh.2015.00023/full

Markkula Center for Applied Ethics, Santa Clara University. (n.d.). *Ethical decision making.* https://www.scu.edu/ethics/ethics-resources/ethical-decision-making/.

Markkula Center for Applied Ethics, Santa Clara University. (2010, January 1). *What is ethics?* https://www.scu.edu/ethics/ethics-resources/ethical-decision-making/what-is-ethics

Monfort College of Business. (n.d.). Daniels Fund ethics initiative. https://mcb.unco.edu/ethics/

National Commission for the Protection of Human Subjects of Biomedical and Behavioral Research. (1979). The Belmont report: Ethical principles and guidelines for the protection of human subjects of research. U.S. Department of Health and Human Services. https://www.hhs.gov/ohrp/regulations-and-policy/belmont-report/read-the-belmont-report/index.html

Open University. (n.d.). *Health management, ethics and research module: 7. Principles of healthcare ethics.* https://www.open.edu/openlearncreate/mod/oucontent/view.php?id=225&printable=1

Pandemic Ethics Dashboard. (n.d.). *APHA public health code of ethics.* https://pandemicethics.org/consensus-documents/apha-public-health-code-of-ethics/

Schröder-Bäck, P., Duncan, P., Sherlaw, W., Brall, C., & Czabanowska, K. (2014, October 7). Teaching seven principles for public health ETHICS: Towards a curriculum for a short course on ethics in public health programmes. *BMC Medical Ethics, 15,* article 73 (2014).https://bmcmedethics.biomedcentral.com/articles/10.1186/1472-6939-15-73

Society for Public Health Education (SOPHE). (2020, April 15). *Professional ethics.* https://www.sophe.org/careerhub/ethics/

Tulchinsky, T. H. (2018, March 30). Ethical issues in public health. *Case Studies in Public Health,* 277–316. https://www.ncbi.nlm.nih.gov/pmc/articles/PMC7149338/

University of Washington Department of Bioethics & Humanities. (n.d.). *Public health ethics.* https://depts.washington.edu/bhdept/ethics-medicine/bioethics-topics/detail/76

QUIZ QUESTIONS

1. In public health, ethics are about
    a. making decisions and upholding standards of behavior based on a common "code."
    b. the rules governing the conduct of lawyers and judges that are adopted by each jurisdiction.
    c. providing professional standards to protect the dignity of clients.
    d. about truth, fairness, and equity in messaging and consumer experience.

2. In reference to a *nonconsequentialist framework*, one would
    a. mutually respect all vulnerable populations to have ethical reasoning.
    b. focus on the future effects of the possible courses of action, considering the people directly or indirectly affected.
    c. deny that the rightness or wrongness of our conduct is determined solely by the goodness or badness of the consequences of our acts or the rules to which those acts conform.
    d. be consistent with particular ideal virtues that provide for the full development of our humanity.

3. In reference to a *consequentialist framework*, one would
    a. mutually respect all vulnerable populations to have ethical reasoning.
    b. focus on the future effects of the possible courses of action, considering the people directly or indirectly affected.
    c. deny that the rightness or wrongness of our conduct is determined solely by the goodness or badness of the consequences of our acts or the rules to which those acts conform.
    d. be consistent with particular ideal virtues that provide for the full development of our humanity.

4. The _____ "emphasizes actions that provide the most good and deals with consequences; it tries both to increase the good done and to reduce the harm done."
    a. common good approach
    b. virtue approach
    c. utilitarian approach
    d. rights approach

5. What is the current order for *A Framework for Making Ethical Decisions* before any decision-making or action taking?
    a. Who is involved? What is the issue between the parties? When did it occur? How did it happen? Why did it happen?
    b. What is the issue? Who is involved? Why did it happen? How do we approach this?

    c. Who is involved? Where does the intervention take place? When does intervention occur? How is this unethical?

    d. How is this unethical? What should be done instead? When do we intervene? Where does the intervention take place? Who is involved in the decision-making?

6. Which of the following would be an example of an environmental change?

    a. Adapting furniture by lowering chairs or securing desks and creating slant boards throughout the classroom for writing support for children with a physical disability or orthopedic impairment.

    b. Changing the amount of lighting or brightening or dimming lights to help children with autism or visual impairment

    c. Increasing access for wheelchair users to get around and thus decreasing the degree to which the condition that led to their use of a wheelchair is disabling

    d. All of the above

7. _____ is an example of system-level change.

    a. Implementing standardized emergency medical personnel training for all emergency medical technicians, medics, nurses, doctors, and all medical personnel

    b. Providing paper shredders to all administrators and assistants in our local hospitals

    c. Marking individual parking spots with clear signs in the parking lots and ramps

    d. Providing complimentary pens and paper when medical personnel attend debriefings on medical procedures and attend conferences related to their field

8. _____ to health promotion emphasizes that health promotion should not only focus on intrapersonal behavioral factors, but also must consider factors at multiple socioecological levels that influence health.

    a. The socioeconomic framework

    b. The systematic process

    c. The socioecological framework

    d. The consequentialism framework

9. If your goal was to ensure access to mental health services in your community, some systems change approaches may include which of the following?

    a. Connecting mental health providers with community outreach centers

    b. Implementing a regional mental health awareness program that would include the local healthcare agencies

    c. Implementing a system of triage for mental health needs

    d. All of the above

10. The *Belmont Report* summarizes ethical principles and guidelines for research involving human subjects. What are the three major ethical principles addressed in this report?

    a. inequitable services, anonymity, respect for all

    b. depravity, do no harm, transgression implementation

    c. respect for persons, beneficence, and the principle of justice

    d. do no harm, inequality, beneficence

ANSWER KEY

1. **A.** Making decisions and upholding standards of behavior based on a common "code."
2. **C.** Deny that the rightness or wrongness of our conduct is determined solely by the goodness or badness of the consequences of our acts or the rules to which those acts conform.
3. **B.** Focus on the future effects of the possible courses of action, considering the people directly or indirectly affected.
4. **C.** Utilitarian approach.
5. **B.** What is the issue? Who is involved? Why did it happen? How do we approach this?
6. **D.** All of the above.
7. **A.** Implementing a standardized emergency medical personnel training for all EMTs, medics, nurses, doctors, and all medical personnel.
8. **C.** The socioecological framework.
9. **D.** All of the above.
10. **C.** Respect for persons, beneficence, and the principle of justice.

5.4 WILLEM VAN ROOSENBEEK

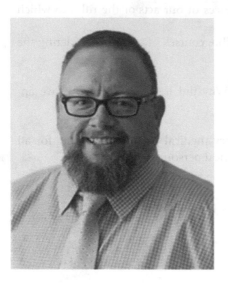

Willem Van Roosenbeek serves as the director of the Pride Center at University of Wisconsin–La Crosse (UWL). Willem provides overall direction for LGBTQ+ (lesbian, gay, bisexual, transgender, and queer; the plus sign indicates an all-encompassing representation of sexual orientation and gender identities) education, programs, training, advocacy, and support. Willem oversees the changing needs of an increasingly diverse student, faculty, and staff population. Willem works on the development, planning, and implementation of services that foster and increase understanding of sexual orientation and gender identity/expression issues in society.

Q. What Led or Inspired You to Become Engaged in LGBTQ+ Advocacy, Specifically as It Relates to Policy Change and Public Health?

While in undergraduate school I had the opportunity to attend an Alternative Spring Break trip. The Freedom Ride was to Atlanta, Georgia. We were going to learn about the civil rights movement and Dr. Martin Luther King Jr. At this time, I was also involved with a student group at the Newman Center. Those experiences introduced me to social justice work; I was confronted with our county's history and the discrimination of underrepresented communities. I did not realize I was part of the LGBTQ+ community until I was in college. Between my new-found identity, the introduction to social justice, the history of our past, and the realization of discrimination against underrepresented people I could no longer be silent or do nothing. I did not know that this would become my career until I was hired into my current position as the director of the Pride Center.

Q. Could You Describe the Work You Have Done With the Pride Center Concerning Policy Campus/Community and Even State or Nationally?

When I started at UWL, the Pride Center was called the Diversity Resource Center. People did not know what we did or who we were. One of the first actions we needed to take was to change the name so that people would know who we are and what we do. This helped change the center to what it is today. I worked with the Office of Residence Life to designate one all-gender bathroom in every hall and to help create gender-inclusive Housing. On campus I helped change procedure to make it possible for trans and nonbinary students to use a preferred name; this included their email address, classroom rosters, and student ID. I worked to help make it a priority to have at least one all-gender bathroom in every building on campus and that any new building would have them on every floor. When COVID hit I reached out to the other LGBTQ+ directors in the University of Wisconsin system, and we began meeting monthly. This meeting helped us all through the challenge of COVID, provided each other support, and helped plan how to keep our student groups going. I currently sit on the Planned Parenthood Wisconsin Transgender Affirming Healthcare Committee, helping them with their introduction of transgender-inclusive healthcare across the state.

Q. What Are Some of the Biggest Challenges You Have Faced as an Advocate?

I have faced hate, people's refusal to see LGBTQ+ identities as legitimate, and the inability of institutions to make change due to money. Whenever there is anything posted about the LGBTQ+ community in the news, just read the comments. They are filled with hateful words. We did a panel in a high school, and a middle school student called us faggots on our way out. Our chalking on campus for Coming Out Day has been defaced several times. An administrator of a local school (the school asked us to provide a panel) interrupted the panel with the question: "Are you here to recruit?" We go into panels today stating that we will not defend our legitimacy. Getting institutions to move when there is a problem is a big one. It took years to get the state insurance to be inclusive of trans and nonbinary employees despite a nondiscrimination policy that included gender identity/expression. Getting all-gender bathrooms in every building on campus is taking years. These are the things that can break you!

Q. What Is One Piece of Advice You Would Like to Offer Emerging Advocates in Public Health?

I would suggest emerging advocates remember the phrase "nothing about us without us," a phrase used by disability rights groups to mean no policy shall be decided by any representative without the full and direct participation of the members of the group affected by the policy. The LGBTQ+ community needs advocates who don't work for us but with us!

The Policy Process

CICILY HAMPTON

In the real world, answers may not be clear cut. There will be messy choices, and you're not going to be able to construct a policy response in a neat and tidy way. Being able to listen to other people, even as you stay true to your principles, that's how you actually succeed.

—JAKE SULLIVAN

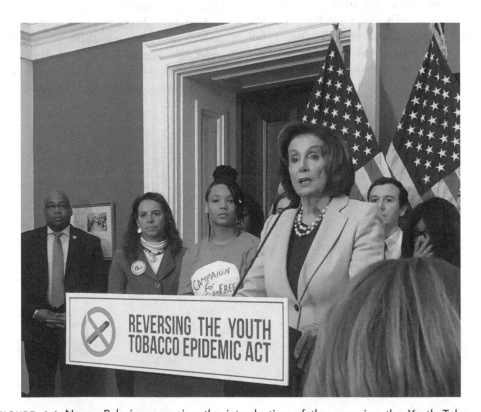

FIGURE 6.1 Nancy Pelosi announcing the introduction of the reversing the Youth Tobacco Epidemic Act on February 28, 2020.
Photo by Cicily Hampton.

Cicily Hampton, *The Policy Process*. In: *Be the Change*. Edited by Keely S. Rees, Jody Early, and Cicily Hampton, Oxford University Press. © Oxford University Press 2023. DOI: 10.1093/oso/9780197570890.003.0006

Objectives

1. Describe the cyclical nature of the policy process.
2. Differentiate a policy problem from other types of problems.
3. Explain dominant theories in public policymaking.
4. Summarize the six steps in the policy cycle.
5. Identify factors that impact policy formation and adoption.

INTRODUCTION

Policy problems are all around us. Take a walk around your neighborhood and take note of things that could be improved. Is there litter in a certain area? Are cars speeding down a certain stretch of road? Is there a dilapidated building that could be put to better use in the community? These could all be considered public policy problems. Identifying these policy problems kicks off the policy process.

There is no one definitive policy process due to differences in the type of policy problems and available solutions, policy arenas, and politics associated with each area of public policymaking (Figure 6.1). Despite the differences, political scientists and public policy scholars alike generally accept that the public policymaking process is cyclical, with six widely accepted steps having been identified. The steps in the policy process are problem identification, agenda setting, policy formulation, policy adoption, policy implementation, and policy evaluation (see Figure 6.2 below). The policy evaluation step serves as the venue to identify any remaining or new public policy problems to begin the cycle again.

The way in which a policy problem is identified and defined can greatly influence whether it is placed on the agenda and resolved in a satisfactory manner. The number and complexity of policy problems limits the number of issues that can be placed on the policymaking agenda. The process by which issues rise to the agenda and remain there to receive policymaker attention is highly competitive and fluid over time, often influenced by outside factors.

DEFINING POLICY PROBLEMS

Think of the policy problems above: litter, speeding cars, and dilapidated buildings. In order to abate the litter, citizens might ask the city for additional money in the budget for clean-up efforts or additional trash cans in that area. You might also ask the city for a traffic study in the area where cars are speeding to determine if speed bumps are necessary. In the case of the dilapidated building, you might petition the local zoning board for a change that would facilitate the building being put to a more desirable use in the community. While these are all examples of local policy problems, policy problems also exist at the state, federal, and even global levels. One example of a policy problem at the state level is deciding whether a state should expand its Medicaid-eligible population as a result of the Affordable Care Act. At the federal level, defining an accountable care organization and designing the payment

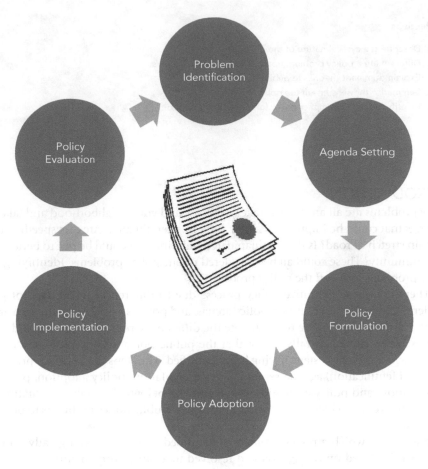

FIGURE 6.2 Six steps in the policy cycle.
Source: Cicily Hampton.

mechanisms to ensure viability of that model is a policy problem also resulting from passage of the Affordable Care Act. While different political systems govern various countries, there are policy problems that must be tackled at the global scale as well. One example of the global policy problem is combating climate change. Multiple countries must come together to agree on carbon reduction targets in order to have a meaningful impact on climate change.

While there are potential policy problems all around us, not all problems are *policy* problems. In order to determine whether a problem is indeed a policy problem, one must understand the structural elements, characteristics, and dimensions of the problem (Anderson, 2014). One example may be with prescription medication costs. Just because one person cannot afford a medication that they have been prescribed does not necessarily mean there is a problem associated with affordability. In this case, it would not be the role of the government to intervene in each case when a private citizen was not able to afford a specific medication. The flip side of this example is the rising price of the life-saving drug insulin. According to the Centers for Disease Control and Prevention (CDC), more than 34 million Americans suffer from diabetes (CDC, 2020), with many of those being dependent on insulin to control their diabetes. In 1996, when man-made insulin was introduced to the market, one vial sold for $25. In 2019, the cost of that same vial has increased 1,200% to $275 though the value of the dollar has only decreased 62% during that interval (Roberts, 2019). The unsustainable price of insulin is a policy problem because it affects millions of Americans directly by making their medication unaffordable and the rest of us in the costs to the healthcare system, decreased productivity, and unnecessary lives lost due to uncontrolled diabetes. This example illustrates the complex nature of adequately defining policy problems. While both examples deal with the affordability of prescription drugs, only one affects large numbers of people, including a large number of people who are not directly involved themselves. Additionally, individualistic solutions available to someone who cannot afford one specific prescription drug such as borrowing money from a friend or family member will not eradicate a policy problem, such as the cost of insulin exponentially outpacing inflation.

There are a few questions to ask to determine ways to tell if a problem you have identified is a policy problem or not.

- Does this problem affect more than one person, or is it unique to one person?
- Is the problem caused by an individual's circumstances or by systemic, institutional, or currently enacted policy?
- Does the problem have a direct policy solution?

Understanding whether the problem is a local, state, federal, or global policy problem or some combination thereof and the mechanisms of the appropriate government solution will determine how an advocate will go about agenda setting.

AGENDA SETTING

Once one has discovered a policy problem, the problem must be moved on to the **policy agenda** at the appropriate venue. In order for a policy problem to be moved on to any policy agenda, a sufficient number of people must have evaluated the problem against a common value standard and determined the continuation of the status quo to be unacceptable. Certain indicators of social or economic performance tend to get policymakers' attention and affect what is ultimately placed on the agenda. Additionally, there must be some sort of government solution readily available to solve the problem before a policy problem can be placed on the agenda. While there are thousands on thousands of public policy problems surrounding each of us every day, only a relatively small number will ever be moved on to the policy agenda for serious consideration by policymakers.

Cobb and Elder (1983) provided two different agenda types for consideration in the policymaking process. The first type of agenda is the **systemic agenda**. The systemic agenda is the discussion agenda of an institution or governmental body. This agenda consists of all of the policy problems that those in the institution have deemed relevant and sufficient for discussion at the current time. A systemic agenda will exist for each and every type of political institution, though most of the items that make it on to the systemic agenda will not result in policy actions. The second type of agenda is the **institutional agenda**. The institutional agenda is the action agenda of policy problems to be acted on by policymakers. The institutional agenda can consist of not only well-known topics and policy problems that legislators and constituents are talking about but also minor issues, technical fixes, or incremental policy changes that may not be known, or even interesting, to the general public. While an item making its way from the systemic agenda on to the institutional agenda is necessary for a policy problem to be acted on, just because a problem makes its way on to the agenda does not necessarily mean it will be acted on.

Particularly with regard to the institutional agenda-setting process, policy inaction *is* a policy action. There may be a number of scenarios where policy problems are being discussed by citizens in the local community or across the nation, and policymakers at the local level and party leaders at the national level are not acting on the concern. One scenario is that the policymakers have evaluated the problem and determined the status quo is acceptable. Policymakers may also recognize a problem and want to place it on the policy agenda but are unable to find an acceptable policy solution to address the problem at this time. Another scenario may be that policymakers have evaluated the problem and agree that something must be done to alleviate the problem, but that there are other problems that must have a higher priority on the agenda at the current time. Last, policymakers may not believe they have authority to take action on a policy problem.

The dominant theory of governmental agenda setting is Professor John Kingdon's policy streams model (Kingdon, 1984). Kingdon's policy streams model consists of three, relatively independent, tracks that converge in a **policy window** for a problem to be placed on the agenda (see Figure 6.3). The problem stream consists of any matter that citizens, policymakers, or interest groups would like policy action on. The policy proposals stream consists of the viable solutions to the policy problem. These possible policy solutions generate from policymakers themselves, their professional staff, advocates and interest groups, think tanks, bureaucrats, and academics. The politics stream consists of all of the political realities associated with a policy problem. It also consists of current and future elections, results of recent elections and the resulting majorities in political institutions, party politics, and public perceptions of the policy problem and how public mood can be utilized in elections.

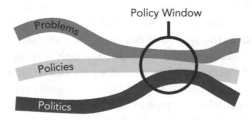

FIGURE 6.3 Policy streams.
Source: Bontje, L., Hallin, C., Wang, Z., & Slinger, J. H. (2016). Coastal erosion and beach nourishment in Scania as issues in Swedish coastal policy. *Journal of Water Management and Research, 73,* 103–115.

While Kingdon's policy streams theory has been criticized for being seen as random, advocates know that there are ample opportunities to influence each of the three streams. Advocates must ensure that they have identified and defined the policy problem to ensure that it is palatable to the agenda given the politics and competing priorities of the policymakers. Policy windows can open predictably due to a scheduled legislative review or when a law is up for reauthorization. Policy windows can also open seemingly randomly, such as in the case of **focusing events**.

Baumgartner and Jones (1993) described focusing events as sudden, relatively rare, attention-grabbing events that act as potential triggers for policy change. While focusing events can be positive, negative events that highlight harms, future harms, or potential harms are most likely to put policymakers in a position where they have to act by moving an issue on to the institutional agenda or further along through the policymaking process (Box 6.1). Focusing events can be the results of natural events or can be manufactured by advocates or opponents of an issue. Whether a focusing event is natural or manufactured, postevent mobilization by advocates or interest groups will still be critical to moving the issue on to and through the policy agenda. Since focusing events are uncommon, advocates should be prepared to highlight the problem, policy failures, and potential policy solutions in the wake of focusing events. It will be particularly important for advocates to be prepared with their issue framing (see Chapter 12) to ensure that acceptable policy solutions are advanced through the policy process.

Once your problem has sufficient public and policymaker attention to be placed on the agenda, it is critically important that advocates continue to draw attention to their issue. This is the time that it is most important to "keep your foot on the gas." It is important to understand that just because a policy problem or issue gets on the policy agenda does not mean that it will be able to stay there, particularly in light of new focusing events around other policy issues that may be arising, that the issue will be acted on, or that the policy problem will be resolved with your preferred policy solution. Advocates want to ensure that they can continue to create support among other policymakers for their champion and momentum for the issue to proceed through the policymaking process. Additionally, advocates must continue to communicate with their champions and supporters to combat any information they may be hearing from opponents. Even if an issue does not have direct opposition in the beginning, once an issue makes it to the policy agenda and begins garnering attention opponents may appear. These opponents may not have direct opposition to solving the particular policy problem or the advocates' preferred policy solution but may be opponents simply because they are arguing for a competing priority or for government resources to be utilized in a different way. Another reason that advocates must continue to communicate with their policymakers on the issue is that the calendar essentially resets every legislation session. In a new Congress, your previous champion may have retired or lost their election or the majority, party leadership, or administration priorities may have changed. Advocates who have cultivated wide support will have less groundwork to lay each time items on the agenda are up for discussion and inclusion. Even when a policy problem has sufficient interest and support to be placed on the agenda, little will be done about a problem that does not have a viable policy solution.

ADVOCACY IN ACTION BOX 6.1	School Shooting as a Focusing Event for Gun Violence Prevention

For many years there has been major tension in the public health advocacy space surrounding gun violence. On the one hand, gun violence is one of the leading causes of death in the United States, and many public health advocates feel that it should receive the same treatment as any other leading cause of death in America, researched, and prevented. On the other hand, gun control policy has typically centered on the Second Amendment, an issue far outside the realm of public health. The resources available to gun rights groups dwarf those available to most public health advocacy campaigns, so many public health advocates do not agree that they can make an impact with the miniscule resources they have compared to some of the other public health issues that could more effectively utilize those resources.

On February 14, 2018, a gunman opened fire at Marjory Stoneman Douglas High School in Parkland, Florida, killing 17 people and injuring 17 others, the deadliest school shooting in U.S. history. Despite the previous numerous mass shootings, the tragedy at Parkland served as a focusing event for many in the public health community. A major advocacy conference was scheduled for October that year centered on the public health approach to gun violence prevention. At this conference, advocates asked Congress for $50 million for the CDC to study the causes of gun violence and to repeal the Dickey Amendment, language in each year's appropriation bill that states that the CDC cannot use any appropriated funds to advocate or promote gun control, which has been manipulated to prevent the CDC from studying gun violence as a leading cause of death.

POLICY FORMULATION

Policy problems are continuously evaluated against a set of social values, as such defining policy problems are inherently political. The defining characteristics of the problem, the acceptable policy solutions, and the government interventions necessary to address the policy problem are also socially constructed. One example is the policy problem of the unhoused. Depending on the dominant social values, this policy problem could be defined as one of affordable housing in which the policy solution might be a housing support voucher system, increased subsidies for developers of affordable housing, or rent control. The policy problem of the unhoused may also be defined by some as primarily a mental illness or substance misuse policy problem for which appropriate policy solutions may range from increased support for mental health services or even increased utilization of the criminal justice system. As illustrated here, how a problem is defined by advocates or their opponents can determine how the root cause of the problem is perceived, the magnitude and severity of the problem, and, ultimately, the amenability of the problem to available policy solutions. Formulating policy solutions is a critical component of an advocate's work.

Radical, innovative policy proposals are scarcely created and even more rarely ever enacted into law. Over time, many different policy alternatives have been created. While not all of them have been enacted, they are all available to be drawn on, perhaps with modifications, to solve a new, different policy problem. These previously created policy solutions offer answers to some important questions that are not readily available with radical new policies, such as: How much will it cost? How many citizens will be affected? Is this policy solution politically viable to the public? What kind of policymakers are likely to be supporters of this policy solution? What are the unintended consequences?

In an effort to make sense of a complex, fluid, and seemingly irrational at times policy process, policy scholars have developed a number of theoretical models to describe how policies are formulated in response to policy problems. These policy tools provide a useful method to link the nature of the problem and the type of action necessary to solve it.

Garbage Can Models

Garbage can models reject any rational approach to policymaking that is underpinned by the reasoning of problem-solving (Tiernan & Burke, 2002). The garbage can model of policymaking (Kingdon) adapted from organizational theory (Cohen et al., 1972) posits that policymaking is essentially a series of solutions in search of policy problems that they could solve. In many cases, organizations, inclusive of advocacy groups, may have a preferred policy solution and are looking for opportunities that would allow those preferred policy solutions to be implemented. The "garbage can" is where the policy solutions reside until a policymaker reaches in to retrieve one in an effort to solve a policy problem. The universe of policymaking, the solutions, problems, interest groups, and advocates flow in and around a garbage can, and the solutions that get attached to a particular problem are largely random. For this reason, policy problems and solutions may be tangentially related at best. Garbage can theories are antithetical to a rational policymaking process.

Incrementalism and Punctuated Equilibrium

Charles Lindblom's **theory of incrementalism** (1959) is one of the most widely cited theories of policy development. Incrementalism is the practice of making policy through a series of relatively small steps (Weiss & Woodhouse, 1992). In incrementalism, the only policies that are considered for adoption are a few, relatively similar, alternatives that differ only slightly from current policy. For this reason, incrementalism has been criticized as being a conservative process that is inherently reactive rather than proactive to address policy problems (Weiss & Woodhouse, 1992), though another school of thought holds that a series of small incremental steps toward a larger goal or moving away from an unacceptable condition can be a purposeful and powerful technique of policy formulation (Quinn, 1982; Weick, 1984). Incrementalism is the primary policy formulation strategy when pursuing policy change through the appropriation process. Incrementalism works well in federal appropriations because the goals of each department and program area are well defined in their authorizing language, and the results of the proposed changes are relatively easy to predict (i.e., a 10% cut or 10% increase to the budget of the CDC).

Incrementalism lends itself well to advanced democracies, particularly democracies with multiple branches of government and political parties, such as the United States, because it is difficult to get partisans to agree on bold policy moves, the influence of interest groups, and the slow change of social values against which policy problems and solutions are evaluated by the general public. Even when society writ large has deemed a policy problem as unacceptable, moving away from it in incremental steps allows the general public a better understanding of what is happening and also reduces the likelihood of major policy errors. Incrementalism is generally not an appropriate strategy of policy formulation in an unstable or crisis environment, such as after a major focusing event. In a crisis situation, policymakers will likely feel increased pressure to act boldly and, as such, will consider additional policy alternatives. Additionally, in a crisis situation, the perceived costs may be too high to risk inaction, so policymakers may be more willing to bear the uncertainty that may come with major policy shifts (Nice, 1987).

These stable periods of incremental policy change that are occasionally broken up by major policy change or complete redirection are known as the punctuated equilibrium theory of public policymaking (Baumgartner & Jones, 2010; True, 2000). In their seminal work, Baumgartner and Jones (1993) discovered patterns of stability dominated by few prominent interest groups, the relevant government agency, and Congressional champions who control the policy agenda in that area and determine the acceptable policy actions. These closed systems, or policy monopolies, operate with relative stability until they become vulnerable to punctuation. As pressure for change builds, the policy problem is redefined, or public opinion and social values change, previously uninvolved people and organizations may become the dominant actors in the policy monopoly in the new stasis (True et al., 2019).

Baumgartner et al. (2014) argued that the pressure for policy change is resolved differently at different levels of government. Additionally, policymaking can shift from one level of government to another and back and still satisfy the theory of punctuated equilibrium. Punctuated equilibrium theory lends itself well to policy areas such as transportation, healthcare, national defense, energy, and education policymaking (True, 2000). Generally, examining these established policy areas for any significant length of time will reveal small changes in policy and budgeting year over year (or decade over decade if the time window is sufficient) interrupted by occasional major policy change.

Systems Theory (Inputs and Outputs)

Systems theory posits that policymaking is a political system's response to the inputs and outputs of the environment in which it operates. The political system is made up of what we typically think of as government institutions as well as the political processes that drive them (Anderson, 2014). The inputs of the political system are the demands for actions consistent with the values of the people that the political system governs, while the outputs of the political system are the rules, laws, and judicial decisions that reflect the values of society. The policy outputs may result in additional inputs that must be addressed by the political system via outputs creating a feedback loop intrinsic to the system (Anyebe, 2018).

Institutionalism and Rational Choice Theory

Institutionalism is the study of how the behavior of political actors is shaped by the institutions of which they are part and the resulting public policy outcomes. In the context of public policymaking, institutions are the established rules, routines, norms, mores, and previous policy legacies (Bell, 2002; Hall, 1986; March & Olsen,2010). Due to all of these factors, institutions tend strongly toward inertia until external pressures on the institution build to the point that change must occur in one form of punctuated equilibrium (Krasner, 1984), though incrementalism in institutions has also been observed (Cortell & Peterson, 1999). There are multiple schools of institutionalism, but they all come down to the basic explanation that the institutions are major factors in explaining political behaviors (Bell, 2002). Institutions both shape and constrain public policy through the decision-making process and actors associated with the dominant institutions in a given policy area. These institutions determine who and how many actors can influence policy; how policy is to be pursued; and what, if any, information is sought and shared among actors in decision-making and subsequently the policy agenda (Reich, 2000).

Lowi (1964) argued that these policy areas dictate the most appropriate institutional form based on the politics specific to each policy area where institutionalism can be applied. Due to the unique nature of each policy area that can be governed by institutionalism, the institutions in that policy area have evolved in a purposive way to solve the policy problems common to that policy area (Reich, 2000). The varying forms of institutionalism in the political science literature simply posit how much influence these institutions have in resulting public policy (Levi, 2008). Institutionalists will design political institutions to disincentivize the worst of self-interested behavior. This guiding principle in policymaking is referred to as **rational choice** institutionalism.

Rational choice theorists argue that these institutions have been constructed by the political actors for their purposes, and, beyond that, these rational actors are actively engaged in shaping these institutions and institutional environments as a means to their policy goals. In this way the institutions are not only a cause of political behavior but also an effect of this political behavior.

Rational choice theory assumes that all political actors behave rationally, but only in their own self-interest. This self-interest drives public policy through the use of incentives and sanctions to drive those governed by the policy either away from behavior or toward it, based on the rational calculation of their self-interest. If the self-interest diverges from the common interest, there is a need for policy interventions (Stewart, 1993). Policy formulation under rational choice theory devises incentive structures so that behavior conforms to the most socially desirable set of circumstances and assumes that most people or organizations will obey the policy voluntarily (Neimun & Stambough, 1998; Stewart, 1993). These assumptions will hold if the costs (economic or social) of not doing something outweigh the benefits. In practice, this looks like taxing behavior that is undesirable and rewarding or subsidizing behavior that is desirable.

Deciding whether to use sanctions, subsidies, or both is typically the result of analysis that takes into account the current state of affairs, including problem definition, the political landscape, as well as social perceptions, and choosing the most efficient policy. As several of these factors may change, there is a greater chance of moving from regulation to deregulation and back again. One recent example is in the Affordable Care Act. The law was originally written with both tax penalties for anyone who could afford health insurance but did not purchase it and subsidies making health insurance purchased on the exchanges more affordable. Both of these worked together to make purchasing health insurance more attractive and to incentivize people to act in their own self-interest, either by increasing the cost of not purchasing health insurance with the tax penalty and by decreasing the cost of purchasing health insurance with the subsidies. This scheme resulted in about 20 million more people purchasing health insurance between the time the law was enacted in 2010 and 2015 (Garrett & Gangopadhyaya, 2016). Perhaps because so many people gained health insurance under the act that social attitudes about the number of uninsured Americans changed, and certainly because of political changes as a result of the 2016 presidential election, the tax penalties for not having health insurance were removed via subsequent legislation.

Elite–Mass Model and Policy Networks

The **elite–mass model** holds that there is a small number of policy elites acting to create policy on behalf of the masses in a top-down approach. This theory of policymaking relies on a largely apathetic and uninformed mass. The masses send signals about policy preferences to the elite through civic engagement activities, but these activities are informed by the elite themselves using resources available to them to shape mass opinion (Dye, 2015). Elites hold influential positions in powerful public and private organizations, business, and social movements. Mappings and social network analyses document the links between the wealthy, directors of major corporations, and foundations, research institutes, and other nonprofit organizations that examine social problems and propose policy solutions. These elites are able to use their positions of influence on these interlocking organizations collectively to shape policy (Knocke, 1993). Elites determine which policy problems to act on or policy areas to influence by virtue of their personal interests, available resources, and both their formal and informal positions within their organization(s) (Knoke, 1993).

These elites often function within the constraints of one or more **policy networks**. Policy networks are structured patterns of interactions between the political actors within a specific policy area, such as health policy (Bell, 2002). Policy networks function as a structured set of behaviors that political actors engage in rather than a set of institutions or even a set of interest groups, though the interactions can be influenced by the institutions within which the behaviors take place. Policies influenced by policy networks tend to be less strategic and more ad hoc and reactive because the actors that make up the policy network typically do not have decisive authority in the policy area and have to manage competing interests with other actors in the policy network. Networks may be based on personal networks between individuals familiar with each other who share beliefs and a common culture. Networks may also be based on the position and role the actors play within a network, rather than the actors themselves (Marsh & Smith, 2000). Network structures have a tendency to reflect the current broader societal structures, such as class and gender structures, to determine who is a member of the network and their positions within it. In this way policy networks tend to mirror and reinforce structural inequalities of the broader society within which they are located. Whether based on personal relationships or formal roles and responsibilities, the network and culture within constrain the policy outcomes available to those in the network. These network constraints determine the role of the actors, which policy problems are discussed, and ultimately, how the policy issues are acted on. The ultimate policy outcomes as dictated by the network feed back into the network and affect the next set of policy considerations and ultimate outcomes (Marsh & Smith, 2000).

Not all of the policy formulation models are conducive to all policy problems or areas of public policy, and some were specifically created to explain a particular area of policy that may act unlike others. Certain policy areas are more fragmented, unstable, or volatile than others and, as such, may be subject to more reactive or ad hoc policymaking than can be explained in the models defined in this chapter. Irrespective of which policy formulation mechanisms are taking place, advocates should always ensure that they present legal and constitutional, viable, and realistic policy solutions to the policy problems that they are moving on to the policy agenda. Presenting policy solutions is particularly important in health policy because these policy solutions nearly always have to be paid for due to budgetary rules. It is always better to determine your own acceptable "pay fors" rather than providing a policy solution and allowing others to determine how to pay for it and if those pay fors are acceptable. If an advocate presents a policy problem and a solution but does not have a way to pay for it, it could be the difference between the issue moving on to the agenda or not. There may also be a case when other advocates, or even opponents, present a policy solution that may exacerbate a different policy problem and leave the advocate or the community in a worse position than when they began. This is particularly important if the policy area is operating under an elite or network structure where inequities may be baked in and there is incentive to continue to operate under the status quo.

POLICY ADOPTION

Once the appropriate process to formulate a policy has been undertaken and alternatives explored, a policy decision will be made by some official person or body to adopt, modify, or reject the policy alternative. If the decision is made to pursue a positive policy action, rather than inaction, the appropriate mechanism will be decided on, whether the policy will be adopted through legislation, regulation, or executive or judicial order.[1] While having a sponsor agree to adopt a policy that addresses an advocate's policy problem is a huge victory, it is not the end of the road for an advocate. Through the policy adoption mechanism, whichever it may be, there may be additional decision points or compromises that must be made in order to gain enough support for passage (in the case of legislation) or to head off legal challenges (in the case of legislation, an executive order, or regulation). It is important to understand that some provisions may be rejected, added, or modified, and the final policy may be remarkably different from what advocates originally envisioned. In this case, it is important to understand the end goal and ensure that the final policy that is adopted actually solves the policy problem as identified by the advocates, no matter what else the policy may do.

POLICY IMPLEMENTATION

One of the most critical next steps to ensure that the policy solution actually addresses an advocate's problem as intended is to continue to follow the regulations associated with

---

1. It is important to note that the judiciary is not a positive policymaker in the way the legislators are. The judicial branch of government may only react to legal challenges brought by persons with standing before the court. By deciding to pursue legal challenges or submitting amicus briefs to the appropriate judicial venue, advocates are able to shape policy as a strategy.

the policy. Legislative and executive actions will often have more in-depth regulations that are created by the agency tasked with implementing the policy and that will explain in great detail how a piece of legislation or executive order will be implemented. There are multiple opportunities for advocates to continue to make their preferences for policy implementation known throughout the rule-making process. A detailed overview of the rule-making process is covered in the next chapter.

Judicial challenges are also likely to have an impact on policy implementation. Controversial and/or high-profile legislation or executive orders will likely have one or more judicial challenges by groups that do not agree with the policy. As an advocate, you can also file a lawsuit to stop implementation of a policy that you do not agree with, provided that you have the resources to access this type of legal representation. If you elect not to file a lawsuit yourself, you can file an **amicus brief** on behalf of your position regarding the policy, providing the court with relevant information from your perspective. Additional information on advocacy in the judicial arena is covered in the next chapter.

POLICY EVALUATION

The last step in the policy development process is policy evaluation. Engaging in policy evaluation once the policy has been adopted and implemented allows you to gauge whether the policy is working as intended and solving the policy problem as identified in the first step of the policy process. In this way the policy evaluation creates a feedback loop and allows opportunities to offer additional policy solutions that may improve the outcomes associated with the policy or address any side effects or unintended consequences that have arisen as a result of the new policy. For this reason you will want to engage in policy evaluation whether your chosen policy alternative was implemented or not. If your preferred policy was implemented, an evaluation may give you additional evidence that the policy is working and should be continued and/or expanded. If your preferred policy was not implemented, a rigorous evaluation may provide evidence that the policy problem should be placed back on the agenda and your preferred policy solution considered for implementation. You don't want to leave policy evaluation to your opponents because they may design and use the analysis in such a way that it is detrimental to your cause. Advocates should ensure that they have enough money left in their budgets to conduct a rigorous evaluation of the policy efforts. Depending on the policy, this kind of analysis may take years and require hiring or contracting with an expert in policy analysis. It is important to understand that any type of policy analysis will always be constrained by time, money, and manpower allocated to the analysis.

When you are analyzing and evaluating policy into the future you should limit your analysis to a carefully selected set of circumstances most likely to occur within your time window, but because you cannot predict the future you do not want to set about trying to include the entire universe of policy possibilities and variables in your analysis. This will lead to what is commonly referred to as "analysis paralysis," and you will never come up with an appropriate course of action to pursue. An extensive overview of policy evaluation is covered in Chapter 13.

CONCLUSION

The policy process is cyclical, always beginning with problem identification and then moving through agenda setting, policy formulation, policy adoption, policy implementation, and policy evaluation, which typically leads to the next round of problem identification, even if the new problem is that the program should be discontinued or more resources should be devoted to it. While a brief overview of the policy process presented here offers a simplistic view of how policy is created in the United States, the policy process may take a number of years to move through all of the stages or may get stalled at any point in the process.

Because policy problems and solutions are socially constructed, their definitions and viable policy solutions may change over time as society's values and conditions change. The more complex the policy problem, the more people affected by the problem itself, and the more people who may be impacted by the policy change indirectly, the more difficult it can be to navigate the policy process. Social and economic indicators that attract media attention are more likely to be placed on the agenda. Generally, it is easy to get a diverse group of people and organizations to agree that a problem exists, but generating consensus about the appropriate policy solution among those same groups can be extraordinarily difficult. Additionally, there are a number of tools that opponents can use to shape the initial policy proposal, veer the implementation away from the original intent, or block implementation of the policy altogether, so it is important for advocates to offer strong policy proposals, cultivate champions and broad-based coalitions, and follow the policy process through to the end. Policy systems are only enduring if they have the capacity to adjust successfully to change. Policies that learn to correct mistakes or use new technology to solve old problems by more efficient means are critical to the policy process.

REFERENCES

Anderson, J. E. (2014). *Public policymaking.* Cengage Learning.

Anyebe, A. A. (2018). An overview of approaches to the study of public policy. *International Journal of Political Science, 4*(1), 8–17.

Baumgartner, F. R., & Jones, B. D. (2010). *Agendas and instability in American politics.* University of Chicago Press.

Baumgartner, F. R., Jones, B. D., & Mortensen, P. B. (2014). Punctuated equilibrium theory: Explaining stability and change in public policymaking. *Theories of the Policy Process, 8,* 59–103.

Bell, S. (2002). Institutionalism. https://d1w qtxts1xzle7.cloudfront.net/32825086/ eserv-with-cover-page-v2.pdf?Expires=165 4134144&Signature=MI8QVBVmIcRcWD8g 0R5W2RVvJHJXKz0VVF1-7FKDD~UlEY-jMJUOrdDtHTA4ps5ej9Kb0ZodAmRn51V 20kU7kRPaP0n5agdBYh~zv4QIVltg~WZMxPy Cyy6mwhpVv9Yjxa~d1CWqiqODcyzKkpJ8Tx l5PcWJlVl8nO2TVTBHmLrmWLhyqgg0RzrN XqwvcJOxNWoicPCEW16~MEZMzwKFRXro7 1DL~pLn9LEyL8~nGt21LKXU8SMGUBxVUR 1sulINiqRBVUq4P-JZ1E0kbpTb~VdZLZ6V4y OmfGQ68hOVuttIv-HLCRSkcytAyb0kTy6e7X oTC~fK8pTECgEABC2GNg__&Key-Pair-Id= APKAJLOHF5GGSLRBV4ZA

Centers for Disease Control and Prevention (CDC). (2020). *National Diabetes Statistics Report, 2020.* Centers for Disease Control and Prevention, U.S. Department of Health and Human Services.

Cobb, R., & Charles, E. (1983). *Participation in American Politics: the Dynamics of Agenda Building.* Baltimore: Johns Hopkins Press.

Cohen, M. D., March, J. G., & Olsen, J. P. (1972). A garbage can model of organizational choice. *Administrative Science Quarterly*, 1–25.

Cortell, A. P., & Peterson, S. (1999). Altered states: Explaining domestic institutional change. *British Journal of Political Science*, 29(1), 177–203.

Domhoff, G. W. (2017). *The power elite and the state: How policy is made in America*. Routledge.

Dye, T. R. (2015). *Who's running America? The Obama reign*. Routledge.

Garrett, A. B., & Gangopadhyaya, A. (2016). *Who gained health insurance coverage under the ACA, and where do they live?* Urban Institute.

Hall, P. A. (1986). *Governing the economy: The politics of state intervention in Britain and France*. Oxford University Press.

Kingdon, J. W. (1984). *Agendas, alternatives and public policies*. Scott, Foresman and Company.

Knoke, D. (1993). Networks of elite structure and decision making. *Sociological Methods & Research*, 22(1), 23–45.

Krasner, S. D. (1984). Approaches to the state: Alternative conceptions and historical dynamics. *Comparative Politics*, 16(2), 223–246.

Levi, M. (2008). A logic of institutional change. In K. S. Cook and M. Levi (Eds.), *The limits of rationality* Chicago University Press.

Lindblom, C. E. (1959). The science of muddling through. *Public Administration Review*, 19(2), 79–88.

Lowi, T. J. (1964). American business, public policy, case-studies, and political theory. *World Politics*, 16(4), 677–715.

Marsh, D., & Smith, M. (2000). Understanding policy networks: Towards a dialectical approach. Political Studies, 48(1), 4–21.

Neimun, M., & Stambough, S. J. (1998). Rational choice theory and the evaluation of public policy. *Policy Studies Journal*, 26(3), 449–465.

Nice, D. C. (1987). Incremental and nonincremental policy responses: The states and the railroads. *Polity*, 20(1), 145–156.

Quinn, J. B. (1982). Managing strategies incrementally. *Omega*, 10(6), 613–627.

Roberts, D. K. (2019). The deadly cost of insulin. Online American Journal of Managed Care. Retrieved from: https://www.ajmc.com/view/the-deadly-costs-of-insulin

Reich, S. (2000). The four faces of institutionalism: public policy and a pluralistic perspective. *Governance*, 13(4), 501–522.

Stewart, J. (1993). Rational choice theory, public policy and the liberal state. *Policy Sciences*, 26(4), 317–330.

Tiernan, A., & Burke, T. (2002). A load of old garbage: Applying garbage–can theory to contemporary housing policy. *Australian Journal of Public Administration*, 61(3), 86–97.

True, J. L. (2000). Avalanches and incrementalism: Making policy and budgets in the United States. *American Review of Public Administration*, 30(1), 3–18.

True, J. L., Jones, B. D., & Baumgartner, F. R. (2019). Punctuated-equilibrium theory: Explaining stability and change in public policymaking. In Weible, C.M. and Sabatier, P. A. (Eds.), *Theories of the policy process* (pp. 155–187). Routledge

Weick, K. E. (1984). Small wins: Redefining the scale of social problems. *American Psychologist*, 39, 40–49.

Weiss, A., & Woodhouse, E. (1992). Reframing incrementalism: A constructive response to the critics. *Policy Sciences*, 25(3), 255–273.

CHAPTER 6: END-OF-CHAPTER ACTIVITIES

DISCUSSION QUESTIONS

1. What are some of the significant focusing events that have occurred in your lifetime?

2. How have these focusing events had an effect on policy?

3. What are some alternative policy solutions (if any) that should be considered now that these policies have been in effect for some time?

APPLICATION ACTIVITIES

1. Based on your personal values, write out a list of policy problems in your local area.

2. Look up the website of a local politician (mayor, city council member, county commissioner, member of Congress, governor, senator) and find their policy priorities to see which of their priorities align with the policy problem(s) you have identified.

3. Using the contact form on their website, write to your elected official expressing concern for the problem, supporting their policy solution (if you agree with it) or offering alternatives to their policy solutions (if you don't agree).

QUIZ QUESTIONS

1. For a policy problem to be moved to a policy agenda, which of the following must occur?
   a. A sufficient number of people must have evaluated the problem against a common value standard and determined the continuation of the status quo to be unacceptable.
   b. A handful of people must have assessed the issue against one standard and decided that the current situation is acceptable.
   c. The government must not have already addressed this problem and will need to explore possible solutions.
   d. Because of the excessive number of issues often moved to the policy agenda, there is a lottery to help determine which one would be moved first.

2. Which of the following is true about *focusing events*?
   a. They often put policymakers in a position to cancel all requested events.
   b. They are considered as rare, attention-grabbing, and sudden events that act as potential triggers for policy change.
   c. They are never a result of natural events and are never manufactured by advocates or opponents of an issue.
   d. They typically result in failed policy solutions and implementations.

3. In connection to policy formulation, which of the following is not true about garbage can models of policymaking?
   a. This model postulates that policymaking is essentially a series of solutions in search of policy problems they could solve.
   b. This model rejects any rational approach to policymaking underpinned by the reasoning of problem-solving.
   c. This model supports that the policy solutions reside until a policymaker reaches in to retrieve one to solve a policy problem.
   d. This model is congruent to a rational policymaking process.

4. The _____ is "the discussion agenda of an institution or governmental body" and "exists for every type of political institution."
   a. institutional agenda
   b. government agenda
   c. systemic agenda
   d. dialogue agenda

5. In connection to policy formulation, the _____ is well done in policy development and is considered a conservative process that is not proactive in addressing policy problems but rather is considered reactive.
   a. theory of incrementalism
   b. theory of policy streams
   c. theory of equilibrium
   d. theory of policy networking

6. The systems theory suggests that policymaking is a political system's response to the _____ of the environment in which it functions.
   a. contributions and outcomes
   b. productions and reductions
   c. value-laden results and benefits
   d. inputs and outputs

7. Policy networks function as
   a. heterogenic since they bring policies together from different countries.
   b. a level of closure among a group of political actors and the incompetence of collective action.
   c. an influence on the institutions within which political actors and incompetence engage.
   d. a structured set of behaviors that political actors engage in rather than a set of institutions or even a set of interest groups.

8. Institutionalists will design political institutions to disincentivize the worst of self-interested behavior. This guiding principle in policymaking is
   a. domestic institutionalism.
   b. decision-making institutionalism.
   c. rational choice institutionalism.
   d. policy networking institutionalism.

9. As an advocate, if you choose to stop implementation of a policy via lawsuit, you personally can file a _____, and you are someone who is not a party to a case. Still, you can assist a court by offering information, expertise, or insight that has a bearing on the issues in the case.
   a. amicus brief
   b. appellate brief
   c. memorandum brief
   d. coalition brief

10. In a political system, the _____ are the laws, rules, and judicial decisions that reflect the values of society, and the _____ are the demands for actions connected to the values of the people.
   a. inputs; outputs
   b. outputs; inputs
   c. contributions; outcomes
   d. outcomes; contributions

ANSWER KEY

1. **A.** A sufficient number of people must have evaluated the problem against a common value standard and determined the continuation of the status quo to be unacceptable.
2. **B.** They are considered as rare, attention-grabbing, and sudden events that act as potential triggers for policy change.
3. **D.** This model is congruent to a rational policymaking process.
4. **C.** Systemic agenda.
5. **A.** Theory of incrementalism.
6. **D.** Inputs and outputs.
7. **D.** A structured set of behaviors that political actors engage in rather than a set of institutions or even a set of interest groups.
8. **C.** Rational choice institutionalism.
9. **A.** Amicus brief.
10. **B.** Outputs; inputs.

Policy Arenas

CICILY HAMPTON

We the people are the rightful masters of both Congress and the courts,
not to overthrow the Constitution but to overthrow the men who pervert
the Constitution.

—ABRAHAM LINCOLN

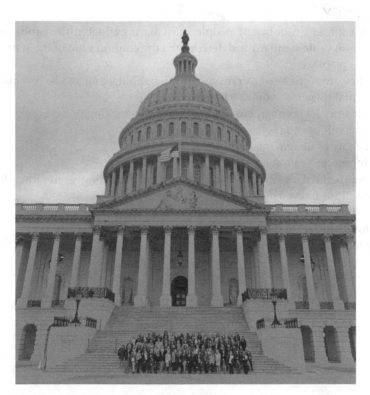

FIGURE 7.1 Advocates on the steps of the U.S. Capitol.
Photo by Cicily Hampton.

Cicily Hampton, *Policy Arenas*. In: *Be the Change*. Edited by Keely S. Rees, Jody Early, and Cicily Hampton, Oxford University Press.
© Oxford University Press 2023. DOI: 10.1093/oso/9780197570890.003.0007

Objectives

1. List the different policy arenas where policy change takes place.
2. Provide an example of an effective advocacy strategy that works best for a particular policy arena.
3. Describe political party structure and party leadership roles.
4. Explain how advocacy strategies are shaped by the norms, rules, and participants of the various policymaking venues.
5. Justify why ballot initiative processes are important to the policy process.

INTRODUCTION

It is impossible to consider advocacy and policy change without considering the venue where that policy change will take place. The institutions where the anticipated policy change will occur are known as **policy arenas**. These policy arenas will dictate the type of policy change that is possible and the most effective types of advocacy strategies that can be targeted at that policy change. The policy arenas may be familiar as they are made up of the three branches of government: legislative, executive, and judicial (Figure 7.1). Each of these policy arenas has its own strengths, weaknesses, advantages, and drawbacks when trying to change policy as well as different procedural processes and timelines for policy change. In addition to the procedural processes and timelines that may determine which policy arenas to target, available resources may dictate which policy arenas advocates are able to target for policy change. Also, depending on resources there may be multiple policy arenas in play at once. Often advocates will want to have a short-term legislative strategy, a long-term regulatory strategy, with the courts as a backup option, if they have the resources.

THE LEGISLATIVE ARENA

Singing along to "I'm Just a Bill, Sitting Here on Capitol Hill" was many young people's introduction to public policymaking, and, even decades after that iconic episode of *School House Rock*, the legislative arena is the policymaking arena that comes to mind first for most people. The lyrics offer a bird's eye view of the federal legislative process inclusive of agenda setting, introduction, referral to committee, committee votes, floor votes, and finally being signed into law by the president (Figure 7.2). While the song focuses solely on the federal level, there are actually legislative arenas at the state and local levels as well. While there are similar structures and processes at the federal, state, and local legislative arenas, there are key differences as well.

WHAT MAKES UP THE LEGISLATIVE ARENA?
Federal Level

At the federal level, the legislative arena is made up of the Congress. Established by the Constitution, Congress is made up of two distinct entities, the House and the Senate. The House is composed of members, elected from their states every 2 years, based on the population, while the Senate is made up of two Senators from each state elected every

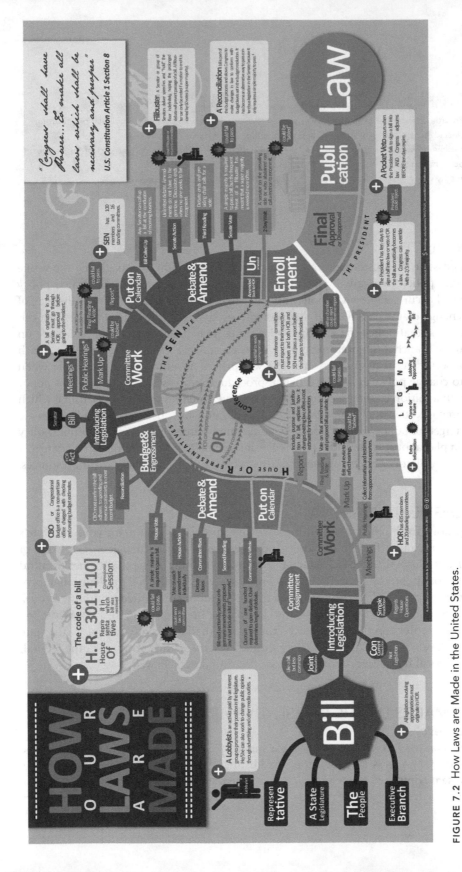

FIGURE 7.2 How Laws are Made in the United States.

Source: How Our Laws Are Made. http://www.ritholtz.com/blog/wp-content/uploads/2010/07/howlawsmadeWIRTH2.jpg

6 years.[1] These 535 members of Congress, 435 in the House and 100 in the Senate, are responsible for introducing and advancing legislation at the federal level.

A legislative body with two houses, typically a House and a Senate, is known as a bi-cameral legislature. A bicameral legislative structure serves many purposes, but one of the main ones is to facilitate different relationships with citizens. Members of the House are meant to be closer to the people who they represent, while the Senate is known as the more "deliberative body"[2] of Congress. With a 6-year term, Senators have more opportunity to build relationships and alliances, direct their committees, and deliver on their chosen legislative agenda. Members of the House and Senate from the same state are able to work together to blend the two perspectives to ensure that the needs of their constituents as a whole are being met and these needs can be considered when legislative decisions are being made.

Congress: House and Senate

Every two years, on January 3 or another date designated by Congress, a new Congress begins and the newly elected members are sworn in (Box 7.1). Once the new members of Congress are sworn in and a quorum is established, the race against the clock begins. There are precious few legislative days[3] on the congressional calendar to get legislation written, introduced, passed through committee, and onto the floor for a vote—with many opportunities for a piece of legislation to die along the way. And, of course, if legislation is not passed during the Congress it is introduced, it must be reintroduced and the process must start all over again in the next Congress.

At the beginning of each year, both the House and Senate release their calendars. The calendars include days in which they are in Washington, D.C., to legislate and hold hearings as well as their district work periods, days when Congress is not in session and legislators are expected to be home in their districts meeting with constituents and holding town halls or other events. For advocates who cannot travel to Washington, these district work periods provide great opportunities to meet with their legislators and advocate on behalf of their issues. While it is important to meet with as many members of Congress as possible to try to get support for your issue, it is also important to understand how your issue falls in the overall priority of both the majority and minority parties in Congress and whether or not the issue is a priority for party leadership to determine how the legislation will move through the legislative process. Next, we examine the party leadership structure and its role in moving legislation in Congress.

1. The vice president serves as president of the Senate, presides when the Senate first convenes every 2 years, as well as serves as a tie-breaker vote on the floor of the Senate.
2. In the Alexandria (VA) *Gazette* on May 3, 1826, the Senate was called the "greatest deliberative body of the nation."
3. From 2001 to 2018, the Senate spent an average of 165 days in session each year, and the House spent an average of 140 days in session.

Party Leadership in Congress

Party leadership positions are not included in the Constitution but have developed gradually over time as the institution of Congress evolved into its current state. Party leadership, whether majority or minority, is ultimately responsible for anything that does or does not happen in the Congress. Below we give a brief overview of the power leadership structure in Congress.

Senate Majority Leader

While the vice president is technically the president of the Senate, the most powerful member of the Senate is the Senate majority leader. The Senate majority leader is a member of the majority party in the Senate elected to the position at the beginning of each Congress. The role of the Senate majority leader is extremely important because they are responsible for the Senate calendar. By having sole discretion over the Senate calendar, the majority leader is ultimately responsible for what legislation comes to the floor in the Senate as well as the unanimous consent agreements necessary to govern the debate of that legislation. The majority leader reserves the right to be recognized before any other Senator and can therefore offer motions and amendments that may ultimately determine a piece of legislation's fate.

Senate Minority Leader

Similar to the Senate majority leader, the Senate minority leader is elected by the members of their party at the beginning of each Congress. The Senate minority leader serves as the official spokesperson for minority party positions in the Senate. Since unanimous consent is necessary to determine the debate structure on legislation and supermajority (60) votes are necessary for some procedural motions, the Senate minority leader can wield his party's votes as a bloc to win concessions in current bill language or amendments or to demand which pieces of legislation the Senate will consider next.

Speaker of the House

The speaker of the House is third in line to the presidency in the line of succession. Each Congress, the speaker is elected to the office by the majority party in the House to be the presiding officer of that body. While the speaker's term expires every 2 years, typically speakers will be elected multiple times to the position, even going from speaker to minority leader and back to speaker if their party loses and then regains the majority in the House. Similar to the Senate majority leader, the speaker of the House is responsible for managing the floor calendar and committee assignments and us the spokesperson for the party's position on issues. Additionally, the speaker of the House is tasked with appointing the leadership of the corresponding (Republican or Democratic) national campaign committee that controls the financing of candidates in the party's House races.

House Majority Leader

The House majority leader is elected by the majority party in the House to manage the legislative business of the House of Representatives. In consultation with members of the majority party and party leadership, the House majority leader moves legislation from introduction to passage.

House Minority Leader

The House minority leader is elected by the minority party in the House to act as spokesperson for the minority party, keep the minority party unified to advance their legislative goals even without a majority in the House, and work toward regaining a majority in the House in the upcoming elections. When the president represents the same party as the minority leader, the leader meets regularly with the president and their aides to advance the president's agenda.

Whips

The party whips are elected by their conference to provide information to members, assuage any concerns members might have with legislation moving forward, and ultimately ensure that the party has enough votes to pass or block legislation.

Committees

Congressional committees are where legislation is considered after its introduction (Table 7.1). Party leadership determines chairmanship and membership on the congressional

TABLE 7.1 Standing Committees in Congress

House		Senate	
Agriculture	Rules	Agriculture, Nutrition, and Forestry	Indian Affairs
Appropriations	Science, Space, and Technology	Appropriations	Joint Committee on Printing
Armed Services	Small Business	Armed Services	Joint Committee on Taxation
Budget	Transportation and Infrastructure	Banking, Housing, and Urban Affairs	Joint Committee on the Library
Education and Labor	Veterans' Affairs	Budget	Joint Economic Committee
Energy and Commerce	Ways and Means	Commerce, Science, and Transportation	Judiciary
Ethics	Permanent Select Committee on Intelligence	Energy and Natural Resources	Rules and Administration
Financial Services	Select Committee on the Climate Crisis	Environment and Public Works	Select Committee on Ethics
Foreign Affairs	Select Committee on Economic Disparity and Fairness in Growth	Finance	Select Committee on Intelligence
Homeland Security	Select Committee on the Modernization of Congress	Foreign Relations	Small Business and Entrepreneurship
House Administration	Joint Economic Committee	Health, Education, Labor, and Pensions	Special Committee on Aging
Judiciary	Joint Committee on the Library	Homeland Security and Governmental Affairs	Veterans' Affairs
Natural Resources	Joint Committee in Printing		
Oversight and Reform	Joint Committee on Taxation		

Source: Cicily Hampton.

committees. Typically long-standing and well-respected members of the chamber are given leadership assignments of the most powerful committees, while new members or those out of favor with party leadership may find themselves appointed to relatively inactive, obscure committees. Depending on the topic of the legislation, it is referred to the relevant committee or committees (when two or more committees have jurisdiction) where the chairperson can schedule hearings on the legislation and decide to bring it for a vote or let it die. Most bills die in committee because there simply is not enough time to consider them all. The committee chairperson will only schedule hearings on legislation in line with party priorities and are expected to have enough support in the caucus to be approved when they come up for a vote.

STATE LEVEL

The chief difference between the federal and state legislative arenas is that the scope of legislation considered by state legislatures is limited to the state. With the exception of Nebraska, each state legislature has the same bicameral structure as the Congress, with a lower house and upper chamber. While the structure of these state legislatures is fundamentally identical to Congress, the details (e.g., number of legislators, committee structure, and electoral and legislative processes) are all determined by the state constitution and state laws. While members of Congress serve in a full-time capacity in either the House or Senate, most state legislators serve in a part-time capacity, so it may be more difficult to reach them or meet with them, particularly when the state legislature is out of session. Additionally, most state legislatures only meet for a limited period of time, with some only meeting for 6 weeks each year, while others may meet for a longer period of time but only every other year. Advocates must become familiar with their state's legislators and the committees on which they serve as well as the legislative calendar in order to effectively advocate at the state level.

While many advocates set their sights on federal legislation in Congress, it may be more effective to target one or a set of states for policy change and then rely on the diffusion of innovation theory to achieve policy goals nationwide. U.S. Supreme Court Justice Brandeis coined the phrase "laboratories of democracy" in a 1932 decision where he observed that a single state's adoption of a novel policy can serve as a social experiment to be tested based on the principles of the scientific method (*New State Ice Co. v. Lieberman*, 285 U.S. 262 (1932)). The **diffusion of innovation theory** posits that state-level policy innovations and programs seen as successful in one or more states are eventually adapted and adopted by other states and/or at the national level (Beyle, 1988). Advocates at the state level should network with their counterparts throughout the states to educate others on the policy innovations in their state as well as learn about policy innovations and strategies that are happening in other states. Bringing in experts from other states where similar policies have been adopted can be incredibly powerful testimony in legislative and budget hearings.

Governors Versus State Legislatures

The governor acts as the executive in each state. The division of powers between the governor and the state legislatures is defined in each state constitution. While the specific powers granted to the governor may differ from state to state, the governor generally has control over the bureaucratic and administrative aspects of the state's business and exercises this power through the powers of appointment and removal of state officials as well as the state budgeting process. Through the appointment of officials to head the state agencies, the governor can control the means and mechanisms of policy at the state level by directing the actions of subordinate bureaucrats as well as program development by controlling state agency budgets (Abney & Lauth, 1983).

While the number of direct appointments has decreased over time and the number of elected boards and commissions out of the purview of the governor has increased over time, the governor still holds significant control over the state budget as a general rule. In most states, the governor's office is responsible for gathering budget requests from state agencies and preparing a final budget proposal to be considered in the bodies that make up the state legislatures (Rosenthal, 1990). Once the budget is approved by the state legislature it is sent to the governor's desk to be signed. The governor has the power to sign the budget, veto the budget in its entirety, or utilize the line item veto[4] to strike portions of the budget that the governor does not agree with. If the governor does use the line item veto, the vetoed items are returned to the state legislature for a veto override, typically requiring a two-thirds majority. The line item veto is one of the most powerful policy tools available to the governor because legislature override of the line item veto is a very rare occurrence.

Ballot Initiative Processes

As of this writing, just over half of states have some sort of ballot initiative or referendum process in place that allows members of the electorate to bypass the state governor and legislature, either entirely or in part. Depending on the state, a private citizen can gather anywhere from a few thousand signatures to close to a million signatures to have their initiative placed on the ballot for a direct vote by the state's electorate.

These initiative or referendum processes can be used when the legislature refuses to take up an issue or votes it down or the governor vetoes a bill after it has been passed by the legislature. Initiatives that can garner broad support throughout the state will be more successful given the amount of signatures needed to get something onto the ballot and then passed in the general election. State advocates should familiarize themselves with their state's ballot initiative process in order to inform their strategy.

THE EXECUTIVE/REGULATORY ARENA

After legislation passes, rule-making commences. It is important for advocates to continue to follow the legislation through the rule-making process to ensure that the legislative intent of the law is maintained as the law is implemented. In some circumstances, rule-making may proceed without a new piece of legislation. In some cases, advocates may use a strategy aimed at urging an agency to use their existing statutory authority

---

4. Variations exist in how a line item veto may be used by the governor as well as the process for overcoming a gubernatorial veto by state.

to tackle a new problem or technology, new interpretation of statutory authority by the judiciary, recommendations by federal advisory committees, or a new perspective on existing regulations, often in the case of a new administration or technological advances.

In the absence of new legislation that prompts the rule-making process, each year agencies publish their "Agenda of Regulatory and Deregulatory Actions" in the fall and spring and the "Regulatory Plan" in the spring. Together these two publications are referred to as an agency's "Unified Agenda." Advocates can look to the *Federal Register* to find an agency's Unified Agenda and prepare their strategy to influence it. Advocates and interest groups may also submit a petition for rule-making in an effort to move a policy issue onto the regulatory agency's agenda.

When Congress passes legislation or the president delegates some presidential authority to solve a policy problem or accomplish a specific goal, the designated agency must follow the Administrative Procedures Act (APA) to ensure that they do not exceed their regulatory authority or violate the Constitution. The APA[5] ensures that the federal agencies utilize a transparent, open, and public process when engaging in the rule-making process.

The first step[6] in a typical rule-making process is for the agency to publish an Advanced Notice of Proposed Rulemaking in the *Federal Register*, although the APA does not include this step and it is therefore not required. This is the formal notice that the agency intends to begin the rule-making process on an issue and is an opportunity for advocates to weigh in on whether the rule is actually needed, to submit their general comments on the policy area, or to point the agency to additional sources of data to consider as they begin to engage in rule-making. Once the comments are received in response to the Advance Notice of Proposed Rulemaking, the agency sets about using the comments and information from the public to craft the proposed rule.

The **Notice of Proposed Rulemaking** is the agency's official plan to address the policy problem and is the first official step included in the APA. The Notice of Proposed Rulemaking will include a summary of the issue, including a synopsis of the policy problem, statutory language that governs the policy area, and any relevant legislative, regulatory, and judicial history.

Throughout the rule-making process, the agency will typically use either a 30- or 60-day comment period. Advocates can comment on the proposed rule, asking for additional time to comment for a particularly complex rule or if for some other reason additional time to consider the proposed rule may be warranted. An agency may extend or reopen the comment period if enough people ask, if not enough high-quality

---

5. 5 U.S.C. §§ 551–559.

6. There are limited circumstances in which an agency can publish a final rule without first issuing a proposed rule and soliciting public comments. In this case, the agency must include its rationale for "good cause" in the preamble of the final rule when published in the *Federal Register*. These interim final rules may be effective on publication but can be altered subject to public comment if the agency finds a compelling reason to do so.

comments are submitted, or if the comments raise new issues that were not addressed in the proposed rule. Advocates may submit their comments in a variety of ways: U.S. postal mail, an agency email address, courier service to the agency, and via the portal at https://www.regulations.gov.

The agency does not use the number of comments in support of or against the rule as a determining factor, but rather uses the substance and quality of the comments in their considerations along with data and expert opinions. This is why form letters are not the most effective tool when commenting on proposed rules, though they work well to show the salience of an issue to a member of Congress. The comments submitted on the proposed rule are considered when the agency is crafting the final rule to be published in the *Federal Register*.

The Final Rule

The final rule will include many of the elements of the proposed rule, including the preamble and relevant history, and may also include a summary of comments received on the proposed rule as well as the agency's efforts to address said comments. The final rule will always have the effective date of the rule as well as the complete regulatory text.

All final rules are sent to Congress as well as the Government Accountability Office for review before they can take effect. In order for this review to take place, final rules must have effective dates 60 days or more from their date of publication in the *Federal Register*, except in very limited circumstances. Both the House and Senate would need to pass a resolution disapproving of the rule and the president would have to sign it or the Congress would need to override a presidential veto in order to void the rule. In that case the agency would be barred from publishing the rule in the same form without express congressional approval.

In addition to establishing the procedures for the rule-making process and governing how the public may engage in that process, the APA dictates, in a process known as "judicial review," when and how the courts can be used by an aggrieved or injured party to the rule.

THE JUDICIAL ARENA

While citizens cannot lobby the courts directly in the same way they can lobby legislators or agencies, the courts remain a powerful arena for advocacy. The concept of **judicial review** was established more than 200 years ago with the case of *Marbury v. Madison* (Prakash & Yoo, 2003). *Marbury v. Madison* established that the courts could intervene in policy when there was a state interest in doing so. While the courts do not engage in direct policymaking, they do so indirectly by ruling on whether legislative, administrative, or executive actions brought before the court are inconsistent with the Constitution. In these rulings, the courts determine if the law may stand and which parts of the law, inconsistent with the Constitution, must be struck down.

The expansive procedures that govern judicial review are codified in the APA. To obtain judicial relief under the APA, an individual or organization must have suffered some sort of wrong by a government agency[7] for which they are seeking redress from the court to right the wrong and be made whole in a concept known as "standing." In order to increase their chances of success, advocates often solicit plaintiffs who have been wronged under a statute and pursue those cases that have the best chance of succeeding. It may be difficult for advocates to have to turn potential plaintiffs away or allow a statute that they fear is unconstitutional to take effect and cause harm prior to seeking relief through the courts, but advocates must understand that striking down a rule or statute will be beneficial to all citizens who have been wronged by the law, even if one potential plaintiff's specific claim of redress is not pursued.

Over time, the concept of judicial review has established the standards under which claims of redress are to be analyzed by the court. These levels of scrutiny determine how the constitutionality of a law will be analyzed as well as which party has the burden of proof (United States v. Carolene Products Co., 1938). **Strict scrutiny** is the highest standard used when there is a threat to equal protection under the law. In order to pass strict scrutiny the government must prove that there is a compelling state interest in regulating the activity *and* that the law has been narrowly tailored to achieve the government's desired result. **Intermediate scrutiny** is the midlevel review typically used when there are claims of sex or gender discrimination. In order to pass intermediate scrutiny, the government must prove that the law serves an important state objective, and the law is substantially related to achieving the government's objectives. The **rational basis** level of scrutiny is the lowest level of judicial review typically used when a plaintiff is arguing that a law is irrational or arbitrary. In order to strike down a law under the rational basis test, a challenger to the law must prove that the government has no legitimate interest in the law or policy or that there is no rational link between the law and a government interest.

Understanding Judicial Review

A careful analysis is necessary to understand whether filing an injunction to stop a new law from going into effect or a lawsuit challenging a law, in whole or in part, will result in the outcome you are anticipating. Ensure that you understand very clearly the level of scrutiny the court will apply, which party has the burden of proof, as well as the potential consequences of the law being struck down, in whole or in part. Even if the government argues that the law is not severable from the unconstitutional provisions, the court has the prerogative to disagree with that assertion and strike down any pieces of the law it deems unfit to stand. There may be tremendous ramifications if an advocate files a lawsuit to get a lawsuit struck down in its entirety and only part of it is found to be unconstitutional. These potential unintended consequences must be explored before any legal action is pursued.

---

7. 5 U.S.C. §§ 701 defines "agency" as each authority of the government of the United States, excluding Congress, the courts, the governments of the territories and Washington, D.C., military courts and commissions, as well as a specific set of functions defined within the APA.

Jurisdictions

When you have conducted the appropriate analysis and determined that a lawsuit is the course of action that will get you to your policy goals, you want to make sure to file the lawsuit in the **jurisdiction** that is most favorable to you. In order to determine the most appropriate venue for your case you need to ensure that the court where you file has both subject matter and personal jurisdiction. Federal courts, rather than state courts, have jurisdiction in matters involving the Constitution.

Advocates must understand who appointed the judges that will eventually rule on their case, in both the circuit court and the district court, and research their past jurisprudence on the issue. Understanding whether the judge was appointed by a Democrat or Republican and who was in the Senate majority during their confirmation is an excellent starting point for advocates when exploring the various personal jurisdictions where your plaintiff may have standing.

Amici Curiae Briefs

Even if an advocate or organization does not have the resources to launch their own legal battle to shape policy in the courts, all is not lost. Advocates are also able to ensure their voices are heard and the courts understand the impact of their ruling on those other than the direct parties to the case. By filing amici curiae or (friend of the court) briefs, advocates can bring their perspective and additional arguments that are relevant to the court case but that may not be included in the initial filing. In this way, advocates with more limited resources can still utilize the courts as a venue for their advocacy. Additionally, filing briefs can further cement relationships in organizations that work together on their advocacy initiatives or that work in service to similar or related populations.

CONCLUSION

Understanding policy arenas is critical to formulating an advocacy strategy. Determining the best policy arena to pursue your policy goals should be one of the first steps when planning for policy change. While the most effective advocacy strategy may involve two or more policy arenas, resources will ultimately determine which policy arena(s) you are able to pursue. As resource constraints dictate, you may need to plan your advocacy strategy around your second best option. Additionally, there are times and circumstances when multiple policy arenas are in play at once. It is not uncommon to be simultaneously engaging in the rulemaking process while advocating for a more advantageous interpretation in Congress. Lastly, remember that just because you may have gotten an outcome in one policy arena, the fight isn't over. Effective advocates must follow their chosen policy through the entirety of the policymaking process as you learned about in Chapter 6.

REFERENCES

Abney, G., & Lauth, T. P. (1983). The governor as chief administrator. *Public Administration Review, 43*(1), 40–49.

Beyle, T. L. (1988). The governor as innovator in the federal system. *Publius: The Journal of Federalism, 18*(3), 131–152.

Prakash, S. B., & Yoo, J. C. (2003). The origins of judicial review. *University of Chicago Law Review, 70*(3), 887–982.

Rosenthal, A. (1990). *Governors and legislatures: Contending powers.* Congressional Quarterly Press.

United States v. Carolene Products Co., 304 U.S. 144 (1938).

CHAPTER 7: END-OF-CHAPTER ACTIVITIES

DISCUSSION QUESTIONS

1. Discuss the benefits and drawbacks of having multiple policy arenas to work with to shape policy

2. Discuss whether or not you think there should be limits on the type of policy change that can be brought forth through the referendum process

3. Determine the advantages and disadvantages to having legislation referred to multiple committees

4. Determine a state law that has been diffused through multiple states in the State Legislature process

APPLICATION ACTIVITIES

1. Using Congress.gov identify the current party leadership of both parties currently in Congress.

2. Look up the Constitution of your state to discover the powers of the Governor where you live.

3. Discuss the pros and cons of allowing citizens to create ballot initiatives using the referendum process.

4. Using FederalRegister.gov identify any proposed or final rules relevant to policy issues you care about.

QUIZ QUESTIONS

1. Who has the right to be called upon first if several senators seek recognition by the presiding officer, enabling him to offer motions or amendments before any other senator?
   a. The Majority Leader
   b. The Minority Leader
   c. Specific Whips
   d. Congressional President

2. Both parties in the Senate elect _____, who mitigate concerns with legislation, provide information to members, and ensure votes.
   a. speakers and lawmakers
   b. the Majority Leader
   c. the Minority Leader
   d. whips

3. Which of the following is not true in reference to the Governor of each state?
   a. has control over the administrative and bureaucratic aspects of the state's business
   b. can control the mechanisms and means of policy at the state level
   c. moves legislation from introduction to passage
   d. acts as the executive of each state

4. Who has a wide range of partisan assignments, all geared toward retaking majority control of the House?
   a. The Majority leader
   b. The Minority Leader
   c. Specific Whips
   d. Congressional President

5. The structure of state legislators are like Congress, and the details such as committee structures, legislative processes, and the number of legislators are determined by:
   a. the state laws and the state constitution
   b. Congress and the party whips
   c. The Majority Leader and the Minority Leader
   d. the speakers and lawmakers

6. Where can advocates locate an agency's Unified Agenda?
   a. within the administrative alcove
   b. applying for a notice of proposed rulemaking
   c. the Federal Register
   d. in the judicial review

7. Which of the following Standing Committees in Congress are under the Senate?
   a. Judiciary Committee, Agriculture Committee, and Armed Services Committee
   b. Select Committee in Ethics, Homeland Security, and Joint Committee on Taxation
   c. Finance Committee, Foreign Relations Committee, and Joint Economic Committee
   d. Foreign Affairs Committee, Ways and Means Committee, and Budget Committee

8. Vot-ER, founded by Dr. Alister Martin, an *emergency medicine physician*, provides which of the following?
   a. a policy solution to address the health problem, and document strong community support for the policy.
   b. digital outreach that helps reach patients beyond the clinic walls and helps them vote in a safe and healthy way.
   c. discouragement to patients to register to vote while under the care of a physician in a hospital or emergency room setting.
   d. HIPAA regulations to help deter political affiliation on all hospitals.

9. In some states, _____ may involve a private citizens obtaining a substantial amount of signatures to have their initiative placed on the ballot for a direct vote by the state's electorate.
   a. the speakers and lawmakers
   b. the Governor and a senate standing committee
   c. poll monitoring or policymaking
   d. ballot initiative or referendum process

10. In reference to budget approval, the Governor has which of the following:
    a. the power to veto the budget in its entirety
    b. utilize the line-item veto to strike portions of the budget
    c. the power to sign the budget
    d. all of the above

ANSWER KEY
1. **A**. The Majority Leader
2. **D**. Whips
3. **C**. Moves legislation from introduction to passage
4. **B**. The Minority Leader
5. **A**. The state laws and the state constitution
6. **C**. The Federal Register
7. **C**. Finance Committee, Foreign Relations Committee, and Joint Economic Committee
8. **B**. Digital outreach that helps reach patients beyond the clinic walls and helps them vote in a safe and healthy way
9. **D**. Ballot initiative or referendum process
10. **D**. All of the above

Advocating for Health Equity

HOLLY MATA, KRISTEN HERNÁNDEZ ORTEGA, AND ADITI SRIVISTAV BUSSELLS

> For while we have our eyes on the future
> History has its eyes on us
>
> —AMANDA GORMAN, 2021

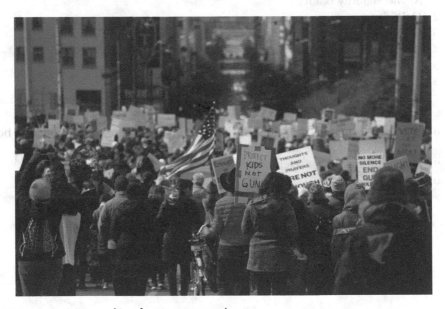

FIGURE 8.1 Activists working for stronger gun laws.
Photo by Ben Mater on Unsplash https://unsplash.com/license provides the license to use without permission.

Objectives

1. Explain how the terms health equity, health literacy, structural racism, and structural competence relate to health advocacy.
2. Discuss the importance of cultural competence, cultural humility, and structural competence.
3. Examine how social and structural determinants of health influence health and health equity.

Holly Mata, Kristen Hernández Ortega, and Aditi Srivistav Bussells, *Advocating for Health Equity*. In: *Be the Change*. Edited by Keely S. Rees, Jody Early, and Cicily Hampton, Oxford University Press. © Oxford University Press 2023. DOI: 10.1093/oso/9780197570890.003.0008

4. Explain how structural racism impacts health and health equity.
5. Identify at least three strategies to increase voter participation.
6. Recommend strategies for advocating for change within an organization.

INTRODUCTION

As public health professionals, we step into large, complex, and deeply rooted community issues, sometimes thinking they're unrelated to health. However, over the years we have come to understand how these determinants of health and structural inequities affect the health of our communities. How do we make sure all people have a fair opportunity to achieve their full health potential? What has been keeping us from advancing the health and well-being of the populations we serve and the communities where we live? Where do we start, and how do we use our voices and our votes to be the change we know we need? It seems like a tall order, and you are not the only one thinking that!

In this chapter, you will discover how public health practitioners and community members are improving the environments in which we live, learn, work, play, and pray by advocating for **health equity**. Health equity means that everyone has a fair and just opportunity to be as healthy as possible—and for that to happen, we need to prioritize action for people and communities historically been excluded from having the resources and opportunities associated with health and healthy environments (Braveman et al., 2017).

HEALTH EQUITY—PRINCIPLES AND POSSIBILITIES

We discuss many terms and concepts in this chapter that advance the well-being of *all* individuals and communities, regardless of their background, the color of their skin, or where they came from. These terms are very important to us as public health professionals, community members, and advocates for policies that support health and health equity. You may have heard of the terms **health disparities** and **health inequities** as they are often used interchangeably. However, it is important to understand that while they are related concepts, they have distinct meanings. Health disparities originally were defined as differences between health and healthcare between groups. Health inequities are the result of health disparities that exist because of structural or institutional practices. As the understanding of inequities has advanced, so has the definition of health disparities.

Health disparities refer to differences in health and health care between groups that stem from broader inequities (Kaiser Family Foundation [KFF], 2021). Specifically, they are "systematic, plausibly avoidable health differences adversely affecting socially disadvantaged groups" (Braveman et al., 2011, p. S151) and "reflect longstanding structural and systemic inequities rooted in racism and discrimination" (KFF, 2021). Some examples of health disparities include the following:

- In the United States, pregnancy-related deaths per 100,000 live births for Black and American Indian/Alaska Native birthing people older than 30 are *four to five times higher than among their White counterparts* (Petersen et al., 2019).

- In Chicago, the average life expectancy at birth is 77.3 years, but life expectancy varies by census tract; in some neighborhoods, the *average life expectancy is only 59 years, while in others it is 90 years* (NYU Langone Health, 2021).

These inequities exist because of the circumstances and environments in which we live. Our health is shaped by the social, environmental, and structural factors around us. That is why we use the term health inequities rather than health disparities to clearly reflect their unjust and unfair impact on people and communities and to acknowledge that these inequities are not only differences, but also inequitable and avoidable differences due to how systems were originally designed to benefit certain groups in our country.

Where we live, learn, work, play, and pray have a profound impact on our health. These social and economic factors are often referred to as **social determinants of health** (Box 8.1) and include housing, employment, education, transportation, community and civic engagement, access to healthy foods and safe places to play and exercise, exposure to violence and trauma, policing and justice systems, access to healthcare, and many others.

As we discuss throughout this chapter, any effort to improve these factors and systems must include identifying and addressing racism, discrimination, and exclusion as root causes of health inequities (KFF, 2021). As public health professionals and as advocates, how we name and frame racism matters (Mata & Roe, 2021). Ra*cism*—not race—is the root of racial inequities in health opportunities and outcomes in the United States (Boyd et al., 2020; Ford et al., 2019). You have likely heard the term **structural racism** and may have wondered how structural racism affects our health and our opportunities across our lifespan. Structural racism has been defined as "the totality of ways in which societies foster racial discrimination through mutually reinforcing systems of housing, education, employment, earnings, benefits, credit, media, health care, and criminal justice" (Bailey et al., 2017, p. 1453). Structural racism impacts individual and population health through inequitable systems and policies in many ways, including but not limited to

---

ADVOCACY IN ACTION BOX 8.1	Social Determinants of Health in Early Childhood: The Concept of Adverse Childhood Experiences

There is a lot of research that examines the impact of social determinants of health (SDOH), such as safety, education, income, housing, or access to services across the lifespan (Bharmal et al., 2015). SDOH influence health at each life stage (childhood health, adult health, family health), with early childhood a critical period in which the exposure to negative social determinants of health can substantially increase risks for poor health outcomes in adulthood (Bharmal et al., 2015). One concept that is receiving widespread attention in public health as a social determinant of health is adverse childhood experiences (ACEs). These traumatic experiences—including witnessing domestic violence, having a parent who is incarcerated, dealing with mental illness or problematic substance use in the home, neglect, physical abuse, sexual abuse, or emotional abuse—are shaped by social factors, including the well-being of older generations. ACEs can affect children's cognitive, behavioral, and physical development and in turn predict current and future health (Bharmal et al., 2015). ACEs are common across populations and are the root cause of many unhealthy behaviors and negative health outcomes we see later in adolescence and adulthood (Srivastav et al., 2020).

"redlining" and racialized residential segregation, mass incarceration, and inequitable healthcare (Bailey et al., 2021).

EXAMPLES OF STRUCTURAL RACISM
Exclusion From Healthcare Coverage
Although the Affordable Care Act expanded healthcare coverage to millions of previously uninsured Americans and narrowed long-standing racial/ethnic inequity in healthcare coverage at a national level, most of the states in the southern United States have not implemented Medicaid Expansion (KFF, 2020). Because more than half of the Black population in the United States lives in the South (Pew Research Center, 2021), the state-level refusal to implement Medicaid Expansion perpetuates inequities in healthcare coverage and access. Additionally, restrictions on undocumented immigrants and other residents who do not have U.S. citizenship that restrict access to Medicaid and other health insurance coverage inequitably impact Hispanic and Asian populations because they represent a larger percentage of nonelderly adults living in the United States who are not citizens (KFF, 2020).

Mass Incarceration
People of color account for 39% of the U.S. population but account for about 60% of people who are incarcerated. The effects of incarceration on people, families, and communities include trauma, limited economic and educational opportunities, negative health consequences that persist for generations (Acker et al., 2019), and being denied the right to vote (Purtle, 2013), all of which impact our health.

HEALTH EQUITY
As we discussed, health equity means that everyone has a "fair and just opportunity to be as healthy as possible. This requires removing obstacles to health such as poverty, discrimination, and their consequences, including powerlessness and lack of access to good jobs with fair pay, quality education and housing, safe environments, and health care" (Braveman et al., 2017, p. 2). Health equity is not the same thing as health equality. Because of the history of our country, which has kept certain groups from reaching their full potential, we know that all populations are not starting at the same place. This means we need to focus on improving access to resources, conditions, and opportunities that support health among populations who have been historically marginalized and excluded from these opportunities. People and communities will need different resources and opportunities to be healthy, and our actions should prioritize meeting those needs. That is why public health focuses on equity and not equality (Figure 8.2).

ADVANCING HEALTH EQUITY
In the next several sections, we cover key approaches and concepts that have been proven to address inequities, specifically within the role of health education. These include

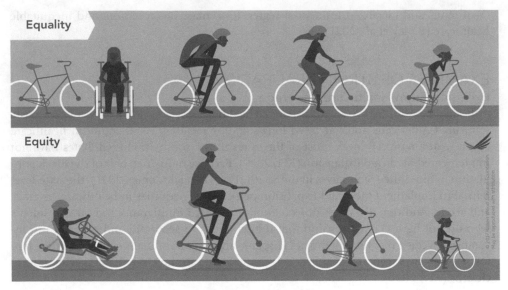

FIGURE 8.2 Visualizing health equity: One size does not fit all.
Source: Robert Wood Johnson Foundation, 2017.

civic engagement, health literacy, health communications, and health equity advocacy. We provide several resources with this chapter to help you build your skills and understanding of these practices.

CIVIC ENGAGEMENT AND HEALTH

Civic engagement and **civic participation** include voting, volunteering, and being part of community groups or activities (e.g., community garden initiatives) that provide a sense of purpose and increase social connections (Office of Disease Prevention and Health Promotion [ODPHP], 2021). All forms of civic engagement and participation can have a positive impact on individual and community health (Nelson et al., 2019) Research on the relationship between voting and health is particularly strong (Ehlinger & Nevarez, 2021). Ensuring that *all* people who are eligible to vote can vote safely and conveniently is imperative in our efforts to advance health equity (Box 8.2).

The Voting Rights Act (VRA) of 1965 was a milestone in the civil rights movement and prohibited racial discrimination in voting. However, in 2013 the Supreme Court ruling in *Shelby v. Holder* decimated the protections of the VRA and set the stage for recent state-level laws and policies that have made it more difficult for people to vote, especially for people and communities of color (Pérez & Lau, 2021). Unfortunately, proposed legislation in recent years have failed to passed the senate. Policymakers and advocates proposed two bills in 2021 that if they had passed, would have strengthened the VRA and addressed voter discrimination, voter suppression, and voter disenfranchisement. The first, the *For the People Act*, was designed to expand voter rights and address election

ADVOCACY IN ACTION BOX 8.2	Proven Strategies to Increase Voter Participation

- Automatic voter registration
- Same-day voter registration
- Preregistration for youth ages 16 and 17
- Online voter registration
- "No excuse" absentee voting
- Early voting

- Vote at home (vote by mail) with community vote centers
- Strengthen civics education in schools
- Invest in voter education and outreach
- Ensure that people who were formerly incarcerated are aware of the process in their state to get their voting rights restored

Source: Root and Kennedy, 2018.

administration and voter suppression issues. The second was the *John Lewis Voting Rights Advancement Act*, which addressed racism and discrimination in our voting systems and processes. Together, these bills would have strengthened and advanced racial equity in our voting systems (Pérez & Lau, 2021) and could have increased civic participation at all levels of government. While these two bills passed in the House (largely on party lines), they failed to pass in the Senate. Therefore, the fight for protecting and expanding voting rights continues.

How do we as public health professionals get involved? Increasing civic participation "is an essential task for anyone interested in advancing health equity . . . part of the job of a public health worker is to help make that happen" (Ehlinger & Nevarez, 2021, p. 46). Public health professionals work in diverse clinical and community settings and have many opportunities to combat voter suppression and discrimination. We can advocate for policies that make it easier and safer to vote, and we can make sure that people in our communities have the information and resources they need to register to vote. One great example is Vote-ER: See how community health centers, hospitals, and other community organizations are advancing voter registration in the places where the people are: emergency rooms, community health centers, and other healthcare and community settings!

HEALTH EQUITY AND HEALTH LITERACY

Health equity is an overarching goal of *Healthy People 2030*, the fifth iteration of the national *Healthy People* initiative in the United States. Updated in 2020 to reflect progress, priorities, and challenges, Healthy People 2030 prioritizes five primary goals (ODPHP, n.d.):

- Attain healthy, thriving lives and well-being free of preventable disease, disability, injury, and premature death.
- Eliminate health disparities, achieve health equity, and attain health literacy to improve the health and well-being of all.
- Create social, physical, and economic environments that promote attaining the full potential for health and well-being for all.
- Promote healthy development, healthy behaviors, and well-being across all life stages.

- Engage leadership, key constituents, and the public across multiple sectors to take action and design policies that improve the health and well-being of all.

Healthy People 2030 includes 355 measurable objectives. Six of these objectives are related to **health literacy** and 19 are related to **health communication**. For many years, the term **health literacy** was typically used only in the context of individuals. For example, a common definition was "the degree to which individuals have the capacity to obtain, process, and understand basic health information and services needed to make appropriate health decisions" (ODPHP, 2020). Our understanding of health literacy has evolved so that we define health literacy at both individual and organizational levels (ODPHP, 2020):

- **Personal health literacy** is the degree to which individuals have the ability to find, understand, and use information and services to inform health-related decisions and actions for themselves and others.
- **Organizational health literacy** is the degree to which organizations equitably enable individuals to find, understand, and use information and services to inform health-related decisions and actions for themselves and others.

Why is health literacy important? Health literacy is central to communities being able to reach their full potential. When individuals can make informed decisions about their health and well-being, we advance health equity along the way.

HEALTH COMMUNICATION

Closely connected to health literacy is **health communication**, which has been defined as "the science and art of using communication to advance the health and well-being of people and populations" (Society for Health Communications [SHC], 2017). As a profession, health communication is "a multidisciplinary field of study and practice that applies communication evidence, strategy, theory, and creativity to promote behaviors, policies, and practices that advance the health and well-being of people and populations" (SHC, 2017).

The Eight Areas of Responsibility for Health Education Specialists (National Commission for Health Education Credentialing, n.d.), which you explored in Chapter 3, include *Area VI: Communications*. Below are some examples of communications competencies and subcompetencies related to health literacy that you will likely use often in your public health practice, whether or not you decide to become a certified health education specialist (CHES) (National Commission for Health Education Credentialing, n.d.)

"6.1.2   Identify the assets, needs, and characteristics of the audience(s) that affect communication and message design (e.g., literacy levels, language, culture, and cognitive and perceptual abilities)

6.1.3   Identify communication channels (e.g., social media and mass media) available to and used by the audience(s)

6.1.4   Identify environmental and other factors that affect communication (e.g., resources and the availability of Internet access)

6.3.3   Tailor message(s) for the audience(s)

6.3.4 Employ media literacy skills (e.g., identifying credible sources and balancing multiple viewpoints)

6.4.2 Select communication channels and current and emerging technologies that are most appropriate for the audience(s) and message(s)

6.5.1 Deliver presentation(s) tailored to the audience(s)

6.5.4 Use current and emerging communication tools and trends (e.g., social media)"

Regardless of the setting in which you work, there are lots of resources to help you develop health communication strategies that are relevant for your priority population, grounded in theory, and likely to reach your intended audience. You'll find several in the Additional Resources section at the end of this chapter. And in Chapter 12 of this text, you will examine the connection between health communication, social marketing, and other forms of media advocacy further.

CULTURAL COMPETENCE, CULTURAL HUMILITY, AND STRUCTURAL COMPETENCE

Cultural competence has gained a lot of notoriety in public health as being an important component in alleviating health disparities that result from systemic inequities (Betancourt et al., 2005). Culturally competent care and practice respects "diversity in the patient population and cultural factors that affect health and health care, such as language, communication styles, beliefs, attitudes and behaviors. Cultural competence is the foundation to reducing disparities by being culturally sensitive and providing unbiased, high-quality care" (American Academy of Family Physicians, 2019, p. 1). In other words, as health educators, embracing and protecting diversity in your practice is key to advancing equity! There are several related terms to cultural competence that you'll encounter often in your public health career—and they are terms that have many definitions and implications for practice. Let's start with some common definitions and then explore how we can integrate our commitment to continued growth in these overlapping and intertwined concepts.

Cultural competence has been defined in many ways, including as "a set of values, behaviors, attitudes, and practices within a system, organization, program or among individuals and which enables them to work effectively cross culturally" (National Center for Cultural Competence, n.d., p. 1). **Culturally and linguistically appropriate services** (CLAS; Office of Minority Health [OMH], n.d.) respect and respond to each person's culture and communication needs. The **National CLAS Standards** provide 15 action steps/standards for CLAS, including the principal standard to "provide effective, equitable, understandable and respectful quality care and services that are responsive to diverse cultural health beliefs and practices, preferred languages, health literacy, and other communication needs (p. 1, https://thinkculturalhealth.hhs.gov/clas/standards). Other examples include "ensure the competence of individuals providing language assistance, recognizing that the use of untrained individuals and/or minors as interpreters should be avoided" and "conduct regular assessments of community health assets and needs and use the results to plan and implement services that respond to the cultural and

linguistic diversity of populations in the service area" (OMH, n.d., p. 1, https://thinkcul
turalhealth.hhs.gov/assets/pdfs/EnhancedNationalCLASStandards.pdf).

Cultural humility was defined by Tervalon and Murray-Garcia (1998,
p. 123) as "a lifelong commitment to self-evaluation and critique, to redressing power
imbalances . . . and to developing mutually beneficial and non-paternalistic partnerships
with communities on behalf of individuals and defined populations" and explicitly
focuses on social justice and equity. In their commentary "Cultural Competence or
Cultural Humility? Moving Beyond the Debate," Greene-Moton and Minkler (2020)
explained:

> While typically focused on building understanding and bridging differences based on
> race/ethnicity, both cultural humility and cultural competence also have been prof-
> itably used to encourage self-reflection and reflective practice with respect to ability/
> disability, sexual orientation and gender identity, and numerous other dimensions
> too often characterized by inequitable power, privilege, and injustice that affect
> health and well-being. Both concepts increasingly have stressed the need to challenge
> the institutions and systems in which we live and work that may, wittingly or unwit-
> tingly, enable these injustices to remain. . . . Finally, as we pursue the path of "both/
> and," we can more effectively partner across a wide range of barriers and divides to
> work collectively toward racial, social, and health equity and the more just and hab-
> itable society and planet on which our work and our future depend. (pp. 144–145)

Structural competency builds on an approach proposed to improve medical education
in the United States (Metzl & Hansen, 2014) and has recently been defined as "the capacity for health professionals to recognize and respond to health and illness as the
downstream effects of broad social, political, and economic structures" (Neff et al., 2020,
p. 2). A structural competency approach not only documents racial health disparities,
but also examines and calls out the structures that created and sustain racial inequity
and structural racism (Neff et al., 2020). In other words, structural competency seeks to
actively dismantle structural racism through our practices and policies.

What might this look like in clinical and community practice settings? These are just
a few examples. What are some others that would make sense in your community or in
your current or future job setting?

- Medical intake and health history forms respect the diversity of gender identity and expression (e.g., providing options for both "sex listed at birth" and
  "gender identity"; providing space for legal name and preferred name; asking for
  pronouns).
- Clinicians screen for adverse childhood experiences (ACEs) to assess the
  risk of toxic stress and respond with evidence-based, trauma-informed care
  across sectors (see ACES Aware in the Additional Resources at the end of this
  chapter).
- Community partners collaborate to improve crisis response systems so that
  people with a mental health crisis or substance-related crisis are connected to
  healthcare and social services instead of the criminal justice system.
- Healthcare organizations and public health departments participate in nonpartisan voter registration initiatives (Vot-ER, 2021).

HEALTH EQUITY ADVOCACY: IT'S UP TO US!

Shifting our conversations from "what can individuals do" to "what can communities do" is key in our efforts to advocate for policies that not only reduce unhealthy substance use but also support healthy eating and active living, educational attainment, economic improvements, and other key social determinants of health.

—ROE and *Mata*, 2019, p. 155

Think about some of the issues that matter to you the most. Maybe you are passionate about all people having access to healthcare. Or perhaps you believe that everyone should have paid family and medical leave. Or you would like to increase high school graduation rates in your community. With all these issues—and with all the factors that influence our health—we have opportunities to advocate at many levels. We can work with individuals and families, providing education and/or connecting them to programs and services. We can work with organizations to advocate for changes in schools and places of employment, these are all important! However, we know that interventions that address social determinants of health and/or improve public policy to change the context to make healthier behaviors easier have the largest impact on population health (Frieden, 2010).

FRAMEWORKS TO SUPPORT HEALTH EQUITY ADVOCACY

There are several action-oriented frameworks that can help you develop your plan for health equity advocacy and ensure that you have the right partners and policy recommendations that will result in the maximum amount of good for the people and communities you serve.

Ten Essential Public Health Services: Centering Equity

Developed in 1994 and revised in 2020, the **10 Essential Public Health Services** (EPHS) provide a framework (Public Health National Center for Innovations, 2020) for public health to protect and promote the health of all people in all communities. To achieve equity, the EPHS actively promote "policies, systems, and overall community conditions that enable optimal health for all and seek to remove systemic and structural barriers that have resulted in health inequities. Such barriers include poverty, racism, gender discrimination, ableism, and other forms of oppression" and emphasize that "everyone should have a fair and just opportunity to achieve optimal health and well-being" (Public Health National Center for Innovations, 2020, p. 155). The framework can help you communicate the role of public health in supporting healthy people and healthy communities.

The Empower Action Model: Preventing ACES

The empower action model (Figure 8.3) provides concrete steps and strategies to prevent ACEs. There is a lot of research that shows that ACEs are a root cause of many health risk behaviors and negative health outcomes across the lifespan, and that children of color are more likely to be impacted by these traumatic experiences early in life (Burke Harris, 2018). The empower action model provides a road map for implementing protective

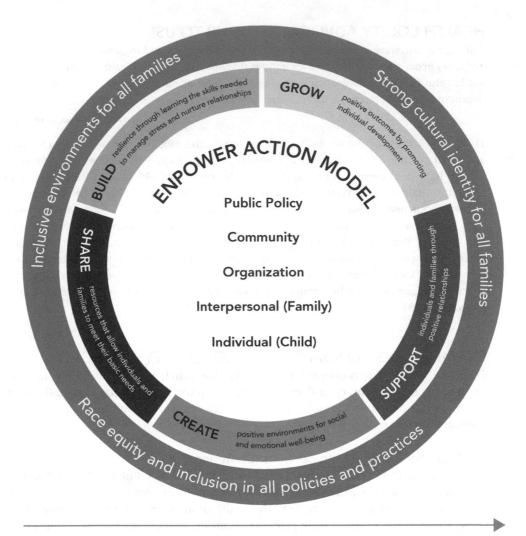

FIGURE 8.3 The empower action model.
Source: Srivastav et al., 2020.

factors, or positive social determinants of health, to build resilience and health equity for individuals, children, and families across multiple levels of influence and across all ages and stages. The model can support families, those who serve families, communities or coalitions, and policy advocates in developing action plans for advocacy in their areas of influence. The model also promotes collaboration across disciplines and sectors (Srivastav et al., 2020). You can read the article, then learn more about the authors and their work through the *Health Promotion Practice* video and podcast series, which you'll find in the Additional Resources at the end of this chapter.

IMPROVING LOCAL POLICY TO IMPROVE HEALTH

As we have discussed throughout the book, advocacy happens at local, state, national, and global levels. We have explored voting rights advocacy and nationwide efforts to increase voter registration and participation. Let's look at some stories from advocates working locally to improve organizational and community-level policies to create healthier environments and reduce substance-related harm.

Our Homes, Our Health: Supporting Smoke-Free Multiunit Housing

El Paso, Texas, implemented a comprehensive smoking ban in public places and workplaces in 2002, which led to reductions in smoking prevalence and was one of the strongest clean air ordinances in the United States (Taylor et al., 2012). In response to emerging tobacco trends, the Paso del Norte Tobacco Control Network and the El Paso Clean Air Coalition have been strengthening tobacco prevention and control policies at university, organizational, and community levels for almost 20 years to support health equity (Garcia et al., 2015). Between 2012 and 2014, community stakeholders, including the local housing authority, a nonprofit health foundation, the local public health department, and a local university, facilitated a "community-engaged process that acknowledged the right of residents to breathe clean air in their own homes, potential challenges residents who choose to smoke may face in adapting to smoke-free policy, and the need for support for those who choose to quit" (Ortega & Mata, 2020, p. 110, 111). In their article, the authors shared the context, process, key milestones, and lessons learned as stakeholders in El Paso implemented smoke-free policy in public housing. Once you've read the article, reflect on the discussion questions you'll find at the end of this chapter.

CONCLUSION

The shift in understanding the social and structural determinants of health equity has broadened much of the conversation in public health practice. Many of us working in the field or in academia also bring our own lived experience coming from marginalized or underrepresented groups. As a diverse workforce, we bring a perspective that shares an understanding of communities that may have historically been excluded and left out of the discussion. Through representation and advocacy, we can contribute to culturally responsive communication and engagement that considers not only the needs but also the assets and strengths of the communities we serve. While we still have much to learn, it is through listening to, engaging with, empowering, and advocating for all communities where our work begins. We hope that you will use your voice to advocate for practices, policies, and systems that support health equity!

We've covered a lot of topics in this chapter. We hope you are inspired to "be the change" and advocate for programs, practices, and policies that support health equity in your community and throughout your career! In all your advocacy work, we encourage you to consider:

- Who is "at the table" and who is not? Are there voices, experiences, and perspectives missing? It is important to ensure that those who are most affected by inequities have a place in decision-making.

- Who might be most affected by policy improvements (or by policies staying the same), and are they able to participate in advocacy efforts? It is important to assess how policies are detrimental or beneficial to the population you are advocating with.

Especially in efforts to address structural racism and exclusion, people who are most affected may have barriers to sharing their stories. Incarceration, immigration status, fear of retribution or retaliation, and many other factors can prevent people from engaging in advocacy. As a health educator, you have a unique opportunity to empower and include and elevate these stories, experiences, and priorities! Many of you will have the opportunity to gain experience through a capstone, practicum, or internship experience as part of your degree. We encourage you to seek opportunities to gain policy advocacy experience. Check out the New Mexico Public Health Association and the Association of State Public Health Nutritionists health equity internship program in the Additional Resources section for ideas and possibilities!

REFERENCES

Acker, J., Braveman, P., Arkin, E., Leviton, L., Parsons, J., & Hobor, G. (2019). Mass incarceration threatens health equity in America. Robert Wood Johnson Foundation. https://www.rwjf.org/en/library/research/2019/01/mass-incarceration-threatens-health-equity-in-america.html

American Academy of Family Physicians. (2019, April 19). Cultural humility is critical to health equity. Leader Voices Blog. https://www.aafp.org/news/blogs/leadervoices/entry/20190418lv-humility.html

Bailey, Z. D., Feldman, J. M., & Bassett, M. T. (2021). How structural racism works—Racist policies as a root cause of US racial health inequities. *New England Journal of Medicine, 384*, 768–773.

Bailey, Z. D., Krieger, N., Agénor, M., Graves, J., Linos, N., & Bassett, M. T. (2017). Structural racism and health inequities in the USA: Evidence and interventions. *Lancet, 389*(10077), 1453–1463.

Betancourt, J. R., Green, A. R., Carrillo, J. E., & Park, E. R. (2005). Cultural competence and health care disparities: Key perspectives and trends. *Health Affairs, 24*(2), 499–505.

Bharmal, N., Derose, K. P., Felician, M., & Weden, M. M. (2015). Understanding the upstream social determinants of health. Rand. https://www.rand.org/content/dam/rand/pubs/working_papers/WR1000/WR1096/RAND_WR1096.pdf

Boyd, R. W., Lindo, E. G., Weeks, L. D., & McLemore, M. R. (2020, July 2). On racism: A new standard for publishing on racial health inequities. *Health Affairs Blog.* https://www.healthaffairs.org/do/10.1377/hblog20200630.939347/full/

Braveman, P., Arkin, E., Orleans, T., Proctor, D., & Plough, A. (2017). What is health equity? And what difference does a definition make? Robert Wood Johnson Foundation. https://www.rwjf.org/en/library/research/2017/05/what-is-health-equity-.html

Braveman, P. A., Kumanyika, S., Fielding, J., LaVeist, T., Borrell, L. N., Manderscheid, R., & Troutman, A. (2011). Health disparities and health equity: The issue is justice. *American Journal of Public Health, 101*(S1), S149–S155.

Burke Harris, N. (2018). *The deepest well: Healing the long-term effects of childhood adversity.* Houghton Mifflin Harcourt.

Centers for Disease Control & Prevention (CDC). (2021) Health literacy. https://www.cdc.gov/healthliteracy/index.html

Cooke, N. A. (2020, May 30). Anti-*racism resources for all ages*: A project of the Augusta Baker Endowed Chair at the University of South Carolina. https://padlet.com/nicolethelibrarian/nbasekqoazt336co

Ehlinger, E. P., & Nevarez, C. R. (2021). Safe and accessible voting: The role of public health. *American Journal of Public Health, 111*(1), 45–46.

Ford, C. L., Griffith, D. M., Bruce, M. A., & Gilbert, K. L. (2019). *Racism: Science and tools for the public health professional*. APHA Press.

Frieden, T. R. (2010). A framework for public health action: The health impact pyramid. *American Journal of Public Health, 100*, 590–595.

Garcia, L., Hernandez, K., & Mata, H. (2015). Professional development through policy advocacy: Communicating and advocating for health and health equity. *Health Promotion Practice, 16*(2), 162–165. https://doi.org/10.1177/1524839914560405

Gorman, A. (2021). *The hill we climb: An inaugural poem for the country*. Viking.

Greene-Moton, E., & Minkler, M. (2020). Cultural competence or cultural humility? Moving beyond the debate. *Health Promotion Practice, 21*(1), 142–145.

Kaiser Family Foundation (KFF). (2020, March 5). *Changes in health coverage by race and ethnicity since the ACA, 2010–2018*. https://www.kff.org/racial-equity-and-health-policy/issue-brief/changes-in-health-coverage-by-race-and-ethnicity-since-the-aca-2010-2018/

Kaiser Family Foundation (KFF). (2021, May 11). Disparities in health and health care: 5 key questions and answers. https://www.kff.org/racial-equity-and-health-policy/issue-brief/disparities-in-health-and-health-care-5-key-question-and-answers/

Mata, H. J., & Roe, K.M. (2021). The power of words 2.0. *Health Promotion Practice, 22*(3), 293–294.

Metzl, J. M., & Hansen, H. (2014). Structural competency: Theorizing a new medical engagement with stigma and inequality. *Social Science & Medicine, 103*, 126–133.

National Center for Cultural Competence. (n.d.). *Definitions of cultural competence*. https://nccc.georgetown.edu/curricula/culturalcompetence.html

National Commission for Health Education Credentialing. (n.d.). Responsibilities and competencies for *health education specialists*. https://www.nchec.org/responsibilities-and-competencies

Neff, J., Holmes, S. M., Knight, K. R., Strong, S., Thompson-Lastad, A., McGuinness, C., . . . Nelson, N. (2020). Structural competency: Curriculum for medical students, residents, and interprofessional teams on the structural factors that produce health disparities. *MedEdPORTAL, 16*. https://www.mededportal.org/doi/10.15766/mep_2374-8265.10888

Nelson, C., Sloan, J., & Chandra, A. (2019). Examining civic engagement: Links to health. Rand.

NYU Langone Health. (2021). *City health dashboard:* Chicago life expectancy in 2015 by census tract. https://www.cityhealthdashboard.com/

Office of Disease Prevention and Health Promotion (ODPHP). (n.d.). Healthy People 2030 Framework. https://health.gov/healthypeople/about/healthy-people-2030-framework

Office of Disease Prevention and Health Promotion (ODPHP). (2020). Health literacy in Healthy People 2030. https://health.gov/our-work/healthy-people/healthy-people-2030/health-literacy-healthy-people-2030

Office of Disease Prevention and Health Promotion (ODPHP). (2021). Healthy People 2030: Civic participation. https://health.gov/healthypeople/objectives-and-data/social-determinants-health/literature-summaries/civic-participation

Office of Minority Health (OMH). (n.d). Think cultural health: *National* CLAS standards. https://thinkculturalhealth.hhs.gov/clas

Ortega, K. E., & Mata, H. (2020). Our homes, our health: Strategies, insight, and resources to support smoke-free multiunit housing. *Health Promotion Practice, 21*(1, Suppl.), 110S–117S.

Pérez, M., & Lau, T. (2021, January 18). How to restore and strengthen the Voting Rights Act. Brennan Center for Justice. https://www.brennancenter.org/our-work/research-reports/how-to-restore-and-strengthen-voting-rights-act

Petersen, E. E., Davis, N. L., Goodman, D., Cox, S., Syverson, C., Seed, K., Shapiro-Mendoza, C., Callaghan, W., & Barfield, W. (2019). Racial/ethnic disparities in pregnancy-related deaths—United States, 2007–2016.

MMWR Morbidity and Mortality Weekly Report, 68(35), 762.

Pew Research Center. (2021, March 25). The growing diversity of Black America. https://www.pewresearch.org/social-trends/2021/03/25/the-growing-diversity-of-black-america/#over-half-of-the-black-population-lives-in-the-south

Public Health National Center for Innovations. (2020, September 9). 10 *essential public health services* toolkit. http://ephs.phnci.org/toolkit

Purtle, J. (2013). Felon disenfranchisement in the United States: A health equity perspective. *American Journal of Public Health, 103*(4), 632–637.

Roe, K. M., & Mata, H. J. (2019). The power of words. *Health Promotion Practice, 20*(2), 153–156. https://doi.org/10.1177/1524839919827900

Root, D., & Kennedy, L. (2018, July 11). *Increasing voter participation in America: Policies to drive participation and make voting more convenient.* Center for American Progress. https://www.americanprogress.org/issues/democracy/reports/2018/07/11/453319/increasing-voter-participation-america/

Society for Health Communications (SHC). (2017). About health communication. https://www.societyforhealthcommunication.org/what-is-health-communication

Srivastav, A., Strompolis, M., Moseley, A., & Daniels, K. (2020). The empower action model: A framework for preventing adverse childhood experiences by promoting health, equity, and well-being across the life span. *Health Promotion Practice, 21*(4), 525–534.

Taylor, T., Cooper, T., Hernandez, N., Kelly, M., Law, J., & Colwell, B. (2012). A smoke-free Paso del Norte: Impact over 10 years on smoking prevalence using the behavioral risk factor surveillance system. *American Journal of Public Health, 102*(5), 899–908.

Tervalon, M., & Murray-Garcia, J. (1998). Cultural humility versus cultural competence: A critical distinction in defining physician training outcomes in multicultural education. *Journal of Health Care for the Poor and Underserved, 9*(2), 117–125.

University of Texas at El Paso (UTEP). (2018, January 11). UTEP public health graduates impact local alcohol policy. https://www.utep.edu/newsfeed/campus/utep-public-health-graduates-impact-alcohol-policy.html

Vot-ER. (2021). About us. https://vot-er.org/aboutus/

CHAPTER 8: END-OF-CHAPTER ACTIVITIES

DISCUSSION QUESTIONS

After reading "Our Homes, Our Health: Strategies, Insight, and Resources to Support Smoke-Free Multiunit Housing" (Ortega & Mata, 2020) and reflect on the following:

- How did community advocates leverage resources and partnerships to implement policy change?
- How important was health literacy in their advocacy efforts? Share an example of how both individual and organizational health literacy was important.
- What role do you think effective health communications played in smoke-free policy advocacy efforts?

APPLICATION ACTIVITIES

1. Envision yourself as a certified health education specialist working in a federally qualified health center. Your supervisor has asked you to develop recommendations for the team that will help them improve organizational health literacy. What are some strategies you might recommend? How would you advocate for these strategies? To help you get started, here are some helpful health literacy resources from the Centers for Disease Control and Prevention (CDC, 2021).
   Culture and health literacy: https://www.cdc.gov/healthliteracy/culture.html
   "Create a Health Literacy Plan": https://www.cdc.gov/healthliteracy/planact/index.html

2. Attend a local government (school board or city or county commission) meeting in your community, in person or virtually. What are some of the issues on the agenda that are important to you? What are some of the issues on the agenda that are related to community health? Who is the representative for your district? If you are already registered to vote, verify that your voter information is correct. If you are not already registered to vote and you are eligible to vote, get registered! You can visit your local county clerk's office, your secretary of state website, or https://www.democracy.works/tools-for-voters.

ADDITIONAL RESOURCES

Health Equity Advocacy and Anti-Racism Tools and Resources: Explore, use, and share!

- **ACES Aware.** Resources to better understand how racism and discrimination are risk factors for toxic stress and how we can use this knowledge to improve health and well-being for all (https://www.acesaware.org/)
- **American Public Health Association** (APHA). APHA health equity factsheets, reports, and infographics (https://www.apha.org/topics-and-issues/health-equity)

- **Antiracism Resources** for all Ages (Cooke, 2020) (https://padlet.com/nicoletheli brarian/nbasekqoazt336co)
- **Association of State Public Health Nutritionists Health Equity Internship Program.** Supporting the diversification of the public health and health-related workforce through paid internships (https://asphn.org/health-equity-internship-program/)
- **CDC Health Communication Gateway.** A one-stop shop for health communicators (https://www.cdc.gov/healthcommunication/index.html)
- **CDC Clear Communication Index.** A research-based tool to help you develop and assess public communication materials (https://www.cdc.gov/ccindex/index.html)
- **ChangeLabSolutions.** Policy solution tools and resources that address many aspects of creating healthier communities for all (https://www.changelabsoluti ons.org/)
- **Community Tool Box** by the University of Kansas. Provides "the basics" in practical tools, examples, and resources for practitioners in any setting (https://ctb.ku.edu/en); be sure to explore their Justice Action Toolkit! https://ctb.ku.edu/en/justice-action-toolkit
- **de Beaumont Foundation**. Practical resources centered on policy, partnership, and people (https://debeaumont.org/)
- **Diversity and Resiliency Institute of El Paso.** Antiracism training, an online, self-paced training to help anyone grow in their understanding of racial justice and allyship (https://www.driep.org/anti-racism-training)
- **Greater Than COVID–The Conversation Between Us, About Us.** Tailored media messages and community tools to address information needs about the new vaccines (https://www.greaterthancovid.org/theconversation/)
- **Health Promotion Practice.** *People and Places* video series (http://healthpromoti onpracticenotes.com/people-and-places/)
- **Health Promotion Practice** podcast series. Authors discussing the robust intersection of their work, lives, identities, and backgrounds (https://anchor.fm/health-promotion-practice)
- **New Mexico Public Health Association.** Promoting public health practice, policies, and systems that support health equity in New Mexico; provides a structured policy advocacy internship for students in public health and related fields (http://www.nmpha.org/)
- **Prevention Institute.** Provides resources and tools around a variety of focus areas in health equity work (https://preventioninstitute.org/)
- **Public Health Communications Collaborative.** A growing collection of resources to support effective health communication resources on a variety of topics (https://publichealthcollaborative.org/)
- **Public Health Law Center.** Health through the power of law and policy; provides tools and resources for everyday practitioners around key focus areas to improve population health and health equity in our communities (https://www.public healthlawcenter.org/)
- **Society for Public Health Education** (SOPHE). Provides the resources and tools for advocating for public health at all levels; yearly hosts an advocacy summit

where public health, advocacy professionals, and students gather to engage in effective advocacy for a common agenda (https://www.sophe.org/advocacy/)

• **Think Cultural Health.** Provides free, continuing education e-learning programs designed to help you provide CLAS (https://thinkculturalhealth.hhs.gov/educat ion). Depending on your interests and career goals, you can choose from trainings tailored for public health and healthcare professionals working in diverse settings. You'll also earn a certificate of completion or continuing education credit for some credentials!

QUIZ QUESTIONS

1. Which of the following is not considered a social determinant of health?
   a. Housing
   b. Transportation
   c. Education
   d. Diabetes

2. Which of the following best reflects a brief definition of health equity?
   a. Everyone has a fair and just opportunity to be as healthy as possible.
   b. Everyone has equal access to healthcare.
   c. Everyone has the same opportunity to be healthy.
   d. Everyone has the same resources.

3. The effects of incarceration on people, families, and communities include
   a. Trauma
   b. Negative health consequences
   c. Voter disenfranchisement
   d. All of the above

4. The primary purpose of the Voting Rights Act of 1965 was to
   a. prohibit racial discrimination in voting.
   b. ensure women have the right to vote.
   c. help people who have been incarcerated get their voting rights back.
   d. make it easy to vote by mail.

5. The "capacity for health professionals to recognize and respond to health and illness as the downstream effects of broad social, political, and economic structures" is a common definition of
   a. cultural competence
   b. structural competence
   c. cultural humility
   d. none of the above

6. All of these are proven strategies to increase voter participation except
   a. allow online voter registration
   b. prohibiting early voting

    c. "no excuse" absentee voting

    d. automatic voter registration

7. Adverse childhood experiences are associated with which of the following in adulthood?

    a. better educational outcomes

    b. negative health outcomes

    c. higher income levels

    d. increased access to healthcare

8. As a health education specialist developing an educational campaign to promote the human papilloma virus vaccine in adolescents, which of these competencies best describe your *first* step in the communication process?

    a. tailor message(s) for the audience(s)

    b. employ media literacy skills (e.g., identifying credible sources and balancing multiple viewpoints)

    c. identify the assets, needs, and characteristics of the audience(s) that affect communication and message design (e.g., literacy levels, language, culture, and cognitive and perceptual abilities)

    d. select communication channels and current and emerging technologies that are most appropriate for the audience(s) and message(s)

9. Which of the following would be most likely to increase fruit and vegetable consumption at the population level?

    a. providing individual counseling and education to support healthy eating

    b. providing brochures on good nutrition in patient waiting room areas

    c. providing cash vouchers for fresh fruits and vegetables in local grocery stores

    d. providing mandatory work site classes to encourage healthy eating .

10. Which of the following are *all* considered structural barriers to health equity?

    a. poverty, racism, gender discrimination

    b. racism, cancer, climate change

    c. mass incarceration, community violence, diabetes

    d. low educational attainment, addiction, ableism

ANSWER KEY

1. **D.** Diabetes
2. **A.** Everyone has a fair and just opportunity to be as healthy as possible
3. **D.** All of the above
4. **A.** Prohibit racial discrimination in voting
5. **B.** Structural competence
6. **B.** Prohibiting early voting
7. **B.** Negative health outcomes
8. **C.** Identify the assets, needs, and characteristics of the audience(s) that affect communication and message design (e.g., literacy levels, language, culture, and cognitive and perceptual abilities)
9. **C.** Providing cash vouchers for fresh fruits and vegetables in local grocery stores
10. **A.** Poverty, racism, gender discrimination

8.5 DR. ALISTER MARTIN AND VOTE-ER

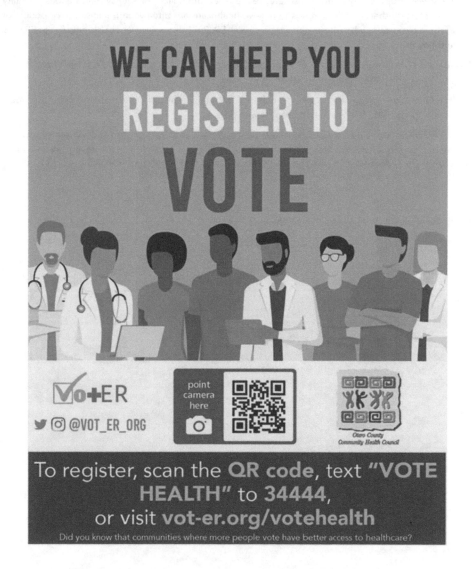

Sample visual of the types of materials VoteER developed for a community organization.
Source: Dr. Holly Mata, Otero County Community Health Council President.

"Dr. Alister Martin is a practicing emergency medicine physician at Massachusetts General Hospital. Like so many nurses, social workers, medical students, and doctors across America, he goes to work every day knowing he'll meet people he can't help through medical care alone. There aren't prescriptions or procedures to fix homelessness, hunger, illiteracy, joblessness, or violence—the larger forces responsible for many people's poor health and reliance on emergency rooms and community health centers. Dr. Martin founded Vot-ER because he believes there's one simple but powerful step we can take immediately: help patients vote. Healthcare providers have a special opportunity to make a difference. Patients who utilize emergency rooms and community health centers as their primary settings to receive healthcare are often young, uninsured, or people of color: the same groups who vote in low numbers" (Vot-ER, 2021, https://vot-er.org/aboutus/). Vot-ER uses these three strategies:

Site-Based Voter Registration: Vot-ER provides posters, discharge paperwork, and patient handouts to hospitals that link patients to a voter registration portal.

Digital Outreach: Vot-ER leverages hospitals and community health centers as trusted messengers about voting via SMS, telehealth, and hospital web pages.

Healthy Democracy Kit: Healthcare providers wear a "Ready to Vote?" lanyard and a voter registration badge backer with a QR code and SMS short code that they can use to help patients register to vote or request an absentee ballot.

8.6 PUBLIC HEALTH STUDENTS IMPROVE LOCAL ALCOHOL POLICY

Evelyn Garcia Thomas and Daniela Marquez

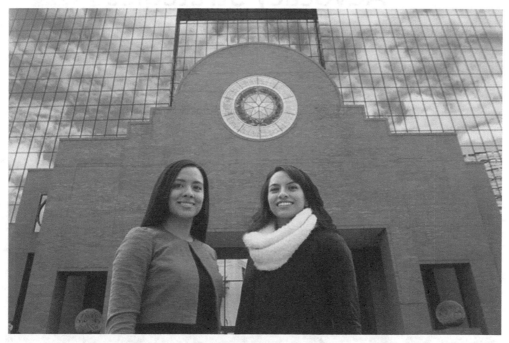

UTEP public health graduate, Evelyn Garcia, left, and Daniela Marquez, right, conducted a survey to assess the support for alcohol restrictions at the El Paso County Sportspark.
Photo by Laura Trejo/UTEP Communications.

As Masters of Public Health (MPH) students at the University of Texas at El Paso (UTEP), Evelyn Garcia Thomas and Daniela Marquez were part of a community coalition advocating for limiting alcohol sales at a county sports park that catered primarily to youth leagues and activities. Their efforts assessing support for and communicating with stakeholders and policymakers resulted in El Paso County commissioners banning alcohol sales at the sports park (UTEP, 2018). What helped this advocacy effort succeed?

- The community group had an established "champion," an elected official who supported their efforts.

- They surveyed a wide range of people who used the sports park, and the results showed strong support for limiting alcohol sales.

- Advocates shared clear and compelling data about the problem, provided a policy solution to address the problem, and documented strong community support for the policy.

- Advocates shared a variety of reasons why the policy would benefit the sports park, including increased safety, reduced spending on security, and increased business revenue from youth sports leagues who prioritized alcohol-free venues.

Advocacy Strategies

ALEXIS BLAVOS AND HOLLY T. MOSES

Do what you can, where you are, with what you have.

—THEODORE ROOSEVELT, autobiography (1913)

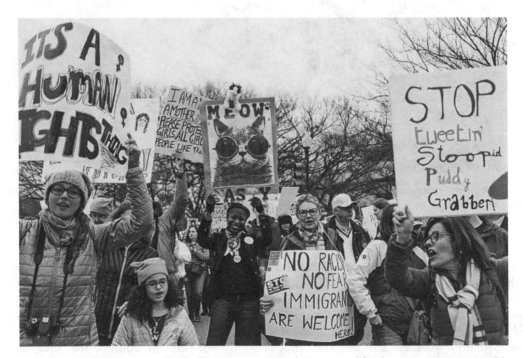

FIGURE 9.1 The Women's March. The Women's March was a worldwide protest on January 21, 2017, to advocate legislation and policies regarding human rights and other issues, including women's rights, immigration reform, healthcare reform, reproductive rights, the natural environment, LGBTQ rights, racial equality, freedom of religion, and workers' rights.
Source: Carol M. Highsmith.

Alexis Blavos and Holly T. Moses, *Advocacy Strategies*. In: *Be the Change*. Edited by Keely S. Rees, Jody Early, and Cicily Hampton, Oxford University Press. © Oxford University Press 2023. DOI: 10.1093/oso/9780197570890.003.0009

Objectives

1. Differentiate between advocacy at the individual, organizational, and community levels.
2. List strategies associated with individual advocacy.
3. Explain the importance of researching organization rules and restrictions prior to engaging in advocacy.
4. Provide examples of community advocacy across multiple government levels.
5. Distinguish between "federal," "state," and "local" governmental levels in the United States.
6. Describe how to find information about congressional and regulatory representatives, voting records, and legislative items.
7. Describe common advocacy tools.
8. List key information to prepare for a meeting with decision makers.

INTRODUCTION

As you have now learned, advocacy can be at the individual, organizational, and community levels (local, state, federal). You are likely wondering exactly HOW to advocate. What can you do as a layperson, and what can you do when you are representing your organization? This chapter focuses on strategies and examples for all of these levels. There are step-by-step examples for finding your legislators and legislation at all levels and how to prepare for these meetings. Common advocacy tools are also discussed.

ADVOCACY AT THE INDIVIDUAL LEVEL

Advocacy can occur at different levels and with different objectives and end goals. Often, advocacy begins at the individual level. This could include self-advocacy, such as standing up for one's self to defend personal rights, views, or interests. **Individual advocacy** could also involve acting on behalf of an individual, or a group of people, to propel their goals and interests. This can include a parent who advocates on behalf of their child. Essentially, individual advocacy involves advocacy efforts as a private citizen. These efforts include voting, signing petitions, attending local government meetings, and testifying at government hearings. Individual advocacy efforts can also include meeting face to face with legislators or communicating with legislators by emails, phone calls, texts, social media outlets, and snail mail.

When local groups and organizations plan a day to meet with legislators (usually referred to as legislative, advocacy, or hill day) to advocate for their organization and mission statement, individuals can support the advocacy efforts of the group by attending the meetings. Many health education and public health students and practitioners attend the Society for Public Health Education (SOPHE) Advocacy Summit, held annually each October in Washington, D.C. The summit engages public health advocates to share advocacy training, materials, and resources (Society for Public Health Education, 2021). This opportunity is appropriate for participants new to advocacy, as well as those who are advocacy veterans. The summit provides a comprehensive opportunity for attendees to also prepare for individual advocacy efforts.

When engaging in individual advocacy, it is important that individuals prepare a statement or disclaimer to ensure that their advocacy efforts are associated with personal views and beliefs. The individual must be certain to explain that their advocacy efforts are separate from their employer and the work that they engage in as a professional. As stated in Chapter 2, unless prohibited by their employer, individuals as constituents may legally participate in lobbying activities of their own volition when using their own resources. It will be important for individuals to review employer policies concerning advocacy and lobbying.

ADVOCACY AT THE ORGANIZATIONAL LEVEL

Advocacy can also occur at the organizational level. At the **organizational advocacy** level, employees are required to engage in advocacy on behalf of the organization that employs them. In this situation, it is critically important for the employee to carefully research organization rules and restrictions prior to engaging in advocacy. It is also important for employees to gather information about government, private, and nonprofit laws and sources of funding for the organization or their position in particular. Depending on the type of organization that they work for, there could be restrictions that limit how information is exchanged with legislators. In some instances, employees will only be permitted to share information with legislators to educate them about the organization's mission and purpose. The employees may be prohibited from requesting change or action ("the ask") from the legislators.

Whatever organization restrictions exist, all employees should prepare a professional folder when meeting with legislators. The folder should be professionally prepared and include the logo of the organization. Information to be shared with the legislators should be prepared as informative and attractive fact sheets. The fact sheets will include content, but it is best to also include graphs/charts, infographics, and pictures to display key information such as shown in Figure 9.1. The folder should always include the names and contact information for employees if the legislator has questions.

ADVOCACY AT THE COMMUNITY LEVEL

Advocacy also occurs at the community level. **Community advocacy** is an important level of advocacy. According to Loue (2006): "Community health advocacy entails advocacy by a community around issues related to health, however, that community is defined or formed" (p. 458). In many instances, the community level is where advocacy originates. Residents with shared values, beliefs, and needs come together for a common purpose. An example could include residents of a community advocating for the addition of speed bumps to slow traffic in the neighborhood. An additional example includes a community of people who advocate for research funding targeting treatments or a cure for a specific disease for which they or a loved one have received a diagnosis.

Community advocacy efforts can be implemented at any of the governmental levels—local, state, or national. The level of government that the advocacy efforts are implemented in is often determined by several factors, including the scope of the issue, the short-term and/or long-term nature of the issue, and the availability of resources (Loue, 2006). There are some situations that require an advocacy issue or effort to move through multiple levels. For example, consider the exorbitant costs associated with medication used to control diabetes. A parent may advocate for their child at an individual level by working to convince pharmaceutical companies to provide these medications at a reasonable price. The parent can also advocate at the community level by rallying support from other parents and community members impacted by the high cost of diabetes medication. As a group, the community members can move through local, state, and national levels of government to seek legislative support to intervene with the pharmaceutical companies and reduce the cost of these required medications.

Several approaches to community advocacy are available to assist community members. Grassroots approaches to advocacy are based on the identification of needs and goals by community members themselves (Loue, 2006). Grassroots efforts usually originate with a group of people in the community who feel passionate about creating a change of some kind. Think of this as the process of collective reflection and action by a group of individuals with the same goal. One of the best strategies to use in grassroots organizing is the development of a coalition with the goal of that particular advocacy effort (Community Tool Box, n.d.). Coalitions can be a very powerful tool for community advocacy efforts. Consider the Washington State Coalition Against Domestic Violence (WSCADV). Operating as a nonprofit 501(c)(3) network, WSCADV was founded by survivors of domestic abuse and their allies and has a clear mission to end domestic violence through advocacy and action for social change. More than 30 years after its establishment, this coalition is considered the primary group working to end domestic violence in Washington State.

Ideally, advocates would develop a coalition with existing partnerships and connections already established within the community and around the advocacy issue being addressed. This should assist with ensuring diversity within the coalition, including influential members of the community, policymakers, and other stakeholders (Community Tool Box, n.d.). More information about grassroots and coalition building is provided in Chapter 10.

Town halls are another approach commonly used in community advocacy. Town halls are public meetings that coalition members can host within their community to share updates on their work/efforts and also to hear from other community members. For the advocates, town halls provide the opportunity to share information about the issue they are advocating for within the community and to gain greater support from members of the community. For participants, attending a town hall is a great way to learn about community priorities and even raise issues that are of importance to them.

The format of a town hall varies and is determined by the person or group hosting the event. Typically, the town hall begins with a short presentation about the advocacy issue and includes updates about the status of the group's advocacy efforts. After the presentation, members of the community engage in dialogue with the advocacy group and also have the opportunity to ask questions. Community advocates can also host town hall meetings with candidates for office as a means for the community to ask questions and engage with the candidates on their particular issue.

After a community group has progressed in their advocacy efforts, it is important to incorporate media advocacy to further push their agenda. Media advocacy is the use of any form of media (television, radio, newspapers, magazines, written materials) to help promote an advocacy group's mission and goals (Community Tool Box, n.d.). Advocating through various forms of media can get a policy message sent across a wide audience in a short amount of time. More information about media advocacy is provided in Chapter 12.

When engaged in community advocacy, it is imperative that strategies are employed to organize the efforts of the community members. One method used to improve the success of community advocacy is community organizing, the process of bringing people together who share a common concern and that want to actively have a say in the decisions that affect their lives. Chapter 11 provides more information about community organizing and introduces five core frameworks to help improve the success of community advocacy efforts.

Helping to Craft Legislation Through Advocacy

In Chapter 7 you learned about how the legislature works and how bills are created and enacted. But what is the role of the health education specialist in crafting and supporting adoption of legislation in Congress? The health education specialists, through their expertise and advocating with members of Congress are able to support legislation in various ways at different levels. These levels include the federal, state, and local levels.

FINDING YOUR CONGRESSIONAL OR REGULATORY REPRESENTATIVES, VOTING RECORDS, AND LEGISLATIVE ITEMS

The first step at the federal level of advocacy for legislation begins by identifying important members of the current Congress. These members might include your house representative and senator, relevant committee chairs, congressional leaders such as the minority or majority whip, those who have signed on as a sponsor or cosponsor for specific legislation, or those who have supported efforts similar to yours in the past. How do you locate this information?

By going to the U.S. Congressional website (https://www.congress.gov/) you not only can locate these important legislators, but also can review their voting history and look up current and past legislative items relevant to your work (Library of Congress, n.d.-b).

Finding your congressional representatives. On the main website for the U.S. Congress (https://www.congress.gov/) you will see an area where you can "contact your member" (Library of Congress, n.d.-b). In this section, you will enter your zip code and select enter. You will be redirected to a new web link that shows all of your senators and representatives. You can also click on their individual names to be taken to another page that includes their contact information and the current legislation they support. This area also includes information on the legislator's committee assignments (Library of Congress, n.d.-b). For example, when typing in your zip code, you will learn who your senators are. Then, if you click on your senator's name, you will be directed to a page that includes their Washington, D.C., office contact information and their senate website. Finding your legislator is not difficult and will help you directly contact them.

Making an appointment with your congressional representative. Making an appointment itself is fairly easy and can be done online, via email, or by calling their office. For example, all congressional members have a Washington, D.C., office phone number that is listed on their U.S. member information page on the U.S. Congress website (Library of Congress, n.d.-b). If you go to your congressional member's direct website, you will find a link to "contact" their office. On the contact page, you have the ability to directly email their office by providing some basic information: name, address, email, phone number, your message, and the subject area that your advocacy initiative best relates to. When the meeting is scheduled, the congressional aide will ask for some basic information about who will attend the meeting. This information includes the number of people attending the meeting (necessary to book an appropriate meeting location) and their specific names. Most meetings are scheduled for 15 minutes but some can be longer and fewer might be shorter.

Finding current committee assignments, legislation, and voting records. The U.S. congressional website (https://www.congress.gov/) includes a link on the legislator's individual pages that shows their committee assignments (Library of Congress, n.d.-b). On each congressperson's specific congressional page, there is a link leading to information on their committee memberships (Library of Congress, n.d.-a). You may find that they are a member of the Committee on Agriculture, Nutrition, and Forestry; Committee on Armed Services; Committee on Intelligence; the Special Committee on Aging; or any number of other committees. Their committee assignments will provide clues about what is important to them.

On the same congressional website, legislation sponsored by a specific representative or senator is available. For example, Senator Gillibrand has cosponsored S.833 (https://www.congress.gov/bill/117th-congress/senate-bill/833?s=1&r=5) in the 117th Congress (2021–2022), a bill that would allow the secretary of Health and Human Services to negotiate prescription drug prices for Part D of Medicare (Library of Congress, n.d.-c). This information suggests that this senator is generally supportive of prescription drug reform.

All congressional members' voting records are public. They can be found on the Congressional Record (https://www.govinfo.gov/app/collection/CREC) website, the official source for recorded floor votes, with voting records located for the years 1994 to the present (U.S. Government Publishing Office, n.d.). How a congressional legislator votes can give insight into how you should craft your message to garner their support. For example, if one votes in support of funding for opioid prevention, but not for full funding for the Centers for Disease Control and Prevention, that suggests that the legislator is in favor of funding specific targeted pieces of legislation. This means when you go to see them, you need to ask for very specific things and not to broadly fund public health.

Finding the correct regulatory representative. This area is a bit trickier than finding a congressional representative; this is because there is no database where names are listed. The advocate has to know who is in charge of implementing a specific policy or law. Then the advocate would go to a search engine and type in a query to find the correct contact information. For example, if the advocacy area of interest was police misconduct and people of color, you could query "US police misconduct" and find out that the U.S. Department of Justice (2020) (https://www.justice.gov/crt/addressing-police-miscond uct-laws-enforced-department-justice) is responsible for implementing these policies and regulations. On the U.S. Department of Justice web page addressing police miscon- duct there is information for who is currently responsible for these laws. That person is currently Kristen Clarke, assistant attorney general (U.S. Department of Justice, 2020), and her contact information is on this same website.

Finding your state representative. Similar to searching for contact information for federal legislators, you can find your own state legislators online easily. There is one big difference: There is no nationwide website to use. Each state has its own website; there- fore, there is no one specific way to find a state representative for all states. In general, start searching by going to your own state legislature website; this can be found easily by typing your "state legislature" into any search engine. For example, by typing "NY legis- lature" into a search browser, the first item from the query is "New York State Assembly" (2021) (https://nyassembly.gov/).

Once you have located the website for a specific state legislature, closely examine the home page. For example, using the query, "Guam legislature," Guam's government website (https://guamlegislature.com/index/) is offered as a search response option (Guam Legislature, 2021a). Searching the home page will offer specific tabs that lead to information, such as the number of seats in the state senate. There is a link to select legislators (https://guamlegislature.com/index/senators/) where we learn that the Hon. Therese M. Terlaje is the speaker of the Senate (Gaum Legislature, 2021b). She serves on the committee on Health, Land, Justice, and Culture. Her contact information is visible and includes a phone number and an email address. Use the state legislature website (https://www.congress.gov/state-legislature-websites) to find your own state legislatures.

Finding your local representatives. Local representatives typically sit on a city council. The impact of advocacy can be high at this level with much quicker impact, so it is important not to overlook this level. Because each community is different, each web- site is different. However, by using search terms such as "NAME OF TOWN/CITY council OR legislature," several search response options will likely be available.

Once locating the website for a specific local council, such as the City of Cortland, New York, Legislature (https://www.cortland-co.org/286/Legislature), look for names of all the representatives, any contact information available, and when they meet (Cortland County, New York, n.d.). Some websites will also include agendas and meeting minutes. By examining the meeting minutes, advocates can learn about each legislator and what kind of efforts they tend to support. The website for the City of North Ridgeville, OH, City Council (https://www.nridgeville.org/Council.aspx) looks a bit different from the website for Cortland, New York. This website includes boards and commissions (City of North Ridgeville, 2021). This could be helpful in locating who would be the best person to contact when looking for support for a specific advocacy initiative.

ADVOCACY AND HEALTH POLICY

Health policy focuses on policy that impacts the health of the public (Wilensky & Teitelbaum, 2020). As discussed in previous chapters, policies include, but are certainly not limited to, healthcare financing, delivery, and access and public health efforts. Advocacy can play a crucial role in the development of health policy through advocate participation in influencing or drafting legislation. Chapter 14 includes a detailed explanation of policy analysis and their uses. The current chapter focuses on researching and drafting a policy analysis. Typically, a **policy analysis** includes a problem statement, background, landscape, options for the legislator to pick from, recommendations, and references (Wilensky & Teitelbaum, 2020).

Problem statement. This is one concise sentence that focuses on the direction of the analysis. For example, "What action should President Biden take to decrease vaccine hesitancy for COVID-19 among underserved populations?"

Background. While there is no defined word limit, it is best to keep work as brief as possible to increase the likelihood of it being read in its entirety. It is best to provide "need to know information" and omit "nice to know" information. For example, need to know information in the scenario for vaccine hesitancy should include data on the disproportionate impact of COVID-19 on underserved populations, the number of vaccine-hesitant individuals in underserved populations, the percentage of people in underserved populations who have already been vaccinated, and data related to why there is hesitancy.

Landscape. The landscape focuses on the current trends in support among key stakeholders. For the example used in this section, these include the president and the president's agencies, the general public, healthcare or other organizations, and Congress. Much of this information may come from popular news sources but should be inclusive of the majority opinion. Using the same vaccine hesitancy example, it is reasonable to state that the president and the president's agencies (Centers for Disease Control and Prevention and the National Institute for Allergy and Infectious Diseases) are supportive of improving vaccine adherence among underserved populations given the almost daily briefings on COVID-19 and vaccination efforts to the nation. It is also reasonable to state that healthcare organizations and Congress are generally supportive of decreasing vaccine hesitancy given their efforts to increase access among all populations. Where this landscape example could get tricky is the general public. The Kaiser Family Foundation reported in December 2020 that while 71% of people in general reported they would get the vaccine, 35% of Black adults said they would not get the vaccine (Kaiser Family Foundation, 2021). If one level of the landscape is adamantly against the policy idea, it can be more challenging to sell a policy idea to the others.

Options. There should be at least two options so the decision maker can consider more than one, which might increase the likelihood that they select at least one. Options should be inclusive of all advantages, disadvantages, the political feasibility, efficiency, timeliness, and financial cost. This is typically able to be accomplished in one long paragraph but might take more room in an analysis if it is a particularly complex issue. Examples of potential options for the president regarding the vaccine hesitancy scenario include directing the Centers for Medicare and Medicaid Services (CMS) to increase educational efforts for those registered with Medicare or Medicaid by mailing information about the vaccine to their homes or signing an executive order that directs all mobile health units (e.g., mammogram vans) to also become mobile vaccine sites in underserved community neighborhoods.

Recommendations. This is where the individual/group writing the policy analysis selects one of the options to recommend to the decision maker. There needs to be a clear explanation why this option is superior to the other(s). This explanation should include a brief description that reiterates advantages and disadvantages, political climes, efficiency, financial burden, and timeliness. For example, it is recommended that President Biden choose Option 2, sign an executive order that directs all mobile health units (e.g., mammogram vans) to also become mobile vaccine sites in underserved community neighborhoods. Due to varied health literacy levels, making vaccines more available in communities through the use of mobile healthcare delivery can increase vaccine visibility, desirability, trust, and, therefore, adherence. While there will be a financial cost associated, by using existing mobile health units, some of this burden can be mitigated.

References. Any facts or information you have gathered from other sources should be properly credited in the reference section and via in-text citations. All sources should be credible, such as the peer-reviewed literature or credible websites. To assess the credibility of a website, use a tool such as the CRAAP test (https://library.csuchico.edu/sites/default/files/craap-test.pdf) developed by Meriam Library at California State University at Chico (2010), which focuses on source currency, relevance, authority, accuracy, and purpose.

ADVOCACY TOOLS

There are a variety of **advocacy tools** that can be used. Each advocate will have a different level of comfort for different types of advocacy. While it is important to push yourself to advocate outside your comfort zone, one should be aware of their capabilities with different tools. Such tools include, but are certainly not limited to, email templates, fact sheets, information folders, phone calls, relevant stories, social media posts, talking points, and voting (Table 9.1).

Email templates. Many organizations/groups create email templates that advocates can use to quickly reach their legislator. The template will have specific information about the current (using the bill number) or potential legislative item. This should also include a specific ask of the legislator. Many organizations use web-based software that allows an advocate to simply enter their personal contact information and then the email will be sent to the advocate's legislators based on the contact information entered. Due to the ability to quickly and consistently advocate for a specific legislative item, these are very effective tools.

Fact sheets. Fact sheets are frequently given to the legislator's office during a personal meeting. More meetings happen via video meeting software; therefore, these fact sheets may be shared electronically or in person at the end of the meeting. Fact sheets include relevant accurate data about specific legislation and how it could/would impact the citizens of a community.

Information folders. Information folders are often part of advocacy days at the federal and state levels. They typically include fact sheets, white papers, resolutions from

TABLE 9.1 Advocacy Tool Usage at the Legislative and Regulatory Branches

Advocacy Tool	Legislative Efforts	Regulatory Efforts
Fact sheets	Used often. Focused on a specific "ask," with factual data supporting the positive impact of the "ask."	Not used as often. But can be useful in advocating for a piece of legislation to be implemented or managed in a specific way. Should be focused on a specific "ask" with data supporting why this is the best way to implement the legislation.
Information folders	These are used often in conjunction with specific advocacy days at the federal or state level. They are useful and typically include a variety of fact sheets, contact information, and other relevant helpful information to craft legislation in the way one is advocating. May include possible policy language.	Not typically used at the regulatory level.
Phone calls	Used frequently and are very easy. Be sure to include your name, if you are a voting constituent, and the specific bill number (if there is one) or the specific topic you are calling to ask the legislator to support.	Used a little less frequently but still effective. Be sure to include your name, the specific policy that is being implemented that you are calling about, and your specific ask.
Email templates	Used frequently. Groups or individuals may make/use email templates that include all relevant information and a specific ask about a specific piece of legislation.	Used frequently. Groups or individuals may make/use email templates that include all relevant information and a specific ask about a specific policy that is being implemented.
Talking points	Necessary and always used during any communication with legislators about potential policy.	Necessary and always used during any communication with those implementing policy.
Social media posts	Used frequently and are visible by others, so they tend to be addressed quickly. Send social media messages by posting on specific legislator's sites, tagging them, or using some other public means to advocate.	Used frequently and visible by others, so they tend to be addressed quickly. Send social media messages by posting to specific regulator branches, tagging them, or using some other public means to advocate.
Relevant stories	Used frequently. Relevant personal stories, especially from someone in the legislator's congressional district, are very effective.	Not often used at the regulatory level.
Voting	Voting directly impacts who represents you and your districts. Vote during every election at all levels.	Voting indirectly impacts who is selected to implement policies as thcse we vote for will appoint, nominate, and hire these public servants.

organizations, and contact information. But they could also include policy analysis or potential policy language. These are often left with the legislator's aide at the end of a meeting; however, if a meeting was not secured, the folder could be dropped off at the legislator's office instead of a meeting.

Phone calls. Phone calls are easy and take only a minute or two. When making an advocacy call, be sure to include the specific bill number or policy, your name, where you live, and if you are a voting constituent. Here is an example:

- Legislative Aide: Hello, this is Senator Gillibrand's office. How can I help you?
- Advocate: Hello, my name is ____ and I am a voting constituent residing at _____. I am calling to ask the senator to support Senate bill _____.

Relevant stories. Relevant stories are essential for any meeting with a legislator. These stories should be true and not made up for effect. The goal is to share with the decision maker how one area of policy has positively or negatively impacted one person or group of people. They are particularly good for legislative meetings because they elicit emotion from the legislator and are often shared in committee while crafting legislation.

Social media posts. Social media posts are very visible; therefore, when communicating accurate information, they typically earn a faster response. The visibility of such posts only works if the poster is able to link their post to the correct decision maker. Posts should be brief, include a specific ask, and offer key relevant accurate data.

Talking points. For any type of advocacy, talking points are essential. Talking points help the advocate stay on task and focus their time. The talking points should be specific and should include a specific ask. All talking points should be grounded in accurate data that are supported by credible resources.

Vote. Voting behavior is directly linked to those who earn seats in government. By electing officials whose values match your own, you increase the likelihood of their supporting your advocacy initiatives. In addition, elected officials, such as the president, nominate and/or appoint individuals whose job it will be to implement approved policy.

MEETING WITH DECISION MAKERS

Before requesting a meeting. Before requesting a meeting, ensure that the person you want to meet with is either your representative or the chair of the relevant committee that crafts policy in the specific advocacy area. Then conduct research to identify if there are specific current, or past, bills that are a natural fit for the area you are advocating. This information is important to give when scheduling the meeting.

Requesting a meeting. When requesting a meeting, share your name and contact information, why you are reaching out to the specific decision maker (are they your representative, the chair of a committee, or the regulatory branch that implements policy/law?), and specifically what you want to discuss (a bill number, the implementation of a new or existing law/policy). It is helpful to have a calendar in front of you to speedily schedule the meeting. If others will be attending the meeting, be sure to share how many will attend and their names.

Before the meeting. Before the meeting takes place, the advocate should conduct research on the decision maker. This research should focus on voting records, how they have implemented similar policy in the past, their political or personal views, or other relevant information that might help inform potential questions they might ask. Being able to prepare for potentially difficult questions can greatly increase confidence and reduce anxiety. All information you may want to leave with the decision maker should also be prepared neatly in a folder. Finally, practice your meeting with those who might go with you or with someone else who can help by asking hard questions. Also, ensure you know exactly where your meeting location is and how to get there; allow extra time for a buffer.

During the meeting. Arrive early or on time for the meeting. Remain professional in the hall and lobby and while engaging with office staff. Once you are in the meeting, begin by thanking the decision maker for taking time to meet with your group and mention the topic of the meeting. Let everyone in attendance introduce themselves and be sure to thank the decision maker for previous votes or policy that are related to your meeting. Begin first by discussing the broader impact of the advocacy area and share relevant data. Next, share specific information about your community and how the legislation has or could impact your life. Then, share a relevant personal story highlighting how specific people or communities are directly impacted by the topic. Finally, summarize the main points, make the ask, and allow for questions. Once all questions have been answered and the meeting is ending, be sure to thank them again for their time and leave them with the prepared folder with additional information, including your contact information. Before walking out, ensure you have the business card of the person you just met with.

After the meeting. Right after the meeting, jot down any additional notes that you have and debrief with your meeting team. During this debrief, ensure a list is made with any items for follow-up and decide who will send an email on behalf of the group thanking the decision maker for their time and offering to serve as a resource person for them in the advocacy area. Further, if the group said they would follow up with information or other action items, indicate in the email who will be doing this and by when.

ADVOCACY CASE STUDY

In 2017 the Kappa chapter of Eta Sigma Gamma at the State University of New York (SUNY) at Cortland began their first advocacy project to have a crosswalk installed at Tompkins Street and Prospect Street. This crosswalk would benefit students coming to class from their off-campus residences and community members using the YMCA for recreation and childcare. When they began their project, there was no safe crossing in more than a half mile of this busy stretch of a state road. The students had no data at the time other than that a current student had been struck and badly injured by a car while attempting to cross the street.

This is when their advocacy committee decided to gather data to support their advocacy efforts. They began by completing an environmental scan of the intersection of Tompkins and Prospect. They each took turns tracking the number of people crossing the street during different times of the day over a 4-day period. After concluding this scan, they recorded 176 individuals crossing the street. To increase the likelihood of the city caring about the issue, they attempted to guess who was a student and who was a

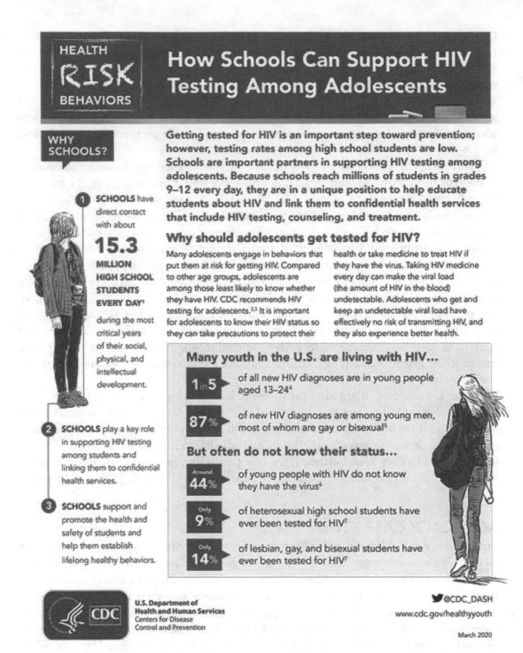

FIGURE 9.2 Fact sheet Example 9.1.

community member. Community member crossings were estimated at 23 with student crossing estimates totaling 153.

Armed with some data, they next sent out a Facebook vote to see if others were potentially interested in this issue. Once they realized this was something that other students, including those in the Student Government Association, were very interested in supporting, they set up an official petition on Change.org (https://www.change.org/).

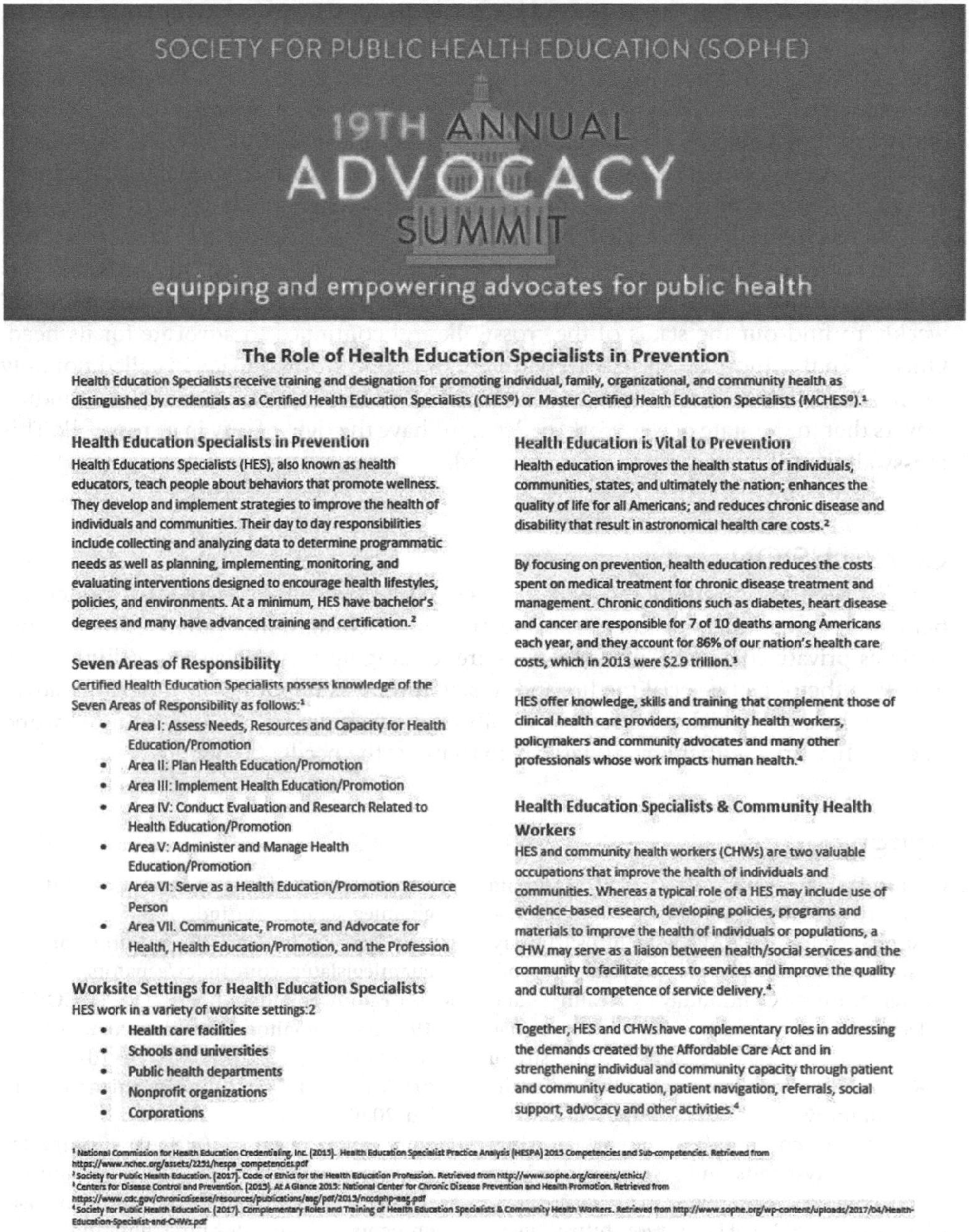
SOCIETY FOR PUBLIC HEALTH EDUCATION (SOPHE)

19TH ANNUAL
ADVOCACY
SUMMIT

equipping and empowering advocates for public health

The Role of Health Education Specialists in Prevention

Health Education Specialists receive training and designation for promoting individual, family, organizational, and community health as distinguished by credentials as a Certified Health Education Specialists (CHES®) or Master Certified Health Education Specialists (MCHES®).[1]

Health Education Specialists in Prevention

Health Educations Specialists (HES), also known as health educators, teach people about behaviors that promote wellness. They develop and implement strategies to improve the health of individuals and communities. Their day to day responsibilities include collecting and analyzing data to determine programmatic needs as well as planning, implementing, monitoring, and evaluating interventions designed to encourage health lifestyles, policies, and environments. At a minimum, HES have bachelor's degrees and many have advanced training and certification.[2]

Seven Areas of Responsibility

Certified Health Education Specialists possess knowledge of the Seven Areas of Responsibility as follows:[1]

- Area I: Assess Needs, Resources and Capacity for Health Education/Promotion
- Area II: Plan Health Education/Promotion
- Area III: Implement Health Education/Promotion
- Area IV: Conduct Evaluation and Research Related to Health Education/Promotion
- Area V: Administer and Manage Health Education/Promotion
- Area VI: Serve as a Health Education/Promotion Resource Person
- Area VII. Communicate, Promote, and Advocate for Health, Health Education/Promotion, and the Profession

Worksite Settings for Health Education Specialists

HES work in a variety of worksite settings:2

- Health care facilities
- Schools and universities
- Public health departments
- Nonprofit organizations
- Corporations

Health Education is Vital to Prevention

Health education improves the health status of individuals, communities, states, and ultimately the nation; enhances the quality of life for all Americans; and reduces chronic disease and disability that result in astronomical health care costs.[2]

By focusing on prevention, health education reduces the costs spent on medical treatment for chronic disease treatment and management. Chronic conditions such as diabetes, heart disease and cancer are responsible for 7 of 10 deaths among Americans each year, and they account for 86% of our nation's health care costs, which in 2013 were $2.9 trillion.[3]

HES offer knowledge, skills and training that complement those of clinical health care providers, community health workers, policymakers and community advocates and many other professionals whose work impacts human health.[4]

Health Education Specialists & Community Health Workers

HES and community health workers (CHWs) are two valuable occupations that improve the health of individuals and communities. Whereas a typical role of a HES may include use of evidence-based research, developing policies, programs and materials to improve the health of individuals or populations, a CHW may serve as a liaison between health/social services and the community to facilitate access to services and improve the quality and cultural competence of service delivery.[4]

Together, HES and CHWs have complementary roles in addressing the demands created by the Affordable Care Act and in strengthening individual and community capacity through patient and community education, patient navigation, referrals, social support, advocacy and other activities.[4]

[1] National Commission for Health Education Credentialing, Inc. (2015). Health Education Specialist Practice Analysis (HESPA) 2015 Competencies and Sub-competencies. Retrieved from https://www.nchec.org/assets/2251/hespa_competencies.pdf
[2] Society for Public Health Education. (2017). Code of Ethics for the Health Education Profession. Retrieved from http://www.sophe.org/careers/ethics/
[3] Centers for Disease Control and Prevention. (2015). At A Glance 2015: National Center for Chronic Disease Prevention and Health Promotion. Retrieved from https://www.cdc.gov/chronicdisease/resources/publications/aag/pdf/2015/nccdphp-aag.pdf
[4] Society for Public Health Education. (2017). Complementary Roles and Training of Health Education Specialists & Community Health Workers. Retrieved from http://www.sophe.org/wp-content/uploads/2017/04/Health-Education-Specialist-and-CHWs.pdf

FIGURE 9.3 Fact sheet Example 9.2.

The petition was quickly signed by 1,500 individuals. This is when the advocacy efforts really began.

Emails and requests for support or meetings were sent to the Student Government Association (supported right away), SUNY Cortland Administration (supported right away), city of Cortland Mayor (supported right away), and the City Department of

Public Works. On discussions with the city Department of Public Works, the students learned that this particular street was officially a state route, which meant that while the city Department of Public Works maintained the street, they did not have authority to make any changes, such as crosswalks. However, they were supportive of the student's efforts, so they helped the group communicate with the New York State Department of Transportation (NYSDOT). In the spring of 2018, the NYSDOT conducted an official survey of the crossing between Tompkins and Prospect Streets and came to the conclusion that a crosswalk was needed.

Advocacy did not stop there. It was not until October 2018 that this crosswalk was officially installed. During those six months in 2018, the group emailed the NYSDOT weekly to find out the status of the crosswalk and continued to advocate for its need. Once given the approval, the city Department of Public Works quickly installed not only the painted crosswalk, but also signs alerting of a new traffic pattern and signs reminding drivers that in the state of New York, pedestrians have the right of way in a crosswalk. This crosswalk is still heavily used and maintained.

CONCLUSION

We all have the opportunity to be advocates. While our employment may hinder our being able to conduct advocacy tasks, we can still be engaged in a variety of ways, especially as private citizens! Daily, advocates are looking up their legislators, calling them, emailing them, using social media, and, yes, voting! It is important to remember advocacy can be small quick tasks such as emails or may require you to do a bit more work, like a policy brief; either way, all tasks help to move the needle on our advocacy goals.

REFERENCES

California State University at Chico, Meriam Library. (2010). Evaluating information—Applying the CRAAP test. https://library.csuchico.edu/sites/default/files/craap-test.pdf

Center for Community Health and Development. (n.d.). *Chapter 3, Section 10: Conducting concerns surveys.* University of Kansas. Retrieved January 2, 2020, from the Community Tool Box: http://ctb.ku.edu/en/table-of-contents/assessment/assessing-community-needs-and-resources/conduct-concerns-surveys/main

Change.org. (2021). Home *page.* https://www.change.org/

City of North Ridgeville, Ohio. (2021). City Council. https://www.nridgeville.org/Council.aspx

Cortland County, New York. (n.d.). Legislature. https://www.cortland-co.org/286/Legislature

Guam Legislature. (2021a). Home *page.* https://guamlegislature.com/index/

Guam Legislature. (2021b). Senators. https://guamlegislature.com/index/senators/

Kaiser Family Foundation. (2021). KFF COVID-19 vaccine monitor: December 2020. https://www.kff.org/coronavirus-covid-19/report/kff-covid-19-vaccine-monitor-december-2020/

Library of Congress. (n.d.-a). Committee assignments of the 117th Congress. https://www.senate.gov/general/committee_assignments/assignments.htm#GillibrandNY

Library of Congress. (n.d.-b). Home *page.* https://www.congress.gov/

Library of Congress. (n.d.-c). S.833—*Empowering Medicare Seniors to Negotiate Drug Prices Act of 2021.* https://www.congress.gov/bill/117th-congress/senate-bill/833?s=1&r=5

Loue, S. (2006). Community health advocacy. *Journal of Epidemiology and Community Health*, *60*(6), 458–463. https://doi.org/10.1136/jech.2004.023044

New York State Assembly. (2021). *About the Congressional Record*. https://www.govinfo.gov/app/collection/CREC

Society for Public Health Education. (2021, March 21). 24th*annual advocacy summit*. https://www.sophe.org/professional-development/conferences_events/advocacy-summit/

U.S. Department of Justice. (2020). Addressing police misconduct laws enforced by the Department of Justice. https://www.justice.gov/crt/addressing-police-misconduct-laws-enforced-department-justice

U.S. Government Publishing Office. (n.d.). Congressional record. https://www.govinfo.gov/app/collection/CREC

Wilensky, S. E., & Teitelbaum, J. B. (2020). *Essentials of health policy and law* (4th ed.). Jones and Bartlett Learning.

CHAPTER 9: END-OF-CHAPTER ACTIVITIES

DISCUSSION QUESTIONS

1. You have been asked to advocate for public health funding as a private citizen. Describe three activities you could participate in at the individual level.

2. Explain why it is important to research organization rules and restrictions prior to engaging in advocacy.

3. Describe how you would prepare for a meeting with decision makers.

APPLICATION ACTIVITIES

1. Prepare a short, 10-minute presentation for a town hall meeting about a particular health or social issue that sparks dialogue for community members and stakeholders representing multiple perspectives. When preparing the presentation, ask yourself: What are multiple perspectives or arguments on the issue that one should consider when preparing for this town hall?; How might the facilitator of this town hall manage the conversation so that all sides felt heard?

2. Conduct research to prepare for a meeting with a representative. For this activity, research the selected congressional representative and identify their current committee assignments. Are they on any committees that might indicate that they might be generally supportive of legislation related to health or social justice?

3. Phone calls are quick and easy ways to advocate. Create your own phone script for a specific legislative bill using the example on page 166 as a guide.

4. Using the CRAAP test discussed in this chapter, do a web search about the public health impact of climate change. Pick the top three websites (not ads) that are presented by the search engine. Open each website and evaluate it for currency, relevance, authority, accuracy, and purpose. Once you have evaluated them, explain why you would or would not trust the sources.

ADDITIONAL RESOURCES

Congressional Management Foundation (CMF). (n.d.). *Home page*. https://www.congressfoundation.org/

Washington State Coalition Against Domestic Violence (WSCADV). (n.d.). *Home page*. https://wscadv.org/

Stanford Social Innovation Review. (n.d.). *Advocacy activities that 501(c)(3) organizations can engage in*. https://ssir.org/images/articles/when_philanthropy_meets_advocacy_updated.jpg

TEMPLATE ON POLICY ANALYSIS:

TO:

FROM:

RE:

Date:

PROBLEM STATEMENT

This is one concise sentence that focuses on the direction of the analysis, for example: "What action should President Biden take to decrease vaccine hesitancy for COVID-19 among underserved populations?"

BACKGROUND

While there is no defined word limit, it is best to keep work as brief as possible to increase the likelihood of it being read in its entirety. It is best to provide "need to know information" and omit "nice to know" information. For example, need to know information in the scenario for vaccine hesitancy should include data on the disproportionate impact of COVID-19 on underserved populations, the number of vaccine-hesitant individuals in underserved populations, the percentage of people in underserved populations who have already been vaccinated, and data related to why there is hesitancy.

LANDSCAPE

The landscape focuses on the current trends in support among key stakeholders. For the example used in this section, these include the president and the president's agencies, the general public, healthcare or other organizations, and Congress. Much of this information may come from popular news sources but should be inclusive of the majority opinion. Using the same vaccine hesitancy example, it is reasonable to state that the president and his agencies (Centers for Disease Control and Prevention and the National Institute for Allergy and Infectious Diseases) are supportive of improving vaccine adherence among underserved populations given the almost daily briefings on COVID-19 and vaccination efforts to the nation. It is also reasonable to state that healthcare organizations and Congress are generally supportive of decreasing vaccine hesitancy given their efforts to increase access among all populations. Where this landscape example could get tricky is the general public. The Kaiser Family Foundation reported in December 2020 that while 71% of people in general reported they would get the vaccine, 35% of Black adults said they would not get the vaccine (Kaiser Family Foundation, 2021). If one level of the landscape is adamantly against the policy idea, it can be more challenging to sell a policy idea to the others.

OPTIONS

There should be at least two options so the decision maker can consider more than one, which might increase the likelihood that they select at least one. Options should be inclusive of all advantages, disadvantages, the political feasibility, efficiency, timeliness, and financial cost. This is typically able to be accomplished in one long paragraph but might take more room in an analysis if it is a particularly complex issue. Examples of potential options for the vaccine hesitancy scenario include directing the Centers for Medicare and Medicaid Services (CMS) to increase educational efforts for those registered with Medicare or Medicaid by mailing information about the vaccine to their homes or sign an executive order that directs all mobile health units (e.g., mammogram vans) to also become mobile vaccine sites in underserved community neighborhoods.

RECOMMENDATION

This is where the individual/group writing the policy analysis selects one of the options to recommend to the decision maker. There needs to be a clear explanation explanation why this option is superior to the other(s). This explanation should include a brief description that reiterates advantages and disadvantages, political climes, efficiency, financial burden, and timeliness. For example, it is recommended that President Biden choose Option 2, sign an executive order that directs all mobile health units (e.g., mammogram vans) to also become mobile vaccine sites in underserved community neighborhoods. Due to varied health literacy levels, making vaccines more available in communities through the use of mobile health care delivery can increase vaccine visibility, desirability, trust, and, therefore, adherence. While there will be a financial cost associated, by using existing mobile health units, some of this burden can be mitigated.

ADDITIONAL INFORMATION

Any facts or information you have gathered from other sources should be properly credited in the reference section and via in-text citations. All sources should be credible, such as peer-reviewed literature or credible websites. To assess the credibility of a website, use a tool such as the CRAAP test (https://library.csuchico.edu/sites/default/files/craap-test.pdf) developed by Meriam Library at California State University at Chico (2010), which focuses on source currency, relevance, authority, accuracy, and purpose.

QUIZ QUESTIONS

1. One of the first steps in federal-level advocacy is knowing important members of the current Congress. Which of the following would be considered important members of the current Congress? (Mark all that apply.)
   a. committee chairs
   b. minority whips
   c. your representative or senator
   d. president of the Senate

2. Congressional member voting records are public. Why is it important to know how your legislator votes before you craft a message and meet with them?
   a. Voting records indicate which type of legislation they are more likely to support.
   b. Voting records indicate who they receive funding from.
   c. Voting records are just public role calls and do not serve much other purpose.
   d. Voting records signify what their constituents want.

3. Policy analysis includes several areas. One such area is the landscape. What is the purpose of the landscape in a policy analysis?
   a. provides current trends among key stakeholders
   b. suggests the likelihood a legislator is going to vote a certain way
   c. includes the most important need to know information
   d. provides the direction for the analysis

4. Recently, Congress passed legislation to increase funding for tobacco cessation programs for pregnant and nursing mothers. You plan to advocate with the regulatory authority to ensure funding is dedicated to evidence-based programming. Which of the following are frequently used advocacy techniques at the regulatory level? (Mark all that apply.)
   a. emails or email templates
   b. creation of talking points
   c. social media posts
   d. fact sheets
   e. information folders
   f. phone calls
   g. relevant stories
   h. voting

5. There are specific activities that advocates participate in before, during, and after meetings with legislators. Which of the following activities occur before the actual meeting takes place? (Mark all that apply.)
   a. Research any current or past bills that support your advocacy area.
   b. Review legislator voting records.
   c. Prepare to answer difficult questions the legislator may ask.
   d. Talk to the legislator about relevant data and statistics.

6. Standing up for one's self to defend personal rights and a parent who advocates on behalf of their child are examples of what level of advocacy?
   a. community
   b. grassroots
   c. individual
   d. organizational

7. When employees are engaged in advocacy on behalf of the organization that employs them, this is an example of which level of advocacy?
   a. community
   b. grassroots

  c. individual
  d. organizational

8. When residents with shared beliefs and needs come together for a common purpose, this is an example of which level of advocacy?
   a. community
   b. grassroots
   c. individual
   d. organizational

9. There are several approaches or strategies used in community advocacy. One approach is holding public meetings that coalition members host within their community to share updates on their efforts while also hearing from other community members. This approach is known as _____.
   a. coalition session
   b. media advocacy
   c. stakeholder report
   d. town hall

10. The use of television, radio, and newspapers to help promote an advocacy group's mission and goals is known as _____.
    a. health communication
    b. media advocacy
    c. skills tool-kit
    d. social marketing

ANSWER KEY

1. **A.** Committee chairs
   B. Minority whips
   C. Your representative or senator
2. **A.** Voting records indicate which type of legislation they are more likely to support
3. **A.** Provides current trends among key stakeholders
4. **A.** Emails or email templates
   B. Creation of talking points
   C. Social media posts
5. **A.** Research any current or past bills that support your advocacy area
   B. Review legislator voting records
   C. Prepare to answer difficult questions the legislator may ask
6. **C.** Individual
7. **D.** Organizational
8. **A.** Community
9. **D.** Town hall
10. **B.** Media advocacy

9.7 MIKKA NYARKO

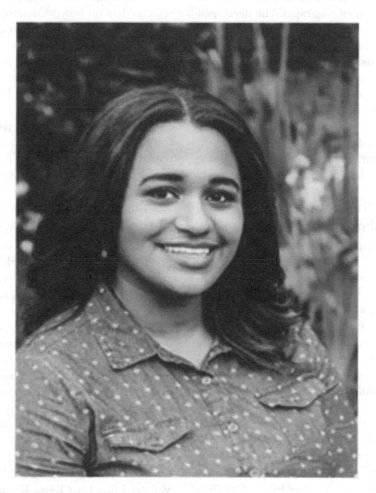

Mikka is currently a Humanitarian Response Fellow at an international relief and development organization, World Concern. She has earned a master of public health (MPH) degree with a global health concentration from Oregon State University and a bachelor of science degree in public health–community health education with a minor in Spanish from the University of Wisconsin–La Crosse. Mikka has a background in cross-cultural public health programs and formal research training in the United States and abroad.

Q. What Led or Inspired You to Become Engaged in Advocacy, Specifically as It Relates to Policy Change and Public Health?

My work and life experiences have inspired me to become engaged in advocacy work. Initially, I became drawn toward advocacy work in the global health field as an undergraduate researcher in the Ronald E. McNair Scholars Program. The research objective was to develop, implement, and evaluate a program to address breast and cervical cancers for women in the Matagalpa region of Nicaragua. The developed program was delivered in the form of mobile clinics to the women in this region. Participants received educational sessions on how to detect and prevent these cancers, followed by a Pap (Papanicolaou) test by medical professionals. For many women, it was their first time learning this information and receiving a screening. Experiences like this, among others, have inspired me to advocate for the development and implementation of culturally sensitive and locally relevant health initiatives.

Q. What Are the Issues or Advocacy-Related Projects You Are Working on Right Now?

In my current role as a Humanitarian Response Fellow, I am involved in projects that work to address humanitarian needs in hard-to-reach places. My organization works in multiple countries where there is little to no infrastructure and resources are limited. What is important in this work is advocating for the communities we serve. We start by listening to the needs of community members, offer support, and provide sustainable and practical tools to address those needs.

I work closely with the disaster response team, which assists communities in disaster mitigation, preparedness, response, and recovery stages. We respond by aiming to meet immediate needs, help families recover and build resilience, and follow a "do no harm" approach. Most of my tasks include researching and writing situation reports in response to natural disasters and neglected crises. Additionally, I assist with the development, planning, and implementation of training modules of various public health topics like drug addiction.

Q. What Is One of Your Greatest Advocacy Triumphs or Successes?

An achievement I am proud to speak of took place during my MPH training, when I interned for a program that worked with a rural community in Botswana. Fellow interns and I employed community-based research to identify multilevel factors that influence the rate of HIV/AIDS in this community. We engaged key community stakeholders on how to develop a comprehensive sexual and reproductive health education program for youth and their families.

Our team communicated preliminary research findings and program components to community members and stakeholders. Findings were also presented to government entities, both local and national in Botswana, to help gain support for the community. When I returned to campus, I continued to disseminate research findings in academic settings such as public health conferences.

Q. What Have Been Some of the Biggest Challenges You Have Faced as They Relate to Your Advocacy Work?

The field of public health is dynamic, and often new challenges arise while you are trying to address other issues. A good example of this is the coronavirus disease (COVID-19) pandemic. This pandemic has caused consequential issues, including, but not limited to economic strain, overwhelmed healthcare systems, and interrupted surveillance of other diseases. Due to the dynamic nature of this field, I have learned how important it is to be adaptable in advocacy work in response to our changing environment.

Q. What's One Piece of Advice You'd Like to Offer Emerging Advocates in Public Health?

My perspective on working with resource-limited communities has been shaped by understanding the importance of cultural humility in public health. Therefore, my advice is to first listen to the needs of the community you serve and utilize sustainable approaches that strengthen local capacities. Another piece of advice is to participate in opportunities where you can practice publicly advocating and sharing an issue. Knowledge sharing can help reach the support of decision makers who can bring resources and solutions.

Partnerships and Coalition Building for Advocacy

JEAN M. BRENY, BREANNA DE LEON, AND ELIZABETH J. SCHWARTZ

> The basic requirement for the understanding of the politics of change is to recognize the world as it is. We must work with it on its terms if we are to change it to the kind of world we would like it to be. We must first see the world as it is and not as we would like it to be.
>
> —SAUL ALINSKY, *Rules for Radicals* (1971)

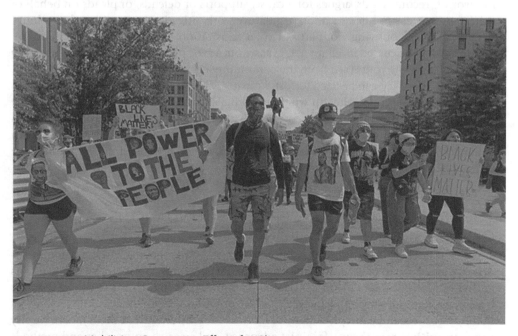

FIGURE 10.1 Mobilizing Community Efforts for Change.
Source: Racial EquityTools.

Jean M. Breny, Breanna De Leon, and Elizabeth J. Schwartz, *Partnerships and Coalition Building for Advocacy*. In: *Be the Change*. Edited by Keely S. Rees, Jody Early, and Cicily Hampton, Oxford University Press. © Oxford University Press 2023. DOI: 10.1093/oso/9780197570890.003.0010

Objectives

1. Define grassroots advocacy.
2. Explain how grassroots advocacy is distinct from other forms of advocacy.
3. Summarize social theories that provide underpinning for advocacy strategies and community engagement.
4. Explain the importance of partnership development as it relates to advocacy.
5. Describe how coalitions can be used to strengthen advocacy efforts.
6. Summarize ways in which professional organizations may be involved with advocacy training efforts.
7. Develop a plan for advocacy on a select issue that starts at the grassroots level.

INTRODUCTION

As public health professionals, we are dedicated to informing, educating, and empowering; mobilizing community partnerships; and aiding in the development of policies that improve the health outcomes and quality of life of the populations we serve (Turnock, 2016). At every intersection of our careers, advocacy is a crucial component and is necessary to achieve health equity. As defined in Chapter 1, advocacy is "any action that speaks in favor of, recommends, argues for a cause, supports or defends, or pleads on behalf of others. It includes public education, regulatory work, litigation, and work before administrative bodies, lobbying, nonpartisan voter registration, nonpartisan voter education, and more." As discussed in Chapter 1, **grassroots advocacy** is a specific form of advocacy that starts from the roots (i.e., from the community itself) and grows upward from there. Grassroots advocacy can be used to foster positive change in all sorts of arenas, and it is commonly used in public health when individuals mobilize collectively to improve the health and safety of those in their community. It involves the people and communities affected by the inequities and policies that need reform (Garcia et al., 2015; Moseley et al., 2008). The collective lived experiences, stories, and actions of the community are utilized as agents of change, which can occur at the local, state, or federal level.

THEORETICAL AND CONCEPTUAL FOUNDATIONS OF GRASSROOTS ORGANIZING

Grassroots advocacy differs from traditional advocacy and lobbying as it is a community-driven movement to educate and inform policy. Effective grassroots advocacy movements are often grounded in a blend of theoretical frameworks and constructs that strive for health equity and social and racial justice (Hampton & Lachenmayr, 2019). Some of these theoretical and conceptual frameworks include **empowerment theory**, **community capacity**, **critical race theory**, **feminist advocacy**, and research approaches and methods such as **Photovoice** and **community-based participatory research** (see Table 10.1). Taken together, this foundation promotes community empowerment, organizing, capacity building, communication, and action with the ultimate goal of cultivating change (Breny & McMorrow, 2021; Hampton & Lachenmayr, 2019; Minkler, 2012).

TABLE 10.1 Social Frameworks, Theories, and Research Approaches Relating to Advocacy

Theory/Approach (Key Authors)	Brief Definition
Critical race theory (Ford & Skrine Jeffers, 2019)	Race is a social construct, and racism is central to all precursors of health disparities and inequities. In order for any advocacy or research work to be truly emancipatory, it must take a "racism-centered orientation."
Feminist advocacy (Evans, 2005)	"Feminist advocacy is concerned with ending injustices throughout the world by advancing women's rights" and the rights of other minority groups.
Empowerment (Minkler, 2012)	Allows for community members to achieve a sense of power over and a mastery of their lives and the political process within which they live.
Community capacity (Goodman, 2009)	Following from a sense of empowerment, a community then exhibits having the tools and resources to mobilize on their own, that is, having the capacity to do so as a unified and empowered group. Also known as community mobilization.
Critical consciousness (Freire, 1970)	A process of self-empowerment grounded in a process of self-reflection and dialogue with others, to come to realize and act on the root causes of their situation.
Community-based participatory research (Israel et al., 1998)	A collaborative approach to conducting research whereby all partners in the research process (i.e., researchers, community members, advocates) have equal power and roles by recognizing the unique strengths that each brings to the table.
Photovoice (Wang & Burris, 1997)	A CBPR-centered, action-oriented, qualitative research methodology that utilizes photographs as codes, or triggers, for critical dialogue (Freire, 1970) to uncover root causes of inequities, like systemic racism. Based in feminist theory and Freirean principles, Photovoice research results are translated into an action for change, such as legislation or policy.

OUR ROLE IN HEALTH ADVOCACY

Despite ongoing work in the field and the major platform for progressive change, systemic health and racial inequities are prevalent and disproportionately burdening disenfranchised communities of color and other marginalized groups across the nation. Because of this burden, advocacy has become a tenet of public health education and practice (Caira et al., 2003; Galer-Unti, 2009; Galer-Unti et al., 2004; Yoo et al., 2004). Grassroots advocacy is employed because there is power in numbers.

Self-awareness of the role we play in the community is critical for successful public health practice and partnerships. Sometimes, we are simultaneously public health practitioners as well as community members ourselves, bringing the insights of our own lived experience to how we conduct our jobs and serve our community. At other times, however, we act only in the role of a public health professional, serving communities of which we ourselves are not a part. When this is the case, public health professionals must understand that we, as onlookers, do not know exactly what is best for the communities we serve (Caira et al., 2003; Moseley et al., 2008). While we may be motivated to save the world, our role as health professionals and advocates is not one of "savior." As public health professionals, we can leverage our education and resources to assist, elevate, and empower communities in ways they identify as useful (Caira et al., 2003; Moseley et al., 2008; Wennerstrom et al., 2022). Therefore, grassroots advocacy is collaborative and academic degrees are not required for participation.

Community members and public health professionals alike can engage in grassroots advocacy. The community's knowledge, experiences, and capacity are invaluable tools in creating awareness and sustaining the long-term process that will lead to change (Blackwell et al., 2018; Hampton & Lachenmayr, 2019; Yoo et al., 2004). This diversity of participants ensures that the community is an active member and that it influences the sought change. Everyone has a voice and a right to use it regarding policy decisions that will impact their life.

Grassroots advocacy can be a driver of policy change at the local, state, and federal levels. Although some sources reserve grassroots advocacy as the last resource for change, it can certainly be employed to address varying and widespread needs. When inequities persist, grassroots advocacy should be used.

PARTNERSHIP DEVELOPMENT AND ITS ROLE IN ADVOCACY

Advocacy is rarely done alone. Finding partners to work with, managing those relationships, and finding common groundwork to advocate for it is the essence of partnership development in advocacy work. In 1993, several organizations working toward the same issues in New Haven, Connecticut, came together to pool their resources for advocacy and policy change, calling themselves "Mothers for Justice." The group was formed by women receiving services from the Christian Community Action, working for welfare reform, who were also members of their local neighborhood advocacy groups. Since then, their purview and membership has grown, and they have changed their name to reflect that. Now, they are Mothers (and Others) for Justice and their advocacy goals include (1) safe and affordable housing, (2) voting access and equity, and (3) access to healthcare (Mothers and (others) for Justice, n.d.).

In Table 10.1, we outline the major tenets and conceptual underpinnings for community work and advocacy, namely, community capacity and empowerment. An empowered community is one that is able to identify its own strengths and utilize those strengths for advocacy, community building, and developing their problem-solving skills (Minkler, 2012). Developing strong partnerships, with the right leadership and planning process, can result in big changes and healthier communities (Community Tool Box, n.d.-c). The example above illustrates how the coming together of existing groups can result in the whole being more than the sum of its parts.

Any organizing effort, especially when a group of partners is being asked to work together, must be organized using a plan and logic model. Goals, objectives, tasks, outcomes, and responsibilities for those tasks must be included in that plan (Community Tool Box, n.d.-b). Although program planning and evaluation are beyond the scope of this chapter, the Mobilizing for Action Through Planning and Partnerships, which was developed by the National Association of County and City Health Officials along with the Centers for Disease Control and Prevention, provides some excellent key strategies for partnership development. These include

- **Dialogue** ensures the inclusion of diverse perspectives and that the voices of all stakeholders are heard in the planning process.

- **Shared vision** guarantees approval and ownership of the process by all concerned, thereby increasing its chances of success.
- **Data**, rather than preconceptions, anecdotes, or intuition, provide a firm basis for planning and action.
- **Partnership** and collaboration make for not only a fairer process, but also increased access to resources and places the responsibility for success on more shoulders.
- **Strategic thinking** makes for a proactive, rather than a reactive, approach to issues and systems.
- **Celebration of successes** keeps enthusiasm high and marks progress and individual and group achievements.

DEVELOPING AN ADVOCACY PLAN

Two of the most commonly identified concerns with grassroots advocacy are "what to do" and "where to begin" (Galer-Unti, 2004, 2009). While there is no absolute answer, many public health professionals begin by developing an advocacy plan (Community Tool Box, n.d.-b; Galer-Unti et al., 2017). The purpose of the advocacy plan is to help advocates identify goals and determine the necessary steps that will help work toward those goals (Community Tool Box, n.d.-b; Galer-Unti et al., 2017). These plans are guides; they are not concrete. It is essential for young public health professionals to understand that flexibility and adaptation are key to successful grassroots advocacy (Blackwell et al., 2018; Community Tool Box, n.d.-b; Hampton & Lachenmayr, 2019).

There are many different ways to structure an advocacy plan. Although the particular sections may vary or be organized in different ways, no matter which plan format you choose, the purpose of advocacy plans is the same: to help you organize information so that you can achieve your goal. Advocacy plans are road maps to help you achieve better health outcomes for your community (Table 10.2). The more fidelity you have to your advocacy plan, the better you'll be able to assess if you're getting where you want to go or what else you might need in order to get there. Like a real road map, they can be used to not only plot your course before you begin on your journey, but also modify along the course along the way if you encounter unexpected roadblocks. It may be helpful for you to think of advocacy plans as delineating the *what* (your goal); *who* (allies, opponents, and audiences); *how* (objectives and activities); and *when* (timeline) of improving your community's health.

Advocacy plans generally start with a goal. This is a broad statement that expresses the end result that you hope to achieve. Goals are outcome oriented rather than action oriented. They are about what you want to accomplish, not about how you're going to get there.

Next, there is one or more objective. Objectives are the "how" or the action that will get you closer to achieving your goal. You can think of them as stepping stones or mile markers along the way. Objectives should be written in "SMART" format, which is to say that they should be specific, measurable, achievable, relevant, and time bound. As an example, if your goal were to be a great student, then one objective could be to increase your grade point average to a 3.5 by the end of the next semester.

TABLE 10.2 Example Advocacy Plan

Goal: Our goal is to eliminate exposure to lead among children living in Centerburg.

Objective 1: By December 31, 2023, at least 70% of homes in Centerburg built before 1990 will have been tested for lead-based paint.

Allies: Parents; local pediatricians; Centerburg Health Department; school board.

Opponents: Landlords; homeowners without children; realtor's association.

Target Audience	Activity	Resources Needed	Resources Available	Timeline
Parents	Organize parents to give testimony at Town Council meeting	—Contact information for parents in Centerburg —Testimony tutorial —Someone to identify which parents are planning to attend	—Zoom account for hosting testimony tutorial —Educational materials —2 volunteers for calls/emails	March 18, 2023
Landlords	Educate about lead abatement tax subsidies	—Pamphlets about tax subsidies —Mailing addresses of landlords —Money for postage	—$400 for print materials and postage —2 volunteers	September 15, 2023

Objective 2: By June 30, 2024, 90% of water sources (including water fountains and sinks in classrooms, bathrooms, and cafeterias) will have been tested for lead.

Allies: Students; parents; teachers; local pediatricians; Centerburg Health Department.

Opponents: School board; principals; taxpayers without children in school system.

Target Audience	Activity	Resources Needed	Resources Available	Timeline
Parent–Teacher Association (PTA)	PTA to raise issue of water testing at next full school board meeting	—Date of next school board meeting —PTA member willing to add this —Information sheet for distribution —$50 for printing of information sheet	—Fact sheet about prevalence of lead in water in Centerburg —1 volunteer to find school board meeting date, print fact sheet, and identify which PTA member will raise this at the meeting —$200 donation	March 1, 2024
Local media	Ask media to cover school board meeting at which this will be an agenda item	—Background info for media representative —Identify at least 2 parents and 2 students who can be interviewed by local news	—Fact sheet about prevalence of lead in water in Centerburg —1 volunteer who has worked with local news before	March 18, 2024

Note: If these were your actual objectives, you'd probably have more activities than are listed here, but this should give you a good idea of how a plan would start.

Even when two objectives are needed to accomplish a single goal, those two objectives can be quite different from one another; therefore, the next steps of the advocacy plan should be completed *per objective*. For example, if the goal were to reduce childhood obesity in your town, the objective of reducing the number of fast food establishments and the objective of increasing the number of students enrolled in afterschool sports would likely encounter different allies and opponents and would be accomplished with different activities, resources, and timeline.

A successful advocacy campaign cannot be done by one person alone, and you should expect that not all stakeholders will necessarily see things your way. In order to rally the most support and prepare for counteractions, it is important to create a list of known or likely allies and of known or likely opponents to your objective.

Allies and opponents are not the only people who need to be considered in an advocacy plan. It is critical to also identify the target audience(s), which is to say, those whose attitudes and behavior you hope to influence through your advocacy efforts. Keep in mind that your target audience may not be only those whose health you are trying to improve or whose behavior you are trying to change.

Once the target audiences have been identified, it is time to think about what actions will be used to engage or communicate with each of them. These actions are like subcomponents of your objective and can include things like meeting with the audience to establish a relationship; providing education or educational materials to them about your cause; attending existing meetings or establishing new forums for conversation around your topic; or engaging media to help you communicate with the key audience. It is common but not necessarily needed to have multiple actions per target audience.

USING GRASSROOTS ADVOCACY EFFECTIVELY

Scholars and activists have written about the power of grassroots advocacy, and there is empirical evidence to support it as an important and necessary strategy for improving health (Cooper & Christens, 2019; Garcia et al., 2015; Rivera et al., 2016). Community member engagement and active participation in advocacy are critical to effectively influence policies that address their needs (Blackwell et al., 2018; Caira et al., 2003; Wennerstrom et al., 2020, 2022). Grassroots advocacy should continue to be utilized in public health practice because it involves the community in a nontokenistic manner. Ideally, community members are respected contributors to the advocacy process and goals (Mondros & Wilson, 1994; Wennerstrom et al., 2020, 2022; Yoo et al., 2004). The work of public health professionals in grassroots advocacy creates an inclusive environment that addresses the community's perceived barriers to involvement, provides resources to improve the community's advocacy skills and knowledge, and increases its capacity to create and sustain future advocacy (Blackwell et al., 2018; Caira et al., 2003; Community Tool Box, n.d.-c). A seemingly small initial grassroots movement can lead to continued education, empowerment, and measurable change over time.

Grassroots advocacy provides a collaboration between communities and public health professionals. As there is a history of distrust between medical and academic institutions and disenfranchised communities, engaging in collective action for a meaningful purpose can help build and maintain lasting relationships between the groups (Galer-Unti, 2009; Yoo et al., 2004).

Finally, grassroots advocacy raises awareness and works to influence and change policy. Because there is power in numbers, grassroots advocacy builds a movement of various stakeholders to influence policymakers (Community Tool Box, n.d.-a; Hampton & Lachenmayr, 2019). Through this form of advocacy, we can hold our policymakers accountable for their constituents' needs (Galer-Unti, 2009; Galer-Unti et al., 2017). We can provide policymakers knowledge they might not have otherwise had when making policy decisions that have lasting effects on health and quality of life. With persistence and over time, grassroots advocacy will create lasting change.

GRASSROOTS ORGANIZING THROUGH COALITION BUILDING

As should be clear by now, one way to ensure a successful advocacy effort is to put together an interdisciplinary and diverse team, where multiple sectors and interests come together on an advocacy effort (Galer-Unti et al., 2017). The added strength that comes with partnerships far exceeds the attempt to do advocacy on one's own. One of the best strategies to use in grassroots organizing would be through development of a **coalition** with the goal of that particular advocacy effort (Community Tool Box, n.d.-a).

Coalitions can be a very powerful tool for community-based work of all kinds, most especially advocacy, though they are like any other relationship and must be nurtured, must be transparent in their work, and rely on excellent communication. An ideal approach to develop a coalition is for advocates to work with existing partnerships and connections that already exist within the community and around the advocacy issue being addressed. Use your networks! Diversity is key in creating coalitions to ensure that multiple voices are heard. This diversity should extend beyond not only differences of demographics of those involved, but also diversity in the rationale for supporting your topic. For example, if you are interested in forming a coalition around passing universal healthcare, having coalition members who, like you, want to see everyone have access to comprehensive medical services and who also come from a variety of ideological and political perspectives will help strengthen your position and help you plan for any dissension when it is time to advocate. Think of how much more persuasive and better prepared to address opposition your group will be if it has a mixture of people who work behind a desk all day and those who work in manual labor; elderly people who want to see their grandkids have access to the same services they themselves used to have, and those college students who want healthcare when they age out of their parents' insurance plans; people who identify as liberal and those who identify as conservative; or those who support universal healthcare because it makes financial sense and those who support it because it makes ethical sense. In sum, you need a variety of people in your coalition, including influential members of the community, young or emerging leaders, policymakers, and other stakeholders (Community Tool Box, n.d.-a).

Many advocacy efforts begin with a small, solid core of dedicated individuals leading the way. This group is key to forging the path, but it is critically important to ensure that your group includes additional participants who may have different perspectives and assets to bring to the task at hand. Work your way outward from your initial network to recruit important voices to the table by using a variety of communication methods. Once your group is established, it will be important to meet to set ground rules, goals, future meetings, and roles and responsibilities for each member. With advocacy work, the benefits of working with a coalition are probably obvious by now, namely, pooled resources, expanded manpower and connections, diversification of opinions and knowledge base, and a community-based approach (Community Tool Box, n.d.-a). Just as there are with many good efforts, coalitions will have their pitfalls and issues. Things to be aware of when working with coalitions are things such as resource allocation (Who will pay for what? How will you distribute work evenly?); turf issues; bad history or reputation with a member/organization in the coalition (How will you handle that); and competing for the same dollars. As with any successful relationship, as we have mentioned above, communication and transparency are key. Once the coalition starts working, if there are issues that arise, they should be addressed immediately and ratified completely.

ADVOCACY TRAINING AT THE GRASSROOTS LEVEL

As mentioned previously, calls to action, building effective and diverse coalitions, and engagement in grassroots advocacy are critical responsibilities of public health professionals. Concurrently public health professionals should purposefully incorporate the community in their work as valued consultants and peers, not merely test subjects. Southern Connecticut State University's (SCSU's) Public Health Department is making significant strides in training the next generation of public health professionals and advocates.

As preliminary work to establish a Center for Health Equity and Eliminating Racism, master of public health (MPH) students collaborated with Black and Brown community members to design and implement three Photovoice-Community-based Participatory Research (CBPR) projects. Photovoice research is a qualitative research that aims to (1) enable people to reflect their community's strengths and concerns, (2) promote critical dialogue and knowledge about root causes through group discussion of photographs, and (3) reach policymakers (Breny & McMorrow, 2021; Wang & Burris, 1997). Through the curriculum at SCSU, MPH students were able to ground their advocacy in critical race theory and the principles of community-based participatory research. The Photovoice projects provided a unique platform for MPH students and community members to train, learn, address health inequities and social determinants of health, and advocate for change.

The framework established through the Photovoice projects served to help empower, enable, and support communities to develop a sustainable and well-rounded foundation for grassroots advocacy and coalition building (see Box 10.1). MPH students were able to translate textbook knowledge and health equity training sessions from the Society for

- *Background:* As we so clearly have seen, the COVID-19 pandemic has intensified inequities in communities of color and highlighted a critical need to investigate needs, build community capacity, and reform policies that maintain cycles of generational poverty, racism, and premature death. The city of New Haven is a small, diverse Connecticut city of 130,000 residents with deep, enduring economic and social disparities. Located on the traditional lands of the Quinnipiac, Paugussett, and Wappinger peoples, New Haven is now home to a diverse population with more than 60% identifying as Black or African American and Latinx (Abraham et al., 2019). The prevalence of chronic disease among New Haven residents is significantly higher than among Connecticut residents. To address social determinants of health, we must deeply understand and demonstrate their impact, including racism as a root cause.

- *Working with the community to identify and understand topics of interest:* Through SCSU's commitment to social and racial justice in the curriculum, public health students could truly understand and value the expertise and experiences of the community. Research dyads, each consisting of one SCSU MPH student and one community member, collaborated to conduct Photovoice research on health inequities heightened during the COVID-19 pandemic. These community-led Photovoice discussions uncovered various topics of concern, including racism, educational barriers, lack of parental involvement, access to healthcare, neighborhood safety, and food insecurity. For this example, we will focus on the topic of food insecurity.

Diving deeper into the concern of food insecurity, community consultants identified living in food deserts as a major health inequity and a cause for reform. They spoke of liquor stores, bodegas, and fast food chains on every corner but only two grocery stores. Community consultants identified that grocery stores are not easily accessible for them, and farmers' markets do not stop in their community and are unwelcoming for nonaffluent people. One specific individual stated, "It's expensive to be poor," when discussing how food stamps are limited, and she cannot afford to get to healthier food options or purchase them.

One community change sought by this specific Photovoice group was increasing access to affordable farmers' markets in low-income neighborhoods.

- *What action or change will occur?* The action was connecting with specific businesses in New Haven known to have the desired healthier food options to arrange a partnership and increased access. One such business identified by the group was City Seed. We have partnered with Mothers (and Others) for Justice to plan and implement advocacy work they have already begun to work on.

- *Who will carry it out?* The Photovoice group, including researchers and community consultants, will carry it out. They identified the necessity to increase awareness of food insecurity among the local community members. The group will work as a whole to gain community support, contact specific businesses, and reach their local government.

- *By when will it take place?* The group will try to have engaged community members and contact the necessary business and government officials over the next year (by the end of 2021), as COVID-19 is still a prevalent health concern for their neighborhoods.

- *What resources are needed to carry out the step?* The Photovoice group will continue to utilize resources and professional connections available through SCSU's Public Health Department. Furthermore, additional funding for continued research and advocacy and projects will be requested through the Connecticut Health Foundation, the Photovoice project's initial funder.

- *Communication about the action step:* All incoming community partners will be provided information on the sought change. Open communication will be continued between SCSU researchers and community members.

Public Health Education (SOPHE) Advocacy Summit to develop a grassroots advocacy plan in the community (Community Tool Box, n.d.-b).

Through their practice, they built trusted relationships in communities of color and among marginalized groups, engaged with various community members and stakeholders, provided training on health equity topics, and created inclusive spaces that encourage critical dialogues. This introduction to public health practice and true community-based grassroots advocacy is a necessary step in the direction of progressive change and health and racial equity.

THE ROLE OF PROFESSIONAL ASSOCIATIONS IN ADVOCACY

In the fields of public health and health promotion, utilizing advocacy as a skill for social change and increasing healthy communities is evident everywhere as a commitment and necessary skill set. This is evident by the inclusion of advocacy as a core public health activity and competency for accrediting schools and programs of public health by the Council on Education in Public Health; in the updated eight areas of responsibilities for health educators (Health Education Specialist Practice Analysis), with advocacy becoming its own area (National Commission for Health Education Credentialing, n.d.); to the inclusion of advocating in the 10 Essential Public Health Services (Centers for Disease Control and Prevention, n.d.). What this means is that public health professional development programs, professional organizations, and practicing professionals must become active organizers and leaders in order to be successful in our health equity work (Breny, 2020).

This increased focus on advocacy opens up great opportunities for health education professional associations, such as SOPHE, Eta Sigma Gamma, and the American School Health Association to provide advocacy training opportunities (Box 10.2). In fact, knowing the power of coalitions in advocacy work, these organizations, along with several of their sister organizations, formed the Coalition of National Health Education Organizations (CNHEO) to do just that. Indeed, the first goal of the CNHEO profession-wide strategic plan is to "advance national, state, and local policies, systems, and environments that support health education and promotion" (CNHEO, 2018, para. 1). To this end, the coalition planned and implemented an annual advocacy summit, drawing hundreds of health education and promotion students and professionals to Washington, D.C., for years, until SOPHE began leading the development, and it continues today. All of these organizations are committed to training their members on how to do quality advocacy campaigns, as well as being leaders in advocacy and testimonials on Capitol Hill. As one example, SOPHE has been a leader in advocacy for more than 70 years.

EXAMPLE: A TWENTY-FIRST-CENTURY GRASSROOTS MOVEMENT: THE #METOO MOVEMENT

Do you know at least three women or four men? If so, chances are that you probably know at least two survivors of sexual violence. Research indicates that approximately one third of women and one quarter of men in America have experienced sexual abuse or assault

ADVOCACY IN ACTION BOX 10.2	The Role of Professional Organizations in Advocacy Training—The Connecticut Public Health Association

Quick! Think about the public health issue you care most about. If you needed to persuade a policymaker to see things your way about that issue right this very moment, how successful do you think you'd be? Let's think about it another way: What's the chance you could write a perfectly polished thesis or win a game of basketball if you had never practiced those activities before? Well, advocacy is no different. Enthusiasm and natural aptitude isn't enough; you need training and practice to become really good at it.

One of the core functions of the Connecticut Public Health Association (CPHA) is to advocate for both the health of the public and the field of public health as a whole. In fact, like most APHA affiliates, the Connecticut Public Health Association has an entire committee dedicated just to advocacy activities. While it's one thing for CPHA to know how to engage in this sort of public health advocacy, health equity can only be achieved when those who are currently marginalized and disenfranchised also have these skills. For each of the last 3 years, CPHA has partnered with public and private educational institutions, Health Equity Solutions, the Connecticut Health Foundation, the New England Public Health Training Center, and others to provide

a free, daylong annual advocacy skills training event to hundreds of community members, students, and representatives of charitable health promotion organizations in the region.

The agenda for each year's training session is roughly the same: First, there is a presentation about ins, outs, and eccentricities of Connecticut's government structure and legislative process; then a break for a free, healthy lunch; a lesson on the basic skills of advocacy; and an opportunity to put those skills into action by practicing elevator pitches and designing advocacy campaigns. Finally, each day ends with one or more local politicians sharing what it's actually like to be on the receiving end of advocacy campaigns and their tips for being a successful public health advocate.

Learning to advocate effectively is a means of empowerment. Professional organizations have an important role to play not only in being advocates for public health but also in training the workforce and communities to advocate as well.

Next Steps: Find out what advocacy activities your state's APHA affiliate engages in. What issue do you think they should prioritize advocating for this year? How can you get involved?

---

at some point in their lifetime (Centers for Disease Control and Prevention, 2021). If you read those statistics and thought to yourself: "There's no way this can be true about the people *I* know," think again! Then ask yourself, "Why is it that something so common is so seldom discussed?" The stigma and isolation surrounding sexual violence mean that victims are often not ready to publicly share their story or even to identify themselves as survivors. The words "advocacy," "organizing," and "coalition building" tend to evoke images of highly visible activities like attending public protests, meeting with groups of like-minded people, giving testimony to policymakers, or maybe even putting a bumper sticker on your car for a cause. When it comes to ending sexual violence, however, this is a conundrum. How can the very visible nature of change-producing activities be reconciled with many survivors' reluctance to tell their stories and make their needs known? Sometimes a new model of social change is what's called for.

The "Me Too" movement started in 2006 when Tarana Burke, an advocate and sexual assault survivor, started using the phrase so that other survivors would know that they aren't alone (Me Too Movement, n.d.). A decade later, the phrase sparked an international movement when millions answered Alyssa Milano's call for those who had experienced sexual harassment or assault respond to her tweet with the words "Me Too" (Me

Too Movement, n.d.). By using the same apps and websites that people already use every day from the relative privacy of their phone or computer, the Me Too movement moved advocacy to a place where survivors could express themselves without exposing themselves to the extent that they might with in-person advocacy.

Traditional methods of advocacy remain critical tools to bring about change. However, when 21st-century advocacy heeds public health's call to meet people where they are by pairing social intelligence with social media, it can solve problems that traditional advocacy hasn't thus far been able to address. Though the solidarity catalyzed by the Me Too movement is itself an antidote to the stigma and isolation felt by so many survivors, the fruits of this movement don't end there. A majority of both women and men reported that the movement has had a positive impact on how sexual harassment is handled in the workplace (Saha, 2020), and within his first 50 days in office, President Biden signed an executive order establishing a Gender Policy Council in the White House (Block, 2021).

CONCLUSION

We hope that after reading this chapter you feel more empowered to take on advocacy efforts either locally or at a national level. We presented you with ways of starting at the grassroots level by either starting your own group or working with an existing one to take on the tough public health and health equity challenges we see every day. From there, you can create an advocacy plan and follow the steps to help new policy or social action come to light! In addition, we encourage you as new professionals to become involved with professional organizations (like American Public Health Association [APHA], SOPHE, American Medical Association) for many reasons, including involving yourself with advocacy efforts and aligning yourself with others working to create systemic change. As the anthropologist and activist Margaret Mead once wrote: "Never doubt what a small group of thoughtful, committed citizens can do to change the world: indeed, it's the only thing that ever has" (Mead, 1978). These small groups can grow to large movements, such as #MeToo and #MomsDemandAction and illustrate how there is also strength in numbers.

REFERENCES

Abraham, M., Seaberry, C., Ankrah, J., Bourdillon, A., Davila, K., Finn, E., Mcgann, S., & Nathan, A. (2019). Greater New Haven community index 2019. https://ctdatahaven.org/sites/ctdatahaven/files/DataHaven_GNH_Community_Index_2019.pdf

Alinsky, S. D. (1971). *Rules for radicals; a practical primer for realistic radicals*. Random House.

Blackwell, A., Thompson, M., Freudenberg, N., Ayers, J., Schrantz, D., & Minkler, M. (2018). Using community organizing and community building to influence public policy. In M. Minkler (Ed.), *Community organizing and community building for health and welfare* (3rd ed., pp. 371–385). Rutgers University Press.

Block, M. (2021). Biden establishes a gender policy council within the White House. https://www.npr.org/2021/03/08/974655385/biden-will-establish-a-gender-policy-council-within-the-white-house

Breny, J. M. (2020). Continuing the journey toward health equity: Becoming antiracist in health promotion research and practice. *Health Education & Behavior*, 47(5), 665–670. https://doi.org/10.1177/1090198120954393

Breny, J., & McMorrow, S. (2021). *Photovoice for social justice: Visual representation in action*. Sage Publishing.

Caira, N. M., Lachenmayr, S., Sheinfeld, J., Goodhart, F. W., Cancialosi, L., & Lewis, C.

(2003). The health educator's role in advocacy and policy: Principles, processes, programs, and partnerships. *Health Promotion Practice*, *4*(3), 303–313. http://doi.org/10.1177/1524 83990325255

Centers for Disease Control and Prevention. (n.d.). *10 essential public health services— CSTLTS*. https://www.cdc.gov/publichealth gateway/publichealthservices/essentialhea lthservices.html

Centers for Disease Control and Prevention. (2021). *Sexual violence is preventable*. https:// www.cdc.gov/injury/features/sexual-viole nce/index.html

Coalition of National Health Education Organizations (CNHEO). (2018). *Profession- wide strategic plan: Goals, objectives, and activi- ties*. https://assets.speakcdn.com/assets/2251/ cnheo_strategic_plan_-_goals_and_objecti ves.pdf

Community Tool Box. (n.d.-a). *Coalition building 1: Starting a coalition*. https://ctb.ku.edu/en/ table-of-contents/assessment/promotion-str ategies/start-a-coaltion/main

Community Tool Box. (n.d.-b). *Section 7: Developing a plan for advocacy*. https://ctb. ku.edu/en/table-of-contents/advocacy/advoc acy-principles/advocacy-plan/main

Community Tool Box. (n.d.-c). *Section 13. MAPP: Mobilizing for action through planning and partnerships*. https://ctb.ku.edu/en/table- of-contents/overview/models-for-commun ity-health-and-development/mapp/main

Cooper, D. G., & Christens, B. D. (2019). Justice system reform for health equity: A mixed methods examination of collaborating for equity and justice principles in a grassroots organizing coalition. *Health Education & Behavior*, *46*(1, Suppl.), 62S–70S. https://doi. org/10.1177/1090198119859411

Evans, K. (2005). A guide to feminist advo- cacy. *Gender and Development*, *13*(3), 10–20. https://doi.org/10.1080/1355207051233 1332293

Ford, C. L., & Skrine Jeffers, K. (2019). Critical race theory's antiracism approaches: Moving from the ivory tower to the front lines of public health. In C. L. Ford, D. M. Griffith, M. A. Bruce, & K. L. Gilbert (Eds.), *Racism: Science*

& *tools for the public health professional* (pp. 327–342). APHA Press.

Freire, P. (1970). *Pedagogy of the oppressed*. Herder and Herder.

Galer-Unti, R. (2009). Guerilla advocacy: Using aggressive marketing techniques for health policy change. *Policy and Politics*, *10*(3), 325– 327. https://doi.org/10.1177/152483990 9334513

Galer-Unti, R., Bishop, K., & Pulliam McCoy, R. (2017). Advocacy. In C. L. Fertman & D. D. Allensworth (Eds.), *Health promotion programs: From theory to practice* (2nd ed., pp. 171–192). Jossey-Bass.

Galer-Unti, R., Tappe, M., & Lachenmayr, S. (2004). Advocacy 101: Getting started in health education advocacy. *Health Promotion Practice*, *5*(3), 280–288. https://doi.org/ 10.1177/1524839903257697

Garcia, L. B., Hernandez, K. E., & Mata, H. (2015). Professional development through policy advocacy: Communicating and advocating for health and health equity. *Health Promotion Practice*, *16*(2), 162–165. https://doi.org/10.1177/1524839914560405

Goodman, R. M. (2009). A construct for building the capacity of community-based initiatives in racial and ethnic communities: A qualita- tive cross-case analysis. *Journal of Public Health Management and Practice*, *15*(2), E1–E8.

Hampton, C., & Lachenmayr, S. (2019). Advocating for health policy. In R. J. Bensley & J. Brookins-Fisher (Eds.), *Community and public health education methods: A practical guide* (4th ed., pp. 243–266). Jones & Bartlett Learning.

Israel, B. A., Schulz, A. J., Parker, E. A., & Becker, A. B. (1998). Review of community-based research: Assessing partnership approaches to improve public health. *Annual Review of Public Health*, *104*(19), 173–202.

Mead, M. (1978). *Culture and commitment: The new relationships between the generations in the 1970s* (Rev. ed.). Anchor Press/Doubleday.

Me Too Movement. (n.d.). History & inception. https://metoomvmt.org/get-to-know-us/hist ory-inception/

Minkler, M. (2012). *Community organizing and community building for health and welfare* (3rd ed.). Rutgers University Press.

Mondros, J. B., & Wilson, S. M. (1994). *Organizing for power and empowerment.* Columbia University Press.

Moseley, C., Melton, L. D., Francisco, V. T. (2008). Grassroots advocacy campaign for HIV/AIDS prevention: Lessons from the field. *Health Promotion Practice, 9*(3), 253–261. https://doi.org/10.1177/1524839906292821

Mothers (and Others) for Justice. Christian Community Action. (n.d.). https://www.cca helping.org/mothers-and-others-justice

National Commission for Health Education Credentialing. (n.d.). Responsibilities and competencies for health education specialists. https://www.nchec.org/responsibilities-and-competencies

Rivera, L., Starry, B., Gangi, C., Lube, L. M., Cedergren, A., Whitney, E., & Rees, K. (2016). From classroom to capitol: Building advocacy capacity through state-level advocacy experiences. *Health Promotion Practice, 17*(6), 771–774. http://doi.org/10.1177/1524839916669131

Saha, S. (2020). 76% of US *employees* say #MeToo *positively impacted the workplace culture, surveys careerarc.* https://www.hrtechnolog ist.com/news/culture/76-of-the-us-employ ees-say-metoo-positively-impacted-the-workplace-culture-surveys-careerarc/

Turnock, B. (2016). *Public health: What it is and how it works* (6th ed.). Jones & Bartlett Learning.

Wang, C., & Burris, M. A. (1997). Photovoice: Concept, methodology, and use for participatory needs assessment. *Health Education & Behavior, 24*(3), 369–387.

Wennerstrom, A., Silver, J., Pollock, M., & Gustat, J. (2020). Training community residents to address social determinants of health in underresourced communities. *Health Promotion Practice, 21*(4), 564–572. http://doi.org/10.1177/1524839918820039

Wennerstrom, A., Silver, J., Pollock, M., & Gustat, J. (2022). Action to improve social determinants of health: Outcomes of leadership and advocacy training for community residents. *Health Promotion Practice, 23*(1), 137–146. http://doi.org/10.1177/1524839920956297

Yoo, S., Weed, N. E., Lempa, M. L., Mbondo, M., Shada, R. E., & Goodman, R. M. (2004). Collaborative community empowerment: An illustration of a six-step process. *Health Promotion Practice, 5*(3), 256–265. http://doi.org/10.1177/1524839903257363

CHAPTER 10: END-OF-CHAPTER ACTIVITIES

DISCUSSION QUESTIONS

1. Discuss how grassroots advocacy is different from other types of advocacy. In what kinds of efforts would grassroots advocacy be the most effective?

2. Research and identify an organization in your area that has engaged in health advocacy. What kinds of advocacy efforts have they supported in the past? What public health issues have not been advocated for?

3. As a future (or current) health advocate and public health professional, what are your strengths as an advocate? Where do you see yourself needing to seek training to hone your advocacy skills?

4. There are many emerging issues needing advocacy and organizing work, such as the health effects of climate change, racism as a public health emergency, and continuing issues around vaccinations for COVID-19 prevention. What are our professional organizations doing with regard to advocacy, resolutions, and member trainings around these issues? What do you think they could do more of to address these issues?

APPLICATION ACTIVITIES

1. *Research a Candidate:* Choose one of the candidates running for office this election year, next year. It can be at the federal level (president or Congress person) or at the state level (governor, state senator, or state representative). Go to their campaign website and read their position on a policy related to health, such as healthcare, gun violence prevention, safe schools, family medical leave, and so on. Explore what organizations or coalitions, if any, are they working with to get policies passed? Write a one- or two-page paper on their position statement, taking a stand yourself on how you see their position helping or hurting the public's health. Include in your position statement ways you could partner and organize with others on this legislation.
   - Write a 2-minute testimony on this statement and practice presenting it with your friends.
   - Bonus points: Schedule yourself to give this testimony in person.

2. *Identify a Pressing Health Issue in Your Community:* Create a list of organizations, agencies, and groups that could align to work on this issue together. What could each bring to the partnership that would help achieve positive change relating to this issue? Contact one of the agencies you've identified and interview them on their advocacy process.
   - Write a one- or two-page reaction paper on how this contact went. Be sure to include the policy you were contacting them about, including any research you did on the topic. This paper will include a summary of the policy and the organization's position, as well as a reaction on how your contact with them went.

3. *Research a Movement:* Research a grassroots movement you would like to know more about. Maybe it is around Black Lives Matter organizing, the #MeToo movement, or a local effort in your area around getting out the vote.
   - Write a one- or two-page reaction paper. Include in the paper a summary of what the advocacy goals of the event/movement are and your reaction to being a part of it. Include any thoughts about how the community was, or could have been, involved.

4. *Develop an Advocacy Plan:*
   - First, form a group of three to five people.
   - Then, choose a public health issue of concern for your community.
   - Next, use the template in Table 10.2 to start developing an advocacy plan. Feel free to add more lines for additional objectives and activities if you need to.

ADDITIONAL RESOURCES

Community Tool Box. https://ctb.ku.edu/en
National Council of Non-Profits. *Everyday advocacy resources.* https://www.councilofnonprofits.org/everyday-advocacy-resources

Society for Public Health Education. *Advocacy summit.* https://www.sophe.org/professional-development/conferences_events/advocacy-summit/

QUIZ QUESTIONS

1. "Following from a sense of empowerment, a community then exhibits having the tools and resources to mobilize on their own" is the definition of what?
   a. critical race theory
   b. Photovoice
   c. community capacity

2. Which of the following is the definition of empowerment?
   a. a process of self-empowerment grounded in a process of self-reflection and dialogue with others
   b. allows for community members to achieve a sense of power over and a mastery of their lives and the political process within which they live
   c. a CBPR-centered, action-oriented, qualitative research methodology that utilizes photographs as codes, or triggers, for critical dialogue

3. How does grassroots advocacy differ from other forms of advocacy?
   a. Starts from the ground and works its way up.
   b. Starts from the top and works its way down.
   c. Grassroots advocacy is more expensive.

4. What do you begin when developing an advocacy plan?
   a. a coalition
   b. a goal
   c. a policy

5. Who knows what is best for the community?
   a. the mayor
   b. the public health professional
   c. the community members themselves

6. If you're using an advocacy plan and you face a roadblock, you should
   a. stop what you are doing and start over.
   b. meet with your planning and advocacy team and use your plan to navigate around the obstacles.
   c. continue forging ahead through the roadblock.

7. What is a common pitfall for professionals engaging in public health advocacy?
   a. having a savior complex
   b. not having enough time in their schedule
   c. being afraid of public speaking

8. SOPHE is an example of a/an _____?
   a. grassroots movement
   b. advocacy plan
   c. professional association that trains members on advocacy

9. What is a coalition's greatest strength when working on an advocacy issue?
   a. the diversity of perspectives and strengths within the membership
   b. that they are paid lobbyists
   c. that they always include politicians

10. The #MeToo movement is an example of _____
    a. feminist theory.
    b. grassroots advocacy.
    c. traditional advocacy.

ANSWER KEY
1. **C.** Community capacity
2. **B.** Allows for community members to achieve a sense of power over and a mastery of their lives and the political process within which they live
3. **A.** Starts from the ground and works its way up.
4. **B.** A goal
5. **C.** The community members themselves
6. **B.** Meet with your planning and advocacy team and use your plan to navigate around the obstacles
7. **A.** Having a savior complex
8. **C.** Professional association that trains members on advocacy
9. **A.** The diversity of perspectives and strengths within the membership
10. **B.** Grassroots advocacy

10.8 VICTORIA BRECKWICH VÁSQUEZ FROM THE BASTA COALITION OF WASHINGTON STATE

Victoria Breckwich Vásquez

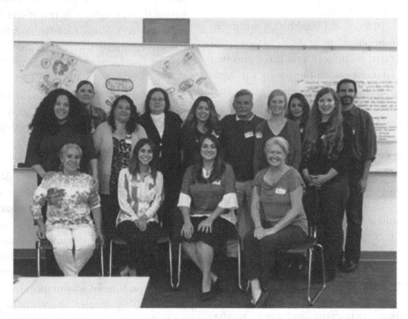

Photo: Dr. Breckwich Vásquez with members of the BASTA Coalition of Washington: Left to right, first row: Paola Zambrano, Stephany Rivas, Dr. Victoria Breckwich Vásquez, Marcy Harrington. Left to right, second row: Giselle Cárcamo, Olga Sánchez, Elizabeth Torres, Carmen Ruela, Dr. Jody Early, Guadalupe Gamboa, Allyson Dimmitt-Gnam, Teresa Mata, Dennise Drury, Andrew Kashyap.

Q. What Was Your Impetus for Cofounding the BASTA Coalition of Washington?

In this spotlight we highlight, the work of the BASTA Coalition of Washingon where their mission is to eliminate farmworke sexual harassment in the workplace. Sexual harassment of farmworkers is a problem that needs greater visibility in the workplace and in the policy sphere. It affects everyone in the workplace. I feel strongly that it be considered an occupational/worker health issue and not just a legal issue for victims/survivors to figure out. Applying a public health and advocacy approach

can lead to improved workplace training, policies, procedures, and greater accountability from those in positions of power. I recognize that training alone cannot fix the problem. There are workplace and community policies that don't go far enough to protect farmworkers from harm. In Washington State, for example, we don't have a mandatory workplace training policy in place in the agricultural sector. All of these factors motivated me to help organize and recruit a statewide coalition with multisector stakeholders that advocate for proactive policies and involve farmworkers as leaders in this work.

Q. How Prevalent Is Workplace Sexual Harassment in Agriculture? How Is the BASTA Coalition Addressing It?

In Washington State, agriculture is a $49 billion cornerstone of the economy, with approximately 200,000 farmworkers at peak times of the year (Ramachandani, 2018; World Health Organization, 1948). Women may represent as much as one third of Washington's farm workforce, and it is estimated that 75%–80% of women employed in the agricultural industry are victims of workplace sexual harassment (Washington State Department of Agriculture, 2018; Washington State Employment Security Department, 2015).

Sexual harassment can have long-lasting and devastating physical and mental health effects. In addition to threats of bodily harm and physical impacts from perpetrators, there are long-lasting psychological and emotional health impacts. Symptoms to recognize are depression, grief, shame, withdrawal, and difficulty trusting others (Department of Labor, 2017). As one can imagine, in addition to the violence, these are stigmatizing experiences for farmworkers. Survivors face gossip, blame from others, ostracism, and often retaliation (Department of Labor, 2017). And farmworker women already experience double the rate of depression as compared to the general public (Okechuku et al., 2013; Waugh, 2010).

We formed the BASTA Coalition of Washington to prevent sexual harassment in agriculture and to improve the safety and security of the agricultural workplace and community. Our primary goal is developing a comprehensive prevention-based approach that involves key stakeholders across sectors (e.g., agriculture, law, human rights, academia, and public health) to promote community awareness, worksite training, and protective policies.

Q. What Are Some of the Achievements of the BASTA Coalition So Far?

In 2012, we heard directly from farmworkers and field outreach workers that farmworkers were experiencing daily trauma from rampant sexual harassment on the job. The following year, we launched an effort to learn more about this from farmworker women themselves in a state-funded, community-based participatory research-to-action project. After several focus group discussions, farmworkers joined us to develop a year-long media advocacy and educational campaign for farmworkers, supervisors, and growers in Yakima County, Washington. Themes for the campaigns were based on our shared analysis of the focus group data. In 2017, we created the Washington Coalition to Eliminate Farmworker Sexual Harassment (since renamed BASTA Coalition of Washington) to stay in touch with advocates, lawyers, farmworkers, and policymakers on what we could do together statewide to bring greater attention to this issue. In 2019, our academic and farmworker partners finalized the BASTA! Preventing Sexual Harassment in Agriculture curriculum and video, and it has been disseminated statewide to hundreds of people. In 2020, this curriculum received national recognition from the American Public Health Association (winning the Health Materials Award). You can learn more about it online (https://deohs.washington.edu/pnash/toolkit).

To bring greater attention to this curriculum and the need for mandatory sexual harassment training in the agricultural industry, in 2021 we proposed, lobbied for, and succeeded in receiving a 2-year budget proviso to fund a statewide program to prevent farmworker sexual harassment through peer training, including (1) peer-to-peer training and evaluation of sexual harassment training curriculum and (2) building a statewide network of peer trainers as farmworker leaders whose primary purpose is to prevent workplace sexual harassment and assault through leadership, education, and other tools.

Q. What Have Been Some of the Biggest Challenges You and the Coalition Have Faced?

There are a few challenges in addressing farmworker sexual harassment. We face the challenge of trying to unite a divided landscape between advocates and growers so that all see that this issue concerns everyone and that we can work together to address this. Also, there is a dearth of available funding to implement our programs so that change can be made and farmworker voices can be heard.

Q. What's One Piece of Advice You'd Like to Offer Emerging Advocates in Public Health?

Never give up! There are multiple ways to bring together stakeholders to understand the issue and your vision. Definitely make sure you have the support of a few policymakers on your team so that you can have a multilayered prevention strategy that includes policy change. Despite the challenge, continue to work in communities and promote effective programs and policies to achieve health equity for those who have not received the protections and services they deserve. Build power and support authentic community leadership by embracing cultural humility as you continue learning and integrating new perspectives.

References

Department of Labor. (2017). *National agricultural workers survey (2015–16)*. https://www.dol.gov/agencies/eta/national-agricultural-workers-survey

Human Rights Watch. (2012). *Cultivating fear: The vulnerability of immigrant farmworkers in the US to sexual violence and sexual harassment*. [16] https://www.hrw.org/report/2012/05/15/cultivating-fear/vulnerability-immigrant-farmworkers-us-sexual-violence-and#_ftn16

Okechuku, C. A., Souza, K., Davis, K. D., de Castro, A.B. (2013). Discrimination, harassment, abuse and bullying in the workplace: Contribution of workplace injustice to occupational health disparities. *American Journal of Industrial Medicine, 57*(5), 573–586.

Ramchandani, A. (2018, January 29). There's a sexual-harassment epidemic on America's farms. *The Atlantic*.

Washington State Department of Agriculture. (2018). *Agriculture—A cornerstone of Washington Economy*. https://agr.wa.gov/getmedia/7ffe2d19-b0d4-42b3-b870-4ed1992c5807/441a-fastfactswsdagen.pdf

Washington State Employment Security Department. (2015, May). 2013 Agricultural Workforce (p. 5).https://esd.wa.gov/labormarketinfo/ag-employment-and-wages

Waugh, I. M. (2010). Examining the sexual harassment experiences of Mexican immigrant farmworking women. *Violence Against Women, 16*(3), 237–261.

World Health Organization. (1948). *Preamble to the Constitution of World Health Organization, as adopted by the International Health Conference, New York, 19 June–22 July 1946*.

Community Organization

JENNIFER DISLA AND MOLLY FLEMING

Every moment is an organizing opportunity, every person a potential
activist, every minute a chance to change the world.

—DOLORES HUERTA

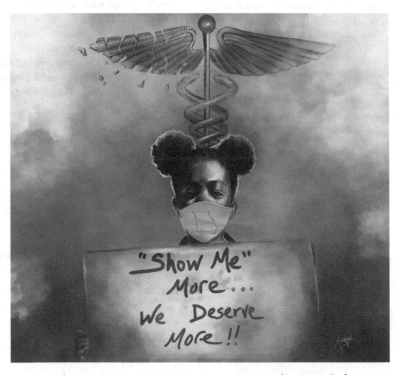

FIGURE 11.1 Artwork captures many Missourian's sentiments who struggle for access to affordable and quality healthcare.
Artist: Marquis Terrell.

Jennifer Disla and Molly Fleming, *Community Organization*. In: *Be the Change*. Edited by Keely S. Rees, Jody Early, and Cicily Hampton, Oxford University Press. © Oxford University Press 2023. DOI: 10.1093/oso/9780197570890.003.0011

Objectives

1. Define community organizing.
2. Compare five frameworks of organizing and their differing analyses and strategies to reach outcomes.
3. Synthesize the five organizing frameworks when applied in a case study.
4. Explain three core challenges in organizing toward health policy: challenges of collaboration, scaling leadership development, and fundraising.

INTRODUCTION

While health advocacy professionals are often guided by a strong sense of al-truism and can provide critical skills and expertise to health policy reform fights, few individuals directly impacted by health policy campaigns are present in their ranks. Millions of Americans choose between putting food on the table and buying prescription drugs or paying medical bills, but their struggles to balance health and welfare rarely influence political decision-making. Without directly impacted individuals, health advocacy can misunderstand the roots of a health crisis or may suggest policy solutions that cannot be accessed by the people who need them most. This chapter considers strategies to advance health policy grounded in communities directly impacted by health access barriers and health inequities through commu-nity organizing (Figure 11.1).

DEFINING COMMUNITY ORGANIZING

Community organizing as defined in Chapter 2 brings ordinary people together to have a say in the decisions that affect their lives. It is developing the leadership skills of grassroots volunteers and mobilizing large numbers of people into action, organizing works to build "people power" to influence decision-makers and create change. **Power**, in this context, is the ability to act. Power is organized people and organized money. Power is the ability to control, create, and, in some cases, prevent unwanted change. How people bring about that change is completely a choice of which tactics and strategy work best in the campaign.

In health policy organizing, many grassroots leaders are directly impacted by gaps and inequities in the nation's healthcare system. Some community leaders may be un-insured, others may have been bankrupted by exorbitant healthcare costs, while others may struggle to access quality mental healthcare. These individuals are united by a shared self-interest in the need to create change in health policy to improve the quality of their lives as well as the lives of others. While any one person harmed by the nation's cur-rent healthcare system may be entirely powerless on their own, community organizing provides a vehicle to take on the system and make it better.

For example, in the Healthcare for America Now Campaign in 2008, community and union organizations came together to change America's healthcare system. Many groups today advocate for universal healthcare systems; this national effort engaged grassroots community members across the country in listening sessions, education about healthcare policy, and massive get out the vote (GOTV) campaigns. Community organizing was not the only strategy to empower the ultimate passage of the Affordable Care Act (ACA), but it was a critical arc of strategy to empower national healthcare reform.

FIVE FRAMEWORKS OF ORGANIZING

There is no one way to organize. Rather, there are several ways to organize campaigns and communities to bring needed change. While there are nearly as many ways to organize as there are community organizers, we suggest five core frameworks for community organizing from which to consider goals, structure, and strategy (Figure 11.2). The frameworks differ vastly on the campaign goals and organizing methods.

Framework: Member Institutions

The first framework represents **member institutions** according to Bhargava (2020). The framework is grounded on a people orientation to power and specifically creating vehicles or containers to build long-term power. One example is unions. Unions use membership as their main organizing vehicle. The membership allows the organization to be fiscally self-sufficient. The goals of unions are to win either union elections (to build membership) or union contracts (to change work environments, both wage and conditions). The organizing methods in union organizing are recruitment, listening sessions, National

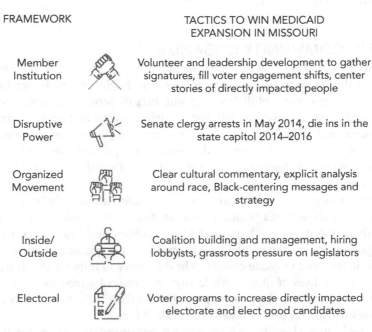

FRAMEWORK		TACTICS TO WIN MEDICAID EXPANSION IN MISSOURI
Member Institution		Volunteer and leadership development to gather signatures, fill voter engagement shifts, center stories of directly impacted people
Disruptive Power		Senate clergy arrests in May 2014, die ins in the state capitol 2014–2016
Organized Movement		Clear cultural commentary, explicit analysis around race, Black-centering messages and strategy
Inside/ Outside		Coalition building and management, hiring lobbyists, grassroots pressure on legislators
Electoral		Voter programs to increase directly impacted electorate and elect good candidates

FIGURE 11.2 The five frameworks of organizing Medicaid expansion in Missouri.
Source: Molly Fleming.

Labor Relations Board (NLRB) election, and building grassroots leaders. Similarly, community organizations utilize this framework as well.

- Goal: Policy demands are specific, immediate, winnable. Issues are chosen and defined in terms of "self-interest."
- Example: Pass a living wage ordinance, clean up a vacant lot, union election or contract.
- Method: 1-1 recruitment, listening sessions, membership organizations that are financially self-sustainable; NLRB election; democratic structure; development of grassroots leaders; "resource mobilization."
- What it means to win: Demands are wholly or partly achieved; organization is stronger at the end of the campaign than at the beginning and gets "credit" for the win.

Framework: Disruptive Power

Another framework is **disruptive power** (Bhargava, 2020). The framework is grounded on short-term power building without necessarily building long-term institutions. A recent example is the Black Lives Matter movement. The organizing method is a loose network of movement activists whose main focus is generating disruption. The organizing method is vastly different from the member institutions for it does not center on the organizer. Rather, it is not orchestrated by organizers with grand strategy. These tend to be short strategic wins such as creating a crisis around mass unemployment or deaths among people living with HIV/AIDS: Elites respond out of fear of losing power. Activities include and are not limited to bringing impacted communities to decision makers' homes/offices or taking over street intersections through civil disobedience.

- Goals: Less policy driven; focus is on forcing a response to a broad set of grievances through raising tension/disruption.
- Method: Loose network of movement activists whose main focus is on generating disruption—rather than on building organizational structures at times of social unrest; NOT orchestrated by organizers with grand strategy.
- What it means to win: Mass disruption and civil unrest results in major concessions from elites to restore order.

Framework: Organized Movement

Additionally, the **organized movement** framework according to Bhargava (2020) is centered on a systematic, premeditated campaign to move major pillars of society to support a deep change in social policy over the long term using a wide range of tactics. This framework is grounded on long-term social–economic narrative. Unlike disruptive power, the organized movement framework has a deeply rooted strategy. Examples include the civil rights movement and marriage equality movement.

- Goals: Big, overarching goal that is not winnable in the short term; may take 10 or 20 years to achieve. Demand seems outlandish at first, then becomes mainstream.

- Methods: Systematic, premeditated campaign to move major pillars of society—business, legal, faith, culture, youth—to support a deep change in social policy over the long term using a wide range of tactics.
- What it means to win: Often after many years of losses, new social consensus is achieved—and is ratified in public policy through the courts or legislation.

Framework: Inside/Outside Strategies

Furthermore, the **inside/outside strategies** framework according to Bhargava (2020) includes coalition-building development around specific policy goals and targets, orchestrated between "insiders" and "outsiders." This framework calls for both power building from within the system and pressure from outside influences. Examples are Health Care for America Now, Fight for $15, and campaigns around rent control in New York City. In this strategic framework, both grasstops and grassroots leaders are engaged in the campaign. Grasstop leaders are those who are heads of organizations, such as faith leaders and grassroots would be their congregation. While utilizing the inside strategy to move stakeholders, like politicians, toward the campaign goal and then putting pressure on the stakeholder with grassroot power, groups are able to win on healthcare issues.

- Goals: Win a concrete, major policy reform in a medium-term time horizon when the balance of forces is nearly equally divided.
- Methods: Coalition building; development of specific policy goals and targets; orchestration between insiders and outsiders.
- What it means to win: Win major policy campaigns delivering significant social change.

Framework: Electoral Strategy

The last framework described by Bhargava (2020) is the **electoral strategy**. This framework is grounded in engaging with the political system and building power by implementing policy and connecting directly with legislators. Examples are the Working Families Party, Rainbow Coalition, and Steve Philips "New American Majority." The organizing method is political party building, electoral mobilization, negotiation among social movements, organizational leaders on priority setting, and aligned action. This strategy has goals to provide a broad, multi-issue platform developed by a combination of social movement, organizational, and party leadership.

- Goals: Broad, multi-issue platform developed by a combination of social movement, organizational, party leadership: State power to enact the agenda is the goal.
- Methods: Political party building; electoral mobilization; negotiation among social movement, organizational leaders on priority setting, aligned action.
- What it means to win: Capture of state power, enactment of governing agenda, stability/growth in party membership.

There can be a default to put these five frameworks into competition—trying to determine which model of organizing is "right" (Table 11.1). However, these frameworks, in

TABLE 11.1 Five Organizing Frameworks

	Organization/Structure	Disruptive Power/Movement Without Design	Momentum-Driven Organizing/Pillars/Movement With Design	Electoral Strategies to Take State Power	Inside/Outside Strategies
Examples: historical and contemporary, including from readings	Unions, community organizations: Congress of Industrial Organizations (CIO), Alinsky's IAF Organizations, Student Nonviolent Coordinating Committee (SNCC); SEIU; MTR NY; Sierra Club; United Auto Workers	ACT UP (AIDS Coalition to Unleash Power)/AIDS movement (1980s/1990s); welfare rights movement (1960s/1970s); unemployed councils (1930s); Occupy Wall Street (2011); Movement for Black Lives	Englers: Civil rights movement Marriage equality movement Serbian freedom struggle	Working Families Party (NYC) Workers Party (Brazil) Harold Washington (Chicago) Rainbow Coalition Steve Phillips: "New American Majority"	Health Care for America Now (HCAN); Campaign to Pass Obamacare; Fight for 15; Recent New York City and New York State campaigns to close Rikers and pass rent control
Goals	Policy demands are specific, immediate, winnable Issues are chosen and defined in terms of "self-interest" Example: pass a living wage ordinance, clean up a vacant lot, union election or contract	Less policy driven; focus is on forcing a response to a broad set of grievances through raising tension/disruption Example: create a crisis around mass unemployment or deaths among people with AIDS—elites respond out of fear	Big, overarching goal that is not winnable in short term—may take 10 or 20 years to achieve; demand seems outlandish at first, then becomes mainstream Example: marriage equality, women's suffrage	Broad, multi-issue platform developed by a combination of social movement, organizational, party leadership—state power to enact the agenda is the goal Example: platform of the Rainbow Coalition	Win a concrete, major policy reform in a medium-term time horizon when the balance of forces is nearly equally divided Example: campaign to pass Affordable Care Act
Organizing methods	1-1 recruitment, listening sessions, membership organizations that are financially self-sustainable; NLRB election; develop grassroots leaders; "resource mobilization"	Loose network of movement activists whose main focus is on generating disruption—rather than on building organizational structures at times of social unrest; NOT orchestrated by organizers with grand strategy	Systematic, premeditated campaign to move major pillars of society—business, legal, faith, culture, youth—to support a deep change in social policy over long term using a wide range of tactics	Political party building; electoral mobilization; negotiation among social movement, organizational leaders on priority setting, aligned action	Coalition building; development of specific policy goals and targets; orchestration between "insiders" and "outsiders"
Examples of theorists/practitioners	Saul Alinsky, John L. Lewis, A. Phillip Randolph, Mary Kay Henry, Theda Skocpol	Frances Fox Piven, George Wiley, Occupy, Movement for Black Lives	Ella Baker, Evan Wolfson, King, Gandhi, Cesar Chavez, Englers	Anthony Thigpenn, Dan Cantor, AOC, DSA, Workers Party (Brazil), Podemos (Spain)	Heather Booth, Bayard Rustin, Frances Perkins

collaboration, are a powerful force to win victories in health advocacy, as seen in the upcoming section. Advocacy groups know that opponents tackle issues from all sides, and groups must be prepared to be ready on all fronts.

CASE STUDY: MEDICAID EXPANSION IN MISSOURI

While the state motto of Missouri is "let the welfare of the people be the supreme law," ordinary Missourians are all but ignored in the policy decisions that affect the quality and longevity of their lives. The very people who should be at the forefront of defining public debate on health policy often cannot get a meeting with their legislators, and the state General Assembly rarely addresses the quality, accessibility, or the affordability of healthcare. Community organizing is a direct response to this inaction—an attempt to correct a power imbalance in Missouri that has devastated its collective health, welfare, and political empowerment (Woolf & Schoomaker, 2017).

The 2010 passage of the ACA expanded eligibility for state Medicaid programs up to 138% of the federal poverty level, about $36,000 for a single parent with three children. The eligibility limit was 22% of the federal poverty level, or $5,550 for a single parent with two children. Childless, nondisabled adults have been deemed ineligible. Research at the time suggested that state expansion would cover at least 230,000 uninsured Missourians, likely saving 300 lives a year according to Woolf and colleagues (2017). But while Medicaid expansion was originally a requirement of the ACA, the June 2012 Supreme Court ruling in *National Federation of Independent Business v. Sebelius* effectively made expansion an option for states. Despite the federal government footing the majority of the cost, the Missouri legislature did not indicate intent to expand eligibility for Medicaid. Missouri's Medicaid eligibility limit remains one of the lowest in the nation. Community-based organizations came together and organizing to expand Medicaid began.

To challenge power imbalances in Missouri and achieve progressive health policy outcomes, community organizations in Missouri have been working together for over a decade to coordinate strategic multicycle and multistrategy campaigns. In doing so, they have utilized each of the five community organizing frameworks previously explored in this chapter.

Member institutions have been at the forefront of the decades-long fight to increase access to quality, affordable healthcare in Missouri. As organizations in deep relationship with directly impacted uninsured Missourians, member institutions have made Medicaid expansion a priority. Organizing a solidarity-based community of workers, Missouri Jobs With Justice recognized the gaps in employer-based healthcare coverage, especially for working class people. For the Missouri Rural Crisis Center, the closure of rural hospitals was a dire threat to the health of rural people—and resources from Medicaid expansion might keep those hospitals open. And as their membership base experienced higher rates of chronic disease and early death than the general population—especially as COVID-19 ravaged communities—the Organization for Black Struggle was an early and ongoing leader in the fight to expand Medicaid.

As they worked together on this shared policy priority, each organizing institution also developed its own power building goals to achieve through this campaign: developing leadership, building a membership base, and growing organizational credentials. As the need for access to healthcare in Missouri transcended race and geography, the campaign to expand Medicaid also afforded the opportunity for organizations from both urban and rural communities to come together to organize for policy that would improve lives across their membership bases. Under the leadership of Jamala Rogers of the Organization for Black Struggle and Rhonda Perry of the Missouri Rural Crisis Center, grassroots organizations across Missouri gathered in a series of Black/rural summits to sharpen clarity about shared fights and to make plans to win together.

In the years immediately following the passage of the ACA, organizations in Missouri developed an **Inside/Outside** strategy grounded in a cross-sector coalition committed to pass Medicaid expansion through the state legislature. The coalition developed a bilegislative strategy, hiring "under-the-dome" lobbyists working in strategic coordination with community organizations engaging legislators and the public in-district.

When hyperpartisan ideological opposition to "Obamacare" doomed a straight path to Medicaid expansion through the state legislature, member institutions then took on a **disruptive power** approach. In 2014 and 2015, they organized escalating direct actions with the goal of raising tension in the state capitol and—if the legislature would not be moved—organizing in the court of public opinion. Tactics included "die ins," capitol protests, and civil disobedience, which led to the arrest of 23 clergy during Senate proceedings. Many of these disruptive actions included demands beyond Medicaid expansion and broader culture shift priorities, like Black Lives Matter.

Membership institutions then turned to the citizens' initiative process, an **electoral** strategy by which Missourians can gather signatures in order to place a policy directly on the ballot for a public vote. Largely through the grassroots bases built by member institutions, a new coalition gathered 340,000 signatures to qualify Medicaid expansion for the ballot and then launched a large-scale GOTV program to ensure turnout and support in the electorate. And in keeping with their goals as member institutions, these Missouri organizations drove their electoral strategy by building volunteer capacity, developing community leaders, and growing their organizational powerbase. Ultimately, Amendment 2—as the Medicaid expansion initiative was named on the ballot—won on the 2020 August primary ballot by a six-point margin according to Smith (2020). Though the legislature had failed to act, community organizing won healthcare for over 2300,000 Missourians.

Though the primary strategy to win expansion policy was electoral, member institutions incorporated **organized movement** strategies as well. As politically opportunistic populist messaging, tinged with racist rhetoric, has gained traction in Missouri, electoral outcomes and voter preferences have shifted. Through the leadership of Black-led organizations like Action St. Louis and the Organization for Black Struggle, Missouri's organizing groups advanced new race-forward narratives to grow support for Medicaid expansion while working toward a shift in electoral preferences and the power of racialized dog whistles. Member institutions continue to work collaboratively to achieve Medicaid implementation while keeping organized movement culture-shift strategies at the forefront of goals. And as the state legislature tried to slow down implementation, these organizations ultimately returned to inside/outside strategies in the capitol, with a broad coalition, hired lobbyists, and bipartisan engagement strategies.

The work of collaborative community organizing to expand Medicaid for over 230,000 Missourians is a success story that showcases the value of each of the five frameworks to achieve progressive health policy. However, Missouri community organizations are clear that nothing short of a political transformation will put the health and well-being of Missourians at the top of the state's policy agenda. That transformation will require many years of coordinated organizing campaigns that engage the very people that the state's health and economic policies impact. They are committed to a long-term social justice agenda utilizing strategies across the five frameworks to shift Missouri's policy landscape and continue to win more radical and impactful reforms.

COMMON CHALLENGES IN HEALTH POLICY ORGANIZING

Organizing is hard work, and most community organizers lose far more fights than they win. Below we summarize three challenges that commonly impact organizational sustainability and policy victories.

Emergent strategy is a framework Adrienne Marie Brown (2017) described as the way in which "complex systems and patterns arise out of a multiplicity of relatively simple interactions" (p. 3). Emergent strategy, she further posited, is "how we intentionally change in ways that grow our capacity to embody the just and liberated worlds we long for" (p. 3). Brown provides concepts that help explain the internal culture of movements, including the need to create deep relationships in movement building. This is a challenge in most organizations. Organizers, leaders, and community members are not encouraged to create authentic relationships, but may lean into transactional relationships. However, true, meaningful relationships are essential to build the world we want to see; the interconnectedness in community organizing and building authentic relationships is evident in the Missouri case study.

Another challenge is leadership development at scale. This is important for member institutions and organizations looking to develop long-term strategy. Long-term strategy calls for community members to be committed to long-view plans. In order to have strong leadership, as discussed previously, you must commit to authentic relationships. Most organizations do not have the capacity for organizers to have more than 100–150 deep member relationships. As organizing evolves, organizations lean on their member-leaders to hold relationships. This is the challenge: How do organizations mobilize people beyond collecting signatures during a ballot initiative and educate and develop, with minimal resources, leaders to build a movement? The most progessive organizations lean into this question, while others respond to the nonprofit complex to meet measurable outcomes and goals. This remains a tension.

More often than not, grassroots community organizations are nonprofits that need to raise revenues to afford staff, rent, travel, and the other daily expenses of keeping an organization running. In difficult situations, the amount of change an organization can empower is limited by its funding. The corporate and legacy foundations that are most likely to provide large-scale grants that can support nonprofit organizations often exist within power structures that benefit from the status quo and that avoid investments in systemic change. Funding can be very narrowly programmatic, which can compromise organizing models away from member priorities and strategy in order to meet the "deliverables" promised to a funder. Some organizations have succeeded at raising general operating support from membership dues or large-scale grassroots fundraising campaigns to derive the bulk of their revenue from the community. Community-based revenue can liberate organizations to make community organizing the priority of an institution.

CONCLUSION

Community organizing puts people directly impacted by health policy at the center of taking action for health policy change. While its practice may not always directly lead to health policy victories, good community organizing also builds power for future campaigns and future victories. This chapter provided five frameworks of community organizing as a summary of the infinite strategies institutions can deploy, and the case study of expanding Medicaid in Missouri illustrates their practice. These frameworks can ultimately work in alignment to ensure the needs of directly impacted people are prioritized in health policy decisions. Though there are many challenges in this work, community organizing is a critical strategic consideration and component to any meaningful health policy campaign.

REFERENCES

Bhargava, D. (2020, October). *Power & strategy.* Harlem; virtual.

Brown, A. M. (2017). *Emergent strategy: Shaping change, changing worlds.* AK Press.

Smith, A. (2020, April 6). Did rural voters nearly sink Missouri Medicaid expansion or boost it to victory? [radio broadcast]. KCUR: NPR. https://www.kcur.org/ 2020-08-06/did-rural-voters-nearly-sink-missouri-medicaid-expansion-or-boost-it-to-victory

Woolf, S. H., & Schoomaker, H. (2019). Life Expectancy and Mortality Rates in the United States, 1959–2017. *JAMA, 322*(20), 1996–2016. https://doi.org/10.1001/jama.2019.16932

CHAPTER 11: END-OF-CHAPTER ACTIVITIES

DISCUSSION

1. How does building authentic relationships in the emergent strategy framework move the different organizing frameworks forward?

2. The five frameworks are grounded in what is strategically the best option for the given campaign. Which frameworks lean toward long-standing base building?

3. How does institutional building play a role in getting organizations to scale?

APPLICATION ACTIVITIES

1. Identify a local or campus issue to organize around in your community that impacts health outcomes (i.e., access to reproductive health, education on coping with stress, prevention for mental health issues, and so on). Once you have decided on the issues, consider the five frameworks and indicate what strategies you will use that relate to these frameworks. Do you think you will be able to move your issue forward successfully after thinking through the factors involved with each of these frameworks? Utilize the case study to gain perspective on which to apply to make your case.

2. Interview a local community organizer or watch or listen to a filmed or radio interview with a famous community organizer, such as Grace Lee Boggs; Martin Luther King, Jr.; Barack Obama; Shannon Watts; Dolores Huerta; Winona Duke; or Alicia Garza. What were the person's organizing goals, and what are two or three tactics or strategies they used to build a movement and achieve their organizing objectives?

ADDITIONAL RESOURCES

Brown, A. M. (n.d.). *Emergent strategy*. https://adr iennemareebrown.net/tag/emergent-strategy/

Building Movement Project. (n.d.). *Alliances for change: Organizing change for the 21st century*. https://drive.google.com/file/d/17xYXvqZZ LSJsS3yLRo0-Aop2KgjtP2MD/view

Midwest Academy. (n.d.). *Training*. http://www. midwestacademy.com/training/

Pastor, M., Terriquez, V., & Lin, M. (2018). How community organizing promotes health equity, and how health equity affects organizing. *Health Affairs*, 3(3). https://www.healthaffa irs.org/doi/10.1377/hlthaff.2017.1285

QUIZ QUESTIONS

1. What are the five frameworks?

2. Define the member institution framework.

3. Which framework focuses on short-term activity and formation?

4. Name a group from the case study that helped with the inside/outside strategy.

5. Working Families Party is an example of
   a. organized movement framework
   b. inside/outside framework
   c. electoral framework
   d. all the above

6. The narrative changed in the Missouri case study. True or false?

7. Authentic relationships foster long-term organizing. True or false?

8. The inside/outside strategy was not used in the Missouri case study. True or false?

9. All five frameworks were used in the Missouri victory case example. True or false?

10. The tension between meeting deliverables and organizing to scale are
    a. nonprofit complex expectations
    b. expectations from community
    c. expectations from the urgent nature of the work
    d. all the above

ANSWER KEY

1. Member institution, disruptive power, electoral, inside/outside, organized movement.
2. Member institution is the framework grounded on a people orientation to power and specifically creating vehicles or containers to build long-term power.
3. Disruptive power.
4. Lobbyist.
5. C. Electoral framework.
6. True.
7. True.
8. False.
9. True.
10. A. Nonprofit complex expectations.

11.9 JENNIFER DISLA

Q1. What Led or Inspired You to Become Engaged in Advocacy— Specifically as It Relates to Policy Change and Public Health?

an issue that needed to be addressed with policy and people power. I also learned that it wasn't an issue only in my community. While working in rural Missouri, I was able to see its impact in rural communities.

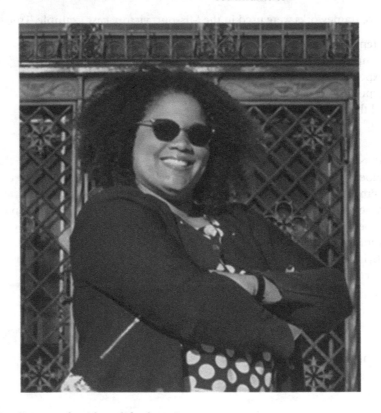

In 2008, I was diagnosed with a life-changing chronic medical condition. I was also faced with a medical bill that was over $10,000. I was already struggling to pay the rent, outpatient medical care, and student loans. Policy, especially around public health, was a lifeline for me. While working for the Healthcare for America Now Campaign, I realized that it was a systemic issue,

Q2. What Are the Issues or Advocacy-Related Projects You Are Working on Right Now?

I am currently working on ensuring electeds from federal to local understand the importance of housing, jobs, and the environment. Currently, I am strongly advocating for a Build Back Better Plan. The Build

Back Better Plan speaks to the human infrastructure that many poor Black and Brown communities needed prior to the pandemic. Families shouldn't have to face a crisis when a member gets sick or they need childcare. Communities shouldn't decide between rent and a prescription. We need more human infrastructure in our country. This needs to be only the beginning.

Q3. What Is One of Your Greatest Advocacy Triumphs or Successes?

My greatest triumph was in St. Louis. While working with Service Employees International Union Local 1, janitors were facing hardships at an Express Scripts facility. We partnered with shareholders, faith leaders, and workers to ensure that when Express Scripts showed support to Black Lives Matter movement, it's more than lip service. Over 100 Black families in St. Louis have access to healthcare, union wages, and protections at this facility.

Q4. What Have Been Some of the Biggest Challenges You Have Faced as It Relates to Your Advocacy Work?

The biggest challenge in the advocacy work is not having enough advocates. The bench is not deep.

In both recruiting and developing the pipeline for leadership, we struggle greatly. We are in a moment where we need bold leadership. We need advocates to think about new paradigms. Also, we need to reimagine the responsibility to advocate on public health issues. Public health impacts the entire community and threads through so many other social issues, like the prison industrial complex. How do we spread more awareness on public health policy needs to everyday people? Most importantly, how do we ensure they take action?

Q5. What's One Piece of Advice You'd Like to Offer Emerging Advocates in Public Health?

Emerging advocates, I encourage you to always center your work on the most impacted and remember their lived experiences. I carry the janitors' stories to every campaign room I am in or when meeting with a legislator. Also, take time to enjoy the beauty in life. This work is hard and a long haul. Change takes time; change is constant.

Media Advocacy and Social Marketing

CHRISTINA JONES AND JULIE COLEHOUR

Journalism is what maintains democracy. It's the force for progressive social change.

—ANDREW VACHSS

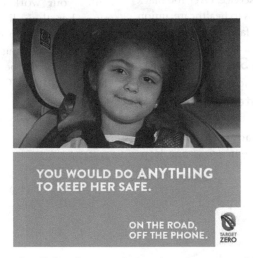

YOU WOULD DO **ANYTHING** TO KEEP HER SAFE.

ON THE ROAD, OFF THE PHONE.

FIGURE 12.1 On the Road, Off the Phone (n.d). Social marketing to address distracted driving in Washington.

Objectives

After reading this chapter, students will feel confident in their ability to
1. Explain the significance of media advocacy and social marketing in social change efforts.
2. Create stories about social change efforts that are likely to be covered by the media.
3. Identify good opportunities in the mass media for sharing your social change efforts.
4. Describe ways to establish trustful relationships with media sources and collaborators.
5. Apply the 10-step social marketing planning process to developing a health advocacy campaign.
6. Differentiate between the terms *media advocacy*, *social marketing*, and *social media*.

Christina Jones and Julie Colehour, *Media Advocacy and Social Marketing*. In: *Be the Change*. Edited by Keely S. Rees, Jody Early, and Cicily Hampton, Oxford University Press. © Oxford University Press 2023. DOI: 10.1093/oso/9780197570890.003.0012

INTRODUCTION

Take a brief moment to consider the time you have spent accessing the media so far today, prior to your reading of this textbook chapter. Have you flipped through the pages of a print or web-accessible newspaper? Did you catch a passing glimpse of the television news as you were preparing your breakfast this morning? How many times did you check your social media feed before you rolled out of bed? We can safely suggest that for most readers, the time you have spent with media so far today has already been quite substantial. While contemporary media consumers are exposed to a wide variety of messages about politics, health, and other current events each day, we far less consider the significant influence that said messages have on health policymaking, legislation, or even community-level support for public health efforts.

George Gerbner, a foundational media studies scholar, once noted that if you can tell a nation's stories, you do not have to worry about who makes its laws (Gerbner, 1992). While television was once considered the nation's most mainstream storyteller, the expansive network of contemporary new media (e.g., social media, digital and online communication) now paints a defined picture of what we, as attentive citizens, are to identify, discuss, and respond to as the most urgent and important issues to address. The act of painting this picture is the work of both **social marketing** and **media advocacy** in deciding what picture to paint and when/where/how to disseminate the picture. When used in conjunction, both media advocacy and social marketing can be used to inform the public in cases where awareness is lacking, to motivate behavior for personal and public good, and to change viewpoints to help guide policy decisions. It is within this context that media advocacy and social marketing are powerful tools for social change.

WHAT IS MEDIA ADVOCACY?

Wallack and colleagues (1993) defined **media advocacy** as "the strategic use of mass media to support community organizers' efforts to advance social or public health policies" (p. 2). Most health communication is crafted with the aim of influencing an intended audience to be persuaded to reduce their risk for illness or injury by providing useful health information or persuasive health messages. In this, individuals themselves serve as the receiver of the communication; information is often provided in a top-down manner. Media advocacy, however, is less about conveying health content to the masses. Instead, media advocacy seeks to encourage community mobilization and the sharing of voices to influence policy and systems change. Media advocacy seeks to even the media playing field by providing community organizations and health advocates with the principles and tools for telling their own stories to the public.

Media advocates work to simultaneously obtain the media's attention while increasing the possibility that the stories told by the media reflect and support the best efforts of public health advocates. In this, media advocacy is a powerful source of influence in encouraging public discourse and debate on public health social change efforts, and, if constructed strategically, media advocacy can be the driving force behind the pressure for policymaking and policy change. For example, Niederdeppe et al. (2007) suggested that the media awareness efforts implemented as part of the Florida Tobacco Control Program were effective in generating news coverage and promoting the passage of the tobacco product placement ordinances, which seek to remove the visual availability of cigarettes by requiring retailers to place tobacco products behind the counter. The study found that a one-unit increase in news coverage regarding pro-policy efforts was associated with a 94% increase in the odds of counties enacting a product placement ordinance.

AGENDA-SETTING THEORY AND MEDIA FRAMING

While media advocacy is a cross-disciplinary practice, with connections in political science, communication studies, and linguistics, the primary theoretical foundation for the study and application of media advocacy rests in the academic discipline of mass communication and media studies. More specifically, media advocacy is driven by two important theoretical concepts: **agenda setting** and **framing**.

Advocates interested in policy change pay close attention to the mass media, largely under the premise that the mass media significantly contributes to what issues we (as a public) think about and how we think about them. Agenda setting is what you accomplish when you influence what the media covers (media agenda) and what people talk about (public agenda) (McCombs & Shaw, 1972; Rogers & Dearing, 1988). More simply, agenda setting suggests that the more coverage and attention an issue receives in the media, the more importance it is given by the public.

It is commonly understood that the public and policymakers do not consider issues to be worthy of attention, or changes worthy of address, unless they are visible in the public domain, and mass media attention is a significant indication of the presence of the issue in broader discourse. For example, Dixon and colleagues (2014) examined the influence of news media coverage of tanning and skin cancer on tanning attitudes and perceptions in a sample of over 6,000 adults, including support for tanning-related policy change. The analysis found that higher potential exposure to news supportive of sun protection was associated with reduced pro–tan attitudes and increased perceived susceptibility to skin cancer. Thus, media advocacy is connected to agenda setting in its focus on ensuring that the mass media attends to (and covers) the issues deemed as significant to a social change effort. Policy change is unlikely to occur if the media fails to recognize the importance of the issue as part of its agenda.

When covering stories, journalists select certain arguments, examples, images, messages, and sources to create a picture of the issue. This selection, or omission, of arguments and voices functions similarly to a frame around a photograph, telling us what information is important and what information we can ignore. Framing argues that the mass media helps to shape the perceived reality of audiences, influencing not only the issues media consumers think about, but also how they think about these issues. In this, the media can affect audience decision-making on matters of public policy and encourage particular conclusions about social phenomena (Fairhurst & Sarr, 1996).

Jashinsky et al. (2017) investigated the national news media's framing of gun violence following a mass shooting. Using the Sandy Hook mass shooting in December 2012 as their case of analysis, the investigators analyzed 375 stories, appearing both before and after the shooting, reported by the *New York Times, Washington Post,* and *Wall Street Journal.* The authors found that individuals were held responsible for gun violence in 63% of pieces before the shooting, yet after the shooting, only 32% of the pieces framed individuals as responsible. Lawmakers were held responsible in 30% of pieces before and 66% after. Additionally, background checks were a proposed gun violence prevention method in 18% of pieces before the shooting, yet 55% of the stories after Sandy Hook proposed background checks as a prevention measure. In this, the authors concluded that following a mass shooting, the media tended to hold the government as primarily responsible for the violence, rather than individuals. The implications for this framing on advancing gun safety policy at the national level are far-reaching. In the context of media advocacy, health and community advocates frame and reframe their issues in hopes that a new presentation will change existing attitudes.

USING MEDIA ADVOCACY AS A SOCIAL CHANGE ADVOCATE

It is clear that the media can increase the public's awareness of issues—about who and what really contribute to health problems, community deterioration, or the choices that individuals make about the behaviors that affect their health and well-being. The media can inform the community of what you are doing and what you have done. Moreover, the media can portray your group and the issues you are standing for in a positive light to the public, or, conversely, the media can portray your opponents in a negative light. You can use the media to pressure policymakers to change or institute policies that affect health and community development and to influence the media to give your organization or coalition extensive coverage, allowing your members to tell their stories in their own words. Media advocacy mobilizes community activities, focusing on collective voices, with the goal of equitable power distribution and social change.

As just one example, although the #Blacklivesmatter hashtag was created in July 2013, it was rarely used through the summer of 2014 and did not come to signify a movement until months after the Ferguson protests (Freelon et al., 2016). On November 24, St. Louis County prosecutor Robert McCullough announced that a grand jury had decided not to indict Darren Wilson for the death of Michael Brown. The previous day, the hashtag appeared in 2,309 tweets; but on that day, the total soared several orders of magnitude to 103,319. Closer inspection of the timing of that day's tweets revealed that 90% of them were posted between the hours of 8 p.m. and midnight central time, coinciding with McCullough's announcement and its immediate aftermath. It is clear that the media can give communities more control by letting public entities who might not otherwise be heard have a clear, unified, and powerful voice in the media. Shining the spotlight on a community can give its members the power and the desire to change the policies and situations that affect their lives.

DEVELOPING YOUR MEDIA ADVOCACY STRATEGY

Just like a political campaign, a media advocacy campaign requires considerable planning and strategic thinking. As you prepare for a media advocacy effort, it is necessary to consider how you will engage in your business with the media and what objectives you hope to achieve throughout that engagement. There are a number of tools and strategies that help in your planning process. However, begin by asking the questions that follow to help guide the development of your media advocacy strategy.

What Is the Best Way to Reach Your Target—The News or Something Else?

Gaining the attention of the public can be a difficult endeavor, particularly in today's crowded message environment. To build attention surrounding your issue or organization, you must consider which of the following tools will be best in attracting the public's eye. What you choose depends on what you have to say, who you want to say it, and, in most cases, what resources you have available. Your choice will largely dictate how you go about engaging with the media as well. One option might include the use of the **news media**, often called **earned media**. Encouraging radio, television, or newspaper journalists to take interest in your issue is one method for providing your perspective. In most cases, information presented in the news is considered highly credible; however, your story is competing with the other "beats" of the day.

Strong connections with the media helps to ensure that your story is featured. Another option might include a **public service announcement**, or PSA. PSAs are free as broadcasting stations use them to fulfill a broader regulation to serve the greater good of the public, and they are used to efficiently convey important information about an issue to the public. However, PSAs are usually very short, and they are often aired whenever the media outlet has extra time to fill—entailing some loss of control. They also cannot address immediate news. Alternatively, **press conferences** are media events in which a representative from your organization presents a statement about something newsworthy and answers questions from invited media outlets. However, while one can invite a number of media representatives to a press conference, there is no guarantee that the media representatives will attend or cover the content that is presented.

Last, **paid media** entails the creation of advertisements that require payment. This might include a paid editorial, a social media "boost" to a post, or out-of-home advertising, like a billboard. In return, one maintains greater control over the places that the ads run, the times that the ads run, and the creative design of the ads. However, paid media is often very costly and requires expertise and resources across creative design and marketing strategy.

What Is Your Message Strategy?

A critical component of your advocacy campaign will be formulating the messages to communicate your policy perspectives to those individuals who are responsible for making changes that will help you reach your goals. Choosing the correct story elements entails selecting those pieces of information that are likely to garner the attention of the media, from an interesting fact to a compelling story from a community member. It is important to develop messages that will resonate with your target audience, encouraging an emotional and intellectual connection with the issue that will move them to action. You might also consider who you want to deliver the information: Would it be useful to include a spokesperson with expertise or an everyday citizen who has a lived experience to share? Strategies for writing stories that news journalists will cover are provided in the next section.

When Might Media Attention Influence Public Perceptions or Policymaking the Most?

While multiple opportunities for engaging with the media might present themselves, selecting an appropriate time to begin your media advocacy effort should be grounded in your overall program strategy and aims. Of course, one should ensure that they possess the appropriate resources, time, and personnel to invest in managing a media campaign before initiating contact with media representatives. Media coverage can be a two-way street; while positive coverage can help an organization or effort, an organization should be prepared to react appropriately and refocus the message should the coverage not be what was expected. The Community Tool Box, a community engagement resource for public health practitioners from the Center for Community Health and Development at the University of Kansas (Community Tool Box, 2021), suggested that good times to engage with the media might include

- *When you are ready to announce a new project.* For example, you may want to recruit more funders to your organization, and publicity given to your effort is a good way to alert the public to your current needs.
- *When you have information that can be tied to community news.* Perhaps your community is grieving after an automobile accident where a child was hit while riding their bike without a helmet. You can tie your efforts to encourage the development of bike trails in your community with news of the accident currently reported in your local paper.
- *When publicity might mean the difference between meeting your goals and your opponent's achieving theirs.* If those against your effort are presented with their own opportunity to tie their viewpoint to a community event, you may want to sway the attention of the media to your side.
- *When your issue presents a crisis*, but community members lack awareness of the depth of the issue. Nursing home residents may be suffering at the hands of poor management and care, but the situation can be invisible to community members without media coverage.
- *When a policy or law you support or disagree with is up for decision and media coverage might significantly influence the outcome.*
- *When you've been successful.* Coverage that focuses on your organization's success can also increase positive perceptions of your work and its influence on the community (Community Tool Box, 2021).

WRITING STORIES THAT THE MEDIA WILL COVER

As noted in previous parts of this chapter, the use of paid media (advertising) for media advocacy in social change efforts is far less common today. Rather, media advocacy efforts work to gain publicity through promotional efforts where space or attention can be earned rather than bought outright. However, the term "earned" entails effort. Media advocacy that seeks to gain attention through means other than paid time must think creatively to sway the interest of media representatives. In the event that you do not have a breaking story to share, you have to make your own news. That often means that you might need to use your imagination to give boring facts or figures and older news a brighter, fresh perspective. A number of strategies for earning media attention are presented below:

- *Choose good media opportunities:* Local/regional events can tie in well to your organization's work, and holidays and other special days may provide a good backdrop to your viewpoint. For example, in October 2018, during national breast cancer awareness month, breast cancer advocates succeeded in lobbying for the passing of "Right to Try" legislation, which provided those diagnosed with a terminal illness greater autonomy in choosing their treatment path (Right to Try, 2020).

- *Present a breakthrough:* What is new or different about this story? One example could be a story on the isolation of a dangerous virus or a new treatment for a disease or birth defect.

- *Attach your effort to a celebrity-supported story or event:* Is there a famous or locally well-known person already with or willing to lend his or her name to the issue? The untimely passing of actor Chadwick Bosemen in August 2020 after a 4-year battle with colon cancer brought a spotlight to the disease, encouraging young adults to alter their perceptions of this form of cancer as something reserved for older adults only. Shortly thereafter, the U.S. Preventive Services Task Force suggested that Americans should begin screening for colon cancer at age 45, not 50, because of an increase in colon cancer among younger adults (Tanne, 2020).

- *Make it a controversy:* Are there opposing sides or conflicts in this story? In the context of the COVID-19 pandemic, a number of media stories reported on the effectiveness of mask wearing as a preventive mechanism for stopping the spread of the disease. Many of these reports painted mask wearing as a controversial issue, focusing on how some citizens protested that their personal freedoms were being infringed on by being told to cover their mouths and noses, while others masked up whenever they left their homes.

- *Right a wrong:* Are there basic inequalities or unfair circumstances to be reported? Health policy advocates focused on issues of health disparity and social justice have long called for racial equity reform based on significant disparities in mortality rates across racial groups. Bringing these inequities to light can result in significant media attention. In the United States, for example, Black women with breast cancer are 40% more likely to die than White women today, even though no such disparity existed 40 years ago. Such disparities have been used to support policies that encourage the collection of better data on the root causes of sickness to better track inequities in cancer care and accelerate reform in clinical trial enrollment and overall survivorship (Whyte, 2020).

- *Make it local:* Why is this story important or meaningful to local residents? Increasing national COVID-19 prevalence rates often took secondary consideration for many local media reporters, who instead chose to focus on the impact of the pandemic on local hospitals and state healthcare systems.

CHANGING MEDIA PERSPECTIVES ON AN ISSUE

In some cases, it may be necessary to generate new media attention to your issue. However, in other situations, the media may have reported some (or much) news on your issue, but perhaps the news is not helpful to your effort. When engaging with the media regarding your policy or social cause of interest, it may be the case that the media does not accurately represent a truth, feature the voices of all relevant audiences, or present the issue in a light that fits your organization's agenda. The media often frames community issues by turning facts and scientific evidence into human interest stories that resonate more closely with their audience. In some cases, this framing may not accurately represent the issue at hand.

For example, instead of writing a story that gives the statistics regarding the total number of sexual assault cases reported at a local college, the media may instead present a picture of a sexual assault survivor who successfully coped with the physical and/or psychological impact of that violence. This imagery fails to consider the countless other victims who struggle with recovery. As a sexual assault prevention advocate, you would need to work to change the media's viewpoint.

One suggested principle to use in changing the media's perspective is to reframe the issue itself in your presentation of that content to the media. The media frequently features and empathizes with the struggles of just one person. Zhang et al. (2016), in their content analysis of print and broadcast media coverage of depression, found that the media presented individuals as more to blame for mental health challenges than social influences. In the rapid media environment, where stories are often very brief (just 30 seconds in some television news media reports), the focus on the struggle itself might disregard the broader complexity in how the community and policy have contributed to that person's situation as well as the best methods for changing the system. The media may not stress the need for community participation to change public health and social conditions, but community input is a significant element of participatory social change.

By bringing the conversation back (as frequently as needed) to basic themes that are easily understood and accepted by the public, rather than the story of just one individual, the media advocate may find success in drawing the public's attention to the bigger social issue at hand. Themes like personal safety, patriotism, fairness, and family are often widely accepted, while drawing attention to violence, oppression, cheating, and lying on behalf of your opposition. The general principle here is to focus your recommendations on community and policy rather than on the personal or individual. Refrain from the inclusion of too many individual stories (e.g., "How Amy overcame her alcohol addiction") in place of a recognition of the sociocultural impact of the community on the broader health narrative (e.g., "How the absence of drug addiction and recovery programs in the community influences the increasing rate of lifelong alcoholism").

SPECIAL CONSIDERATIONS: ESTABLISHING TRUST WITH THE MEDIA

Media representatives have to believe that what you tell them is true, or at least the truth as far as you know it. They can't stake their reputations on stories that aren't accurate or on facts that haven't been checked carefully. Be trustworthy. Always tell the truth to the media. It's best to be polite about it and to imply that you'll talk about the subject when you can. ("I am sorry, but I cannot comment on that right now.") Make sure you have the facts before you make a statement. If you do not have the answer to a question, promise to get it and get back to the reporter with it and do.

Last, alert the media to stories relating to your issue that they might be interested in. These include human interest stories, awards or funding given to your organization, information about the issue itself (a national initiative relating to it, e.g., or new statistics issued about it), or local or national events (an open house or fundraising concert, a national day devoted to the issue). Your help is a gesture that builds goodwill with the media, and in time, a strong relationship can entail the positive coverage your issue needs to find success.

WHAT IS SOCIAL MARKETING, AND WHY IS IT IMPORTANT FOR CHANGING BEHAVIORS FOR GOOD?

Social marketing is a discipline that seeks to change behaviors for the good of society, communities, and people. Said in a simpler way, it is changing behaviors for good. The practice of social marketing is built on a significant base of research that shows awareness and education alone rarely change behaviors. In order to create meaningful, sustainable behavior change, social marketing must use strategies that aim to overcome barriers and provide people with personal, relevant motivators to act. This approach increases the efficiency and effectiveness of marketing efforts by identifying the specific behaviors that must change to achieve a program's goals, segmenting audiences based on who has the highest probability of changing the desired behavior, identifying the barriers preventing the behavior and the benefits to the audience, and the motivators that are most likely to overcome barriers and spur change (Box 12.1).

It is often assumed that social marketing only employs communications strategies to change behavior when, in fact, the main premise of social marketing is to use a strategic planning process to determine the tools that will have the biggest impact on spurring desired behavior changes. The social marketer's tools include strategies such as incentives, policy changes, social diffusion, feedback, commitments, and also often communications. But communications is not always a part of the mix or might just compliment other strategies. For example, dog poop pickup programs learned early on that a key barrier for dog owners was forgetting to bring a bag. Dog owners knew what the correct behavior was and did not need to be convinced. The installation of signage and bag receptacles on trails and in parks is an example of overcoming this barrier by providing a prompt and the needed tool in convenient locations. Communication tools were not needed in this social marketing mix.

SOCIAL MARKETING PLANNING PROCESS

Creating a social marketing strategy can be achieved by following a prescribed process that allows you to make deliberate decisions about the framework of your program. The process relies on using research and other strategies to narrow your approach to what will be most effective in achieving your program's goals.

| ADVOCACY IN ACTION BOX 12.1 | Social Marketing to Address Distracted Driving in Washington |

With the rise of smartphones and social media, distracted driving has become an increasing concern. Many states that had been seeing decreasing trends in traffic-related fatalities have started seeing deaths and serious injury increasing largely due to people interacting with their phones while behind the wheel. According to the National Highway Traffic Safety Administration, cell phones now cause 1 in 4 crashes and 3 in 10 crash fatalities. People are three times more likely to crash while using a cell phone due to slowed reaction time, reduced peripheral vision, and less focus on speed and following distance. Their research showed that drivers on cell phones are as dangerous as a drunk driver that registers a 0.08 on a breathalyzer test.

Communities across the country have begun to address this issue using a variety of social marketing interventions. In most cases, policy and law changes combined with communications approaches have been used to influence the behavior of cell phone use in cars. In Washington State, the Washington Traffic Safety Commission launched the state's new distracted driving law in July 2017. They created the "On the Road, Off the Phone" social marketing campaign to make all Washington drivers aware of the new law and its consequences. The On the Road, Off the Phone campaign content is featured as the introductory photo of this chapter.

The initial campaign focused on trying to reach all Washington drivers. It was created in seven different languages and included advertising, media

advocacy, a media event with Washington's governor at the state capitol, and a partner toolkit.

The launch campaign was followed with a targeted cross-cultural distracted driving campaign targeting moms with young children. Research showed a primary motivator for female drivers who were also parents was to role model good behavior for their children. Using these insights, campaign messaging focused on speaking to the protective instinct of mothers. The strategy focused on identifying a universal moment that moms can connect to, which is that first ride home with their child as a baby not only connecting with their strong feeling of protecting their newborn but also connecting the idea of not using their phone as the continuation of their protection of their child. This campaign was created in English and Spanish using a process called transcreation to ensure that cultural considerations and nuances were included throughout the messaging and visuals used in the campaign.

The On the Road, Off the Phone campaign successfully reached a large swath of Washington State drivers, engaging them about the topic of distracted driving. Data from TrueMotion, an app that monitored actual Washington driver cell phone use 2 weeks before and 2 weeks after the law took effect, showed a 13% reduction in distracted driving as a result of the campaign. An observational study in 2019 showed a 40% decrease of people in Washington using their cell phones while driving, proving that the campaign continued to influence behaviors.

The 10-step process adapted from Kotler and Lee (2016) to develop a social marketing campaign should be followed to create the framework for a campaign before development begins (see Sidebar 12.1). You can use the *Planning for Effective Social Marketing Campaigns* workbook included in the references section (C + C, 2021) to help guide you through the 10-step process and identify pitfalls to avoid as you go.

Step 1: Identify project purpose, goals, and objectives. In order to achieve a successful social marketing campaign, you need a clear vision and articulation of your desired end destination. Your project purpose is why you are doing what you are doing (e.g., prevent HIV infections), your goal is what you want to achieve (e.g., increase HIV testing among high-risk people), and your objectives are how you know if you've gotten there (increase HIV testing by X%, by when). Defining these variables provides the

SIDEBAR 12.1	Social Media and Its Role in Both Media Advocacy and Social Marketing

Digital tools have become a central component of almost any movement. Some of the most used digital advocacy tools include websites, blogs, Facebook, Twitter, email, and texts. Literally hundreds of social media applications exist that could be used for digital advocacy. If using social media as part of your media advocacy effort, it is important to consider your purposes for engaging with the public using social media tools. Is your goal to rebrand your organization as the most knowledgeable? Gather supporters and volunteers who may know little about your work? Share information about your issue with the public or stories to help garner additional support? Or, are you encouraging them to provide donations or to attend an event? Social media's interactive, decentralized environment offers a low-cost way for organizations to mobilize supporters, foster dialogic interactions with large audiences, and attract attention to issues that might otherwise be ignored in more traditional mass media.

With the rise of social media, the terms "social media" and "social marketing" have become widely confused. But they are VERY different things. Social media is one tool in the toolbox of the social marketer. It can be part of Step 7 as a communications social marketing tool and in Step 9 as part of the marketing plan. It should only be used if it can engage the priority audience to overcome behaviors and spur behavior change. It may be helpful to think of social marketing as a discipline and social media as one tool that can be used as part of that discipline.

---

compass for your project. Everything you do in Steps 2–10 should point you toward your purpose, goals, and objectives. This is the most important step in the planning process.

Pitfall: Objectives are not measurable. It is important to ensure that you set measurable objectives up front. You need to figure out how you are going to measure against your objectives. What data do you need? How will you collect the data? If your objective is not measurable, you need to redefine it and find one that is.

Step 2: Research. Good campaigns and materials are grounded in research. Research should be used to understand priority audiences' current actions and identify what they think and feel about the subject matter and behaviors. It can also be used to help evaluate a program's effectiveness. There is a variety of research that can be employed, including the following:

- Secondary research should always be your first step. Look around and see if someone else has already done the research you need. There is no need to recreate the wheel if the data exist from another credible source. There is often very good research already available for public health issues.
- Quantitative studies to develop baseline data, define priority audience groups, and gather information about barriers, benefits, and motivators.
- Qualitative studies to delve deeper with audience groups and to test messaging and concepts.
- Observational studies are useful when there is a concern that the audience groups might not accurately report on their own behaviors. This is the case when working on social issues where people answer how they think they are supposed to answer instead of accurately reporting what they think/do. These studies are an option for understanding behavior and evaluating behavior change.

Pitfall: Failing to trust the research. There is a strong bias to believe that our own assumptions are an accurate reflection of how others feel. This can lead people to insert bias into the interpretation of research results. It is critical that you trust the research and don't let your opinions or the opinions of others (who are not part of the priority audience group) influence decisions in a way that is counter to what you learned in the research. One way to help you do this is to create a research brief document and make sure you share that up through your approval chain. You should also refer to it throughout the development of the project to ensure you aren't making decisions that are counter to what you learned in the research.

Step 3: Identify desired behavior changes. In this step you want to determine the specific desired behavior changes that are the most direct path to achieving the program's goals. This is often done by mapping behaviors on a grid like the one shown in Figure 12.2 based on which will have the highest impact on the goal and the highest probability of change.

Behaviors should be as specific as possible and nondivisible. Rather than telling people to get vaccinated, you want to tell people to get a specific vaccine. The reason for this is that each vaccine may have different audiences as well as unique barriers and motivators that need to be addressed to get people to act. It is also important to note that there can often be multiple behavior changes needed along the path to the ultimate desired outcome for your campaign. It can be a useful exercise to map the steps your audience needs to take to get to the desired behavior. Keeping with the vaccine analogy, when the COVID vaccine was launched, people had to (1) decide to get the vaccine, (2) determine if they were eligible, (3) make an appointment, and (4) show up and get the vaccine. Each of these steps required unique communications and instruction, and each step is a possible place where the audience may drop out and not follow through with the behavior.

Pitfall: Choosing too many behaviors. We know that if you try to tell people too many things, they are likely to do nothing. It is important to focus on one behavior at a time. And, yes, this can be hard. As social marketeers, we have so many things we

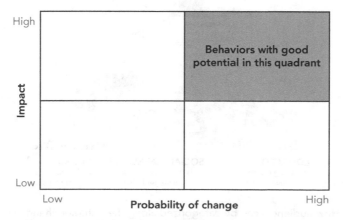

FIGURE 12.2 Understanding probability of change and potential for impact.

want people to do that it is tempting to try and "get it all in" at once. Avoid the urge and do a good job at addressing one behavior at a time. In the long run you will be more successful at changing behavior.

Step 4: Define priority audiences. Your priority audiences are those that are most likely to be receptive to changing their behaviors. It is hoped you were able to identify audience segments in the research you conducted in Step 2. Audiences can be defined as

- Primary—People that you want to change their behaviors
- Influencer—People that can influence your primary audience to change their behavior

You can generally think of audiences in three groups related to any particular behavior change (Figure 12.3).

Those in the "show me" group are people who are the early adopters of your desired behavior. They are going to adopt it right away with no or little intervention. The second group is the "help me" group. These are the people that a social marketing campaign usually targets. They need help understanding the issue and overcoming the barriers they have to changing their behavior. The third group is the "make me" group. This group is very resistant to the behavior and may require a law or regulation before they will make the change. You can think of mapping these three groups on a typical social diffusion curve with the help me group typically representing the middle section of the bell curve.

Once you have your priority audiences chosen, develop a document (an audience profile document or "persona" profile) that summarizes everything you know about them from your research or other sources. This document can help guide you as you develop campaign messaging and materials.

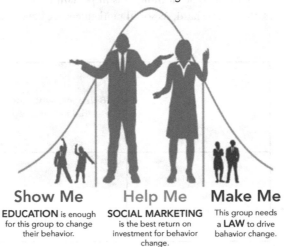

Citizen Behavior Change
Education • Marketing • Law

Show Me
EDUCATION is enough for this group to change their behavior.

Help Me
SOCIAL MARKETING is the best return on investment for behavior change.

Make Me
This group needs a **LAW** to drive behavior change.

FIGURE 12.3 How audiences can be categorized along the behavior change curve.
Source: Adapted from Everett Rogers, Jay Kassirer, Mike Rothchild, Dave Ward, and Kristen Cooley.

Pitfall: Thinking your audience is "everyone." Your audience is NOT "everyone" or the "general public." If you try to be everything to everybody, you will not be anything to anybody. To be effective you must define who your audience is in terms of the barriers, benefits, and motivators related to your desired behavior change. This will never apply to everyone. To be effective, you need to segment your audiences so you can create custom strategies with unique barriers and unique motivators.

Step 5: Identify barriers, benefits, and motivators for the desired behavior changes. Once you know what behaviors you want people to adopt, the next step is to analyze the barriers that are preventing them from doing the desired behaviors and the possible benefits and motivators that could overcome those barriers. Each of these elements is defined as follows:

- Barrier: What is stopping your audience from doing the desired behavior?
- Benefit: What benefit will be delivered to the audience if they practice the behavior? What's in it for them?
- Motivator: What will motivate the audience to act to change their behavior?

This is a key part of the process and one that often provides a reality check. If the motivators for a particular behavior change are not strong enough to overcome the barriers, you will want to rethink that behavior change. The goal here is to set you up for success—pick the achievable behaviors and focus your efforts there.

Pitfall: Buried in barriers. Sometimes it is too easy to come up with a long list of barriers that are preventing the desired behavior change. The key is to really narrow down to the top one or two things that are preventing change for your audience. Since you will be working to overcome key barriers through the strategies you chose and your messaging, you need to be singularly focused on overcoming the primary barrier that is in the way of change for your audience.

Step 6: Create a messaging strategy. A succinct and compelling message strategy is critical to help ensure the success of social marketing efforts. We live in a world where the average person is exposed to between 2,000 and 3,000 marketing messages each day. We have about three to five seconds to catch someone's attention so that they continue reading or viewing to learn more. Once you've caught their attention, the average millennial will spend 14 seconds more on the content. For Gen Z, it's 8 seconds. This highlights the need to be compelling and very succinct in your message strategy. One way to help you do this is to create key value propositions. A value proposition has the following structure (framed in the first person from the perspective of the priority audience):

If I [desire behavior change], I will [benefits/motivators] because [proof points/ support].

Example: "If I purchase ENERGY STAR products, I will be making a smart decision that helps protect the environment and saves money on my energy bills because ENERGY STAR is a simple way I can know that a product uses less energy."

A good message strategy finds the "key insight" that will drive behavior change. It ties back to earlier steps in the process. If you have a well-developed profile of your priority audience's barriers, benefits, and motivators, this step should flow naturally from the work you've already done. Additionally, good messaging involves keeping things simple (can the audience understand the main message in 3–5 seconds?) and striving to create an emotional connection with the audience. An emotional connection helps catch attention and drives message retention.

> **Pitfall: Selling features instead of benefits.** People buy benefits, not features. They don't want to hear about how something works, they want to hear about what it will do for them. Make sure your messaging strategy is focusing on benefits and resist the urge to explain features. Here are a few examples of headlines that illustrate focusing on benefits:
>
> - "Our 9 p.m. news is like their 10 p.m. news only you're awake" (news channel)
> - "No One Ever Went to Their Deathbed Saying 'You Know, I Wish I'd Eaten More Rice Cakes'" (chocolate company)
> - "Save the crabs, then eat 'em" (government agency focused on water quality)

Step 7: Choose your social marketing intervention. This step is the culmination of the process where you prioritize and choose what social marketing tools will work best to influence behaviors among the priority audience groups. Below is a list of common social marketing tools.

- **Commitments:** Making a commitment to change a behavior makes it more likely that people will follow through. The more visible and durable the commitment is, the more likely the audience is to follow through. A visible commitment is one that is publicly shared. A durable commitment is one that persists and can be witnessed over time. It is also important to note that commitments that are made in writing are more effective than verbal.
- **Social Norms:** People will change their behaviors if they believe everyone else has done so. If your issue has a social norm present—most people already do the desired behavior—it can be a powerful strategy to point that out to the priority audience group you are trying to influence.
- **Social Diffusion:** Peer and referent groups (friends/family, people they work/go to school with, people in their geographic vicinity) spread behavior change through conversations, interactions, and observation of each other. Looking for ways to spur social diffusions within your priority audience groups is an effective social marketing tool for many campaigns.
- **Prompts:** Placing reminders to act as close to the location of behavior as possible (e.g., signage or mobile/text reminders).
- **Policy/Regulation:** Creating policies can help throughout the behavior adoption curve. Early on with the show me group, policies can build momentum for the desired behavior change. For the help me group, they can help overcome barriers and build momentum for a social norm. For the make me group, they can provide strong incentives or disincentives for not practicing the behavior.
- **Communication:** There are many communications tools that can be employed by social marketers (Sidebar 12.2). These tools seek to capture attention, overcome barriers with motivators, and highlight benefits. Examples include advertising, media relations, social media and digital media. It is important to pick the tools/channels that have the best reach to your priority audiences.

SIDEBAR 12.2	Social media and its role in both media advocacy and social marketing

Digital tools have become a central component of almost any movement. Some of the most-used digital advocacy tools include websites, blogs, Facebook, Twitter, email, and texts. Literally hundreds of social media applications exist that could be used for digital advocacy. If using social media as part of your media advocacy effort, it is important to consider your purposes for engaging with the public using social media tools. Is your goal to rebrand your organization as the most knowledgeable? Gather supporters and volunteers who may know little about your work? Share information about your issue with the public or stories to help garner additional support? Or, are you encouraging them to provide donations or to attend an event? Social media's interactive, decentralized environment offers a low-cost way for organizations to mobilize supporters, foster dialogic interactions with large audiences, and attract attention to issues that might otherwise be ignored in more traditional mass media.

With the rise of social media, the terms "social media" and "social marketing" have become widely confused. But they are VERY different things. Social media is one tool in the toolbox of the social marketer. It can be part of Step #7 as a communications social marketing tool and in Step #9 as part of the marketing plan. It should only be used if it can engage the priority audience to overcome behaviors and spur behavior change. It may be helpful to think of social marketing as a discipline and social media as one tool that can be used as part of that discipline.

- **Incentives:** Providing a tool or discount that helps overcome a barrier to trying the behavior. Incentives can be monetary (e.g., rebates on energy-efficient products) or nonmonetary (e.g., dog poop bags at parks).
- **Convenience:** This stems around making it easy to do the desired behavior. For example, providing free masks and sanitizing stations in public locations is one example of convenience. Automatic scheduling of your second COVID-19 vaccine appointment is another. Opt-out versus opt-in strategies are another example of a convenience tool. Many programs have shown that if people are asked to opt-out rather than asked to opt-in there is a much higher rate of participation. This is illustrated with automatic enrollment in 401K programs or organ donation programs.
- **Cognitive Dissonance:** Many social issues have cognitive dissonance at play. This is when people's values and beliefs do not match their behaviors. If this is the case, a first step in a campaign can be to point out the dissonance to your audience.
- **Recognition/Feedback:** People want to know that their behavior is making a difference. Report back with messages like, "XX% of people or groups have committed the behavior" or "Thank you; you're helping make a difference." This feedback acts to solidify the behavior habit among your audience by confirming that they made the right choice and their behavior is making a difference.

Every program will use a different combination of the tools listed above. Your challenge in this step of the planning process is to pick the tools that will most efficiently help get you to your program's goals.

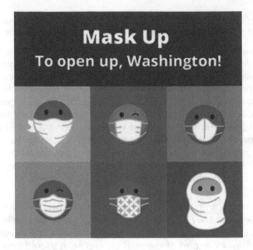

FIGURE 12.4 Mask Up campaign.
Source: Washington State Department of Health.

Pitfall: Thinking awareness leads to behavior change. It is the logical assumption to make the conclusion that if someone knows about a social issue or a problem, they will change their behavior to try to address it. This is not true. Behavioral science research has shown over and over again that awareness alone has no correlation to changing behaviors. This finding is the foundation that the social marketing discipline is built on. Instead, you need to define the specific barriers for your audience to change their behavior, the benefits the behavior will provide them, and the motivators you can offer to get them to act.

Step 8: Identify partners. Partnerships can help create demand for a program by providing access to a larger audience, incentives for program participants, and addition of credibility to the cause. Good potential partnerships have the following characteristics:

- **Complementary missions:** You should have complementary goals or at least goals that are not in conflict.
- **Audience alignment:** The partner's audiences should overlap with your campaign's priority audiences.
- **A balance of value:** It is important to make sure the potential partner has something of value to offer/bring to the table, and that in turn, you have something of value to offer to them.
- **Collaborative history:** It is also good to look for partners with a history of collaboration and community involvement. A good partnership makes things easier, not harder.

You can consider partners in the private, public, and/or nonprofit sectors. For some programs, working with local media partners can provide added exposure and value to the program. To get started identifying your partnership strategy, make a list of all potential partners and then rank them based on the criteria listed above.

Pitfall: Telling a partner why you need them instead of why they need you. When you approach a partner, always start with their perspective. Learn as much as you can about them before you reach out. Then, craft the conversation around their needs. Think of this as a mini social marketing plan. What are you asking the partner to do? What barriers are in the way for them? What benefits and motivators can you offer the partner?

Step 9: Develop a marketing plan. A fully developed marketing plan is crucial to the success of social marketing efforts. This plan shares how to operationalize social marketing tools and deliver the program's message to priority audiences, as well as define outreach strategies and tactics that will deliver on the program's goals and objectives. When you think about your plan, strategies are broad and tactics are specific. So, if you decide in Step 7 that commitments are going to be part of your strategy, in this step you define how that will work (the tactics). Is it an online commitment? How will you make it visible? How will you promote it? You will likely have several marketing strategies with a variety of tactics supporting each strategy. Make sure that you do a check back at this point to confirm that your marketing strategy is going to help you achieve your program goals and objectives as defined in Step 1.

It is always better to start with a pilot and then scale larger. This allows you to learn from a smaller scale (in terms of audiences or geography) implementation and then make adjustments before you invest in a full rollout.

Pitfall: Starting with this step. The main pitfall here is that people start with this step! They jump straight to figuring out how they want to communicate and tools they are excited about using rather than taking the time to complete Steps 1–8 first. If you do start here, it is guaranteed that your program will not be as effective as it could be. It is critically important that you create your framework by completing the earlier steps before jumping into your marketing strategy.

Step 10: Create an evaluation plan. The evaluation plan is designed to track the program's progress, celebrate successes, and make necessary changes along the way. It includes measurements of campaign inputs, outputs, outcomes, and overall campaign impact. Inputs are the resources (budget, staff time, etc.) that you put into a campaign. Outputs are the reach and engagement of your campaign (people reached, events held, social media engagements, etc.). Outcomes are what happened as a result, such as the number of people that changed their behavior or changed awareness levels or attitudes. Impact maps back to your campaign's purpose (see Step 1).

If your purpose is to reduce deaths through vaccination, did that happen? Did you reduce carbon emissions through energy efficiency adoption? Reduce waste going to the landfill through recycling? At the end of the day, impact is the ultimate thing you want to measure in a social marketing program. However, having all four elements (inputs, outputs, outcomes, impact) included in your evaluation plan gives you a good look at what needs to happen at first and also allows you to analyze what you might want to change or adjust as your program continues. For a deeper look at evaluation, see Chapter 14.

Pitfall: Self-reporting bias: Failing to account for self-reporting bias in the evaluation strategy is a common pitfall for this step. Self-reporting bias is when people answer a question based on what they think they should do instead of accurately reporting their true behaviors. One perfect example of this issue is with recycling. If you ask people if they always recycle, more than 80% will say yes. Yet, in many communities more than 50% of what is in garbage cans is still recyclable. Wherever possible, you can avoid self-reporting in your evaluation strategy by figuring out how to instead measure actual behavior changes rather than surveying people. For recycling, this could mean measuring actual recycling rates by looking in cans before and after your campaign. If you have to use self-reported data, ensure you have a baseline and measure the amount of change, not absolute numbers, so that you can isolate the impact of self-reporting bias.

HOW DOES MEDIA ADVOCACY DIFFER FROM SOCIAL MARKETING?

Media advocacy is a tool sometimes integrated in social marketing campaigns, but media advocacy doesn't have to be an integral part in the effort to change awareness or health behaviors. Primarily, media advocacy makes the most sense when public awareness of your issue or organization's purpose is misguided or when the media is misleading the public regarding an important element of your strategy. For example, if an important partner in your social marketing campaign is presented by the media as acting counter to your program objectives, you may need to engage with the media to ensure that future representations more accurately represent their work or position.

In light of the coronavirus pandemic, the mass media, in their effort to gain and sustain the attention of the public, presented the COVID vaccine as risky, focusing on the limited number of side effects and adverse reactions experienced by those who chose to get vaccinated. Conversely, many social marketing and public health professionals across the United States sought out to reframe the media's presentation and public's perception of the COVID vaccination as necessary and harm reducing. In this way, media advocacy was used as a tool for countering the misleading information that was prohibiting the success of vaccination campaigns. Understanding how the potential for media misinformation may impact your program's implementation is an important task to consider in the planning stages of a social marketing effort. If reframing media discourse is necessary, it would be pertinent to insert your media advocacy tasks as part of your broader implementation plan.

Engaging in media advocacy within a social marketing campaign also makes sense when policymaking discourse is impeding the progress of the social marketing effort. Media advocacy is commonly used to enlighten the public regarding the influence of community factors, health systems, and policy on their everyday health. A social marketing campaign may make use of media advocacy when discourse surrounding a policy is getting in the way of the public's ability to access, comprehend, or make use of important information. In January 2019, the Defund Planned Parenthood Act threatened to cease all federal funding to the Planned Parenthood organization. Discourse surrounding the bill shifted the public's focus away from the positive influence of the women's health and family services offered by the organization, leaving many young women to wonder how they would go about accessing contraceptives and other health resources. Social marketing professionals recognized the need to address the broader policy discourse surrounding the defunding of Planned Parenthood as part of their sexual health awareness programming.

The H1N1 virus vaccine is a great example of a social marketing effort that did not use media advocacy. Instead it used a product- and distribution-based social marketing strategy/approach to get people vaccinated without needing communications. The approach was to add the H1N1 vaccine to the seasonal flu vaccine. By doing this, there was no need to conduct any communications or media advocacy to overcome a unique set of barriers beyond what is done for the flu vaccine.

BOTH MEDIA ADVOCACY AND SOCIAL MARKETING IN ACTION

COVID-19 Response in Washington State

At the onset of the COVID-19 pandemic, the Washington State Department of Health (WA DOH) launched a social marketing campaign with the purpose to "save lives and reduce serious illness related to COVID-19." They moved quickly to engage with people who live and work in Washington about COVID-19 and to counteract the spread of misinformation and influence their behavior through a statewide "Spread the Facts" media campaign. The media plan included ads on social, Google search, digital display, video/audio, TV and radio, print, and in-language community media. The campaign was initially translated into 7 languages and later expanded to 36 languages.

As the COVID-19 pandemic progressed, WA DOH began infusing more social marketing research and planning into the effort. To do this, the campaign employed a phased approach to address critical messaging and behaviors over time—from an emphasis on the Stay Home, Stay Healthy order; to promoting healthy coping strategies; to an effort to encourage wearing masks, smaller gatherings, and physical distancing; as well as highlighting the harsh realities of the virus. Research informed efforts to create campaigns to reach young adults, and partnered with local health jurisdictions (LHJs) to support communications in their communities with localized approaches. All creative assets and tools were made available to LHJs around the state via an online partner toolkit.

The ultimate goal of this campaign was to help flatten the curve of COVID-19 cases and deaths in Washington and drive traffic to coronavirus.wa.gov, where people could get accurate information and resources. As of the end of 2020, the campaign had generated 3.8 million clicks to the website and 1.1 billion completed video views (examples of output evaluation metrics). In terms of meeting the campaign's purpose to save lives, as of January 12, 2021, the Washington curve performed better than most other states, ranking 46th out of 50 states in terms of cases and 44th out of 50 in terms of deaths per 100,000. While the social marketing and media advocacy campaign cannot take all the credit for this success, it was certainly one important piece of the puzzle (Figure 12.5).

Golden Gate Suicide Barrier

For years, advocates had been asking the Golden Gate Bridge Highway and Transit District to construct a suicide barrier on the bridge. Since 1937, more than 1,700 people have jumped to their death. Formal discussions began in 1970 when the bridge district directors commissioned an architectural firm to develop feasible designs for a barrier, but the directors never settled on a design, and the plans were set aside. The San Francisco Suicide Prevention hotline decided it was time to revive that discussion and advocate for a barrier in the mid-1990s. In 1996, it formed the Golden Gate Suicide Barrier Coalition, focused on educating the public about the bridge's unfortunate status as the last suicide icon without a barrier. Coalition members began attending bridge district board meetings to emphasize the number of people who had died jumping off the bridge and the need for a barrier. Still, the directors were unmoved, arguing that the suicidal people would simply find another spot to commit suicide.

Approaching the 60th anniversary of the building of the Golden Gate Bridge on May 27, 1997, the coalition refocused its efforts, focusing on the idea that the many stories about the anniversary should also consider the dark side of the bridge. The coalition sponsored a contest for local civil engineering students to create a suicide barrier for the bridge, with plans to unveil the winning model at a news conference at the School of Public Health on the anniversary. The model would give the TV cameras a way to picture the barrier, and the contest would give the reporters a story to tell. Ultimately, every local news outlet covered the bridge's 60th anniversary, and every one included a story about the struggle for a suicide barrier (Quintero, 2014). While the decision to construct a barrier was still put aside, in 2019, the city of San Francisco finally voted to construct the world's largest suicide deterrent in the world. At a size of more than 380,000 square feet and costing over $200 million, the barrier is set to be completed in 2023 (Houston, 2020).

CONCLUSION

As was suggested in the introduction to this chapter, capturing the "power of the press" is an exceptionally useful tool in the promotion of social change. Whether the goal is to increase the public's awareness of an issue (agenda setting), inform the community about one's on-the-ground efforts, portray one's image in a specific light (framing), or pressure decision makers to initiate change, establishing a positive relationship with the media will be essential to gaining the favor of important stakeholders. Strategic consideration of the purposes, timing, and content of one's media engagement should entail a recognition of the public's relationship with and trust in media sources. Strategic planning also serves as a foundation to a social marketing campaign, in the work of identifying a behavioral focus, segmenting audiences, identifying barriers, and highlighting motivators to change. Moreover, media advocacy and social marketing can work together when specific viewpoints get in the way of the public's ability to understand or use information that might guide a policy decision.

In a 2008 blog post, Craig Lefebvres, a leading social marketing scholar, noted: "What media advocacy and social marketing do together is provide a broader framework for thinking about the context and determinants of behaviors among groups of people, identify the leverage points through a marketing analysis, and then focus public attention (through media engagement) to the audiences that are critical for success (public opinion leaders, media gatekeepers, elected officials)" (para. 4). Regardless of application, used together or uniquely, both media advocacy and social marketing serve an important role in social change efforts in their ability to move beyond downstream persuasion of individual change to instead empowering communities to become advocates for their own well-being. In this chapter, we hope to have supported George Gerbner's assertion that with the media's help, an informed public can be more powerful than its lawmakers. It is with this power that citizens themselves can become the driving force behind lasting, meaningful change.

REFERENCES

C + C. (2021). *Planning for effective social marketing campaigns: A step by step guide and workbook.* https://cplusc.com/social-marketing-workbook/

Community Tool Box. (2021). Center for Community Health and Development, University of Kansas. http://ctb.k

Center for Community Health and Development. (n.d.). University of Kansas. Retrieved June 2, 2022, from the Community Tool Box: https://ctb.ku.edu/en

Dixon, H., Warne, C., Scully, M., Dobbinson, S., & Wakefield, M. (2014). Agenda-setting effects of sun-related news coverage on public attitudes and beliefs about tanning and skin cancer. *Health Communication, 29*(2), 173–181. https://doi.org/10.1080/10410236.2012.732027

Fairhurst, G., & Sarr, R. (1996). *The art of framing.* Jossey-Bass.

Freelon, D., McIlwain, C. D., & Clark, M. (2016). *Beyond the hashtags: #Ferguson, #Blacklivesmatter, and the online struggle for offline justice.* Center for Media & Social Impact, American University. http://archive.cmsimpact.org/sites/default/files/beyond_the_hashtags_2016.pdf

Gerbner, G. (1992). Society's storyteller: How television creates the myths by which we live. *Media & Values, 59*(60), 8–9.

Houston, W. (2020, April 8). Golden Gate Bridge suicide barrier work continues during pandemic. *Marin Independent Journal.* https://www.marinij.com/2020/04/08/golden-gate-bridge-suicide-barrier-work-continues-during-pandemic/

Jashinsky, J. M., Magnusson, B., Hanson, C., & Barnes, M. (2017). Media agenda setting regarding gun violence before and after a mass shooting. *Frontiers in Public Health, 4,* 291. https://doi.org/10.3389/fpubh.2016.00291

Kotler, P., & Lee, N. (2016). *Social marketing: Influencing behaviors for good* (5th ed.). Sage Publications.

Lefebvres, C. (2008). Social marketing and tobacco control policy. https://socialmarketing.blogs.com/r_craiig_lefebvres_social/2008/10/social-marketing-for-tobacco-control.html

McCombs, M. E., & Shaw, D. L. (1972). The agenda-setting function of mass media. *Public Opinion Quarterly, 36*(2), 176–187. https://doi.org/10.1086/267990

Niederdeppe, J., Farrelly, M. C., & Wenter, D. (2007). Media advocacy, tobacco control policy change and teen smoking in Florida. *Tobacco Control, 16*(1), 47–52. https://doi.org/10.1136/tc.2005.015289

Quintero, F. (2014). *Why the stigma of suicide should not sway the debate about news under the Golden Gate Bridge.* Berkeley Media Studies Group. http://www.bmsg.org/blog/why-the-stigma-of-suicide-should-not-sway-the-debate-about-nets-under-the-golden-gate-bridge/

Right to Try. (2020, January 14). Food and Drug Administration. https://www.fda.gov/patients/learn-about-expanded-access-and-other-treatment-options/right-try

Rogers, E., & Dearing, J. (1988). Agenda-setting research: Where has it been, where is it going. *Communication Yearbook, 11*(1), 555–594. https://doi.org/10.1080/23808985.1988.11678708

Tanne, J. (2020). Colon cancer screening should begin at 45, says US task force. *BMJ, 371,* m4188. https://doi.org/10.1136/bmj.m4188

Wallack, L., Dorfman, L., Jernigan, D., & Themba-Nixon, M. (1993). *Media advocacy and public health: Power for prevention*. Sage.

Whyte, W. (2020, December 15). Racial disparities in COVID-19 are bad. They've even worse in Cancer. *STAT*. https://www.statnews.com/2020/12/15/racial-disparities-covid-19-are-bad-worse-in-cancer/

Zhang, Y., Jin, Y., Stewart, S., & Porter, J. (2016). Framing responsibility for depression: How US news media attribute causal and problem-solving responsibilities when covering a major public health problem. *Journal of Applied Communication Research*, *44*(2), 118–135. https://doi.org/10.1080/00909882.2016.1155728

CHAPTER 12: END-OF-CHAPTER ACTIVITIES

DISCUSSION QUESTIONS

1. How can media advocacy influence the perceptions of the public regarding an individual or community health issue?

2. How are media framing and agenda setting different? What real problems have you seen framed inaccurately in the mass media?

3. Why is it so important to establish trust with the media? What challenges might you face in establishing trust in today's current media environment?

4. What are the key differences between media advocacy and social marketing? In what sort of cases might the two be used in conjunction with one another?

5. Does making people aware of an issue cause them to change their behavior? Why or why not?

6. What should you do if you have multiple behaviors you are trying to influence?

7. Why is it important to define priority audiences for a social marketing program or campaign?

8. What are the best ways to measure the impact of a behavior change campaign?

APPLICATION ACTIVITIES
Good Media Opportunities for Media Advocacy

Objective: To identify a variety of potential "good media opportunities" in your local/ regional news environment with which you could partner your media advocacy efforts.

Utilize: The website or social media account of a local/regional news source, including web, print, and/or television news.

Directions:

1. Visit the web page or social media account for a local or regional news source. Review the news stories that are presented at the top of the page, those that seem to have received the most interest (in comments, views), and/or those that seem to be the most controversial or timely.

2. Select two to four stories that have the potential to be connected to a social change for public health effort. For example, was there a recent automobile accident that involved a texting teenager?

3. Once you have selected your story, answer the following questions:
   a. What public health issues or topics might you be able to partner with this news? Why does this partnership make sense?
   b. In crafting the content of your media, will you need to change an existing public viewpoint? Inform the public about something new? Make "old news" more fresh?

   c. What challenges could you face from the community, policymakers, or other stakeholders as you work to build on the existing news in support of your view?

Mapping Behavior Change Framework

Objective: To learn to think about barriers, motivators, and benefits in the context of behavior change.

Utilize: Pick a nonprofit that works on an issue that you are passionate about.

Directions:

1. Research the nonprofit and the issues they work on. Choose a behavior change to focus on using the grid in Figure 12.2.

2. Pick a priority audience that you think should be the focus for changing your chosen behavior.

3. List the top three barriers you think are stopping the audience from doing the behavior.

4. For each barrier, list the benefits (what's in it for them) and motivator (what will spur action) that you think will overcome the barrier.

ADDITIONAL RESOURCES

Media Advocacy Resources

Berkley Media Studies Group. (n.d.). *Media advocacy 101.* http://www.bmsg.org/resources/media-advocacy-101/

Social Marketing Resources

C + C. (2021). *Planning for effective social marketing campaigns: A step by step guide and workbook.* https://cplusc.com/social-marketing-workbook/

Community-Based Social Marketing. (n.d.). *Health.* https://cbsm.com/terms/health

Tools of Change. (n.d.). *Home page.* https://toolsofchange.com/en/home/

QUIZ QUESTIONS

1. Which of the following terms best describes "the strategic use of mass media to support community organizers' efforts to advance social or public health policies":
   a. media advocacy
   b. social media
   c. social marketing
   d. media literacy

2. In considering recent television news coverage, one might notice that coronavirus incidence and prevalence rates are discussed at the beginning of news programs on almost every major news network. Simultaneously, coronavirus has been perceived as the most important health issue by many U.S. citizens. This

connection between news coverage and perceived importance is a good example of which media theory?

   a. health belief model

   b. agenda-setting theory

   c. media framing

   d. social marketing theory

3. One might notice that many television dramas tend to portray characters who experience mental health challenges as weak, self-absorbed, or abnormal. These perceptions may lead individuals to perceive real-world instances of mental illness similarly, leading to less community-level support for mental health resources and policies. One might argue that this is a good example of which media theory?

   a. media framing

   b. social marketing theory

   c. cultivation theory

   d. agenda-setting theory

4. Which of the following is NOT a consideration as you develop your media advocacy strategy?

   a. What is the best way to reach your target—through the news, a public service announcement, earned media?

   b. When might media attention influence policymaking the most?

   c. What story elements will do the best job in getting the attention of the media?

   d. What are the benefits, barriers, and motivators to engaging in your target behavior?

5. Per discussion in Chapter 12, which of the following opportunities might be a good time to engage with the mass media regarding your efforts to lobby for crossing guards at a busy intersection near a local elementary school?

   a. When the town council is deciding on the personnel budget for town employees for the upcoming year.

   b. When a story was published in the local newspaper about three students who were injured by vehicles as pedestrians at the intersection.

   c. When you are beginning a new project to raise funds for hiring crossing guards.

   d. All of the above would be good times to engage with the mass media.

6. What do you do if you have multiple behaviors you want to target?

   a. Pick the one that will most quickly and efficiently get to your goal.

   b. Pick the top three and focus on them.

   c. Do research to determine which one the audience is most likely to act on.

   d. Focus on them all, just make sure you overcome barriers for each in messaging.

   e. a and c.

7. What are some guidelines to follow when developing a priority audience profile?

   a. It's best to make your audience as big as possible.

   b. You should always define a specific priority audience for the behavior you are trying to change and then test messages with members of your audience.

    c. If you want a cheap way to test your messaging, ask the people you work with or your friends and family.

    d. Your priority audience is likely to have the same opinions and beliefs that you do.

8. What are some tools to help get value from research?

    a. Create a research brief that articulates the key takeaways for your campaign. Refer to this often.

    b. Share the research up through the approval chain.

    c. Point back to the research when you are getting requests to change the campaign in a way that is counter to research findings.

    d. All of the above.

9. Cognitive dissonance in social marketing is when?

    a. The audience does not believe your messaging.

    b. The audience disagrees with what you are asking them to do because of their values.

    c. The audience's values do not match their behaviors.

    d. a and c.

10. What is the best way to avoid self-reporting bias?

    a. Change your survey questions to avoid bias.

    b. Use observational or behavioral tracking evaluation strategies instead of surveys.

    c. Make sure your survey sample size is really large.

    d. Use online instead of telephone surveys to collect data.

ANSWER KEY

1. **A.** Media advocacy.
2. **B.** Agenda-setting theory.
3. **A.** Media framing.
4. **D.** What are the benefits, barriers, and motivators to engaging in your target behavior?
5. **D.** All of the above would be good times to engage with the mass media.
6. **E.** A and C.
7. **B.** You should always define a specific priority audience for the behavior you are trying to change and then test messages with members of your audience.
8. **D.** All of the above.
9. **C.** The audience's values do not match their behaviors.
10. **B.** Use observational or behavioral tracking evaluation strategies instead of surveys.

Evaluation

An Essential Skill in Policy & Advocacy

ANDERS CEDERGREN AND MONTRECE MCNEILL RANSOM

> What is significant in the evaluative process is thus not so much ultimate success and failure, but that policy actors and the organizations and institutions they represent can *learn* from the formal and informal evaluation . . . in which they are engaged.
>
> —GIEST & HOWLETT, 2015

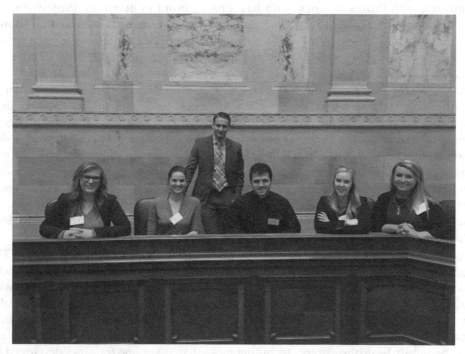

FIGURE 13.1 Students and faculty engaged in Wisconsin State advocacy experience and evaluation project. L to R: Carly Emmel, Lindsay Worley, Dr. Anders Cedergren, Shawn Verbeten, Ashley Heim, Natalie Frederickson

Photo credit: Keely Rees

Anders Cedergren and Montrece McNeill Ransom, *Evaluation*. In: *Be the Change*. Edited by Keely S. Rees, Jody Early, and Cicily Hampton, Oxford University Press. © Oxford University Press 2023. DOI: 10.1093/oso/9780197570890.003.0013

Objectives

1. Compare health program, policy, and advocacy evaluation.
2. Describe why various stakeholders may want to evaluate a health program, policy, or advocacy campaign.
3. Explain how evaluation is an essential part in every step, including early phases of health program, policy, or advocacy efforts.
4. Recommend qualitative and quantitative processes to collect evaluation data for a health program, policy, or advocacy campaign.
5. Suggest ways to identify and overcome barriers to health program, policy, or advocacy evaluation.

INTRODUCTION

Imagine that you are a public health student at a local university. You have been learning about the impact of healthy vending machines on eating habits and stress reduction for students. You realize that your university has very limited healthy vending options available, and conversations with your peers convince you that student health and academic achievement is being negatively impacted by this gap. You raise your concerns with Professor Jones, who has a background in nutrition. Professor Jones readily agrees that limited access to healthy snacks on campus is an issue that should be addressed. After several meetings, the two of you decide to lead an advocacy campaign for a university-wide healthy vending machine policy. Following Centers for Disease Control and Prevention (CDC) guidance, you create a plan. To start, you and Professor Jones convene a working group, a collection of interested students, faculty, and staff, to help determine key audiences and stakeholders. You conduct two surveys, both of which indicate that students, faculty, and staff desire access to vending machines with healthier options. Through your research, you have also discovered that a university in a neighboring county has adopted a healthy vending machine policy just like the one you propose. Using these data, you and the working group create key messages and determine communication activities to deliver those messages. You and the group have worked hard to launch your advocacy campaign and mobilize your base. But how will you know if your advocacy campaign is working? The answer is through *evaluation*.

Evaluation is an essential skill for the 21st-century public health workforce. The complexities of public health practice coupled with the constant changes in the social and political environment in which public health operates necessitate a workforce with strong evaluation skills. In fact, evaluation is among the top areas that public health practitioners identify as potentially helpful for improving job performance (Mid Atlantic Regional Public Health Training Center, 2017). Evaluation training and development for the public health workforce, including more than 20 online trainings developed by the 10 Health Resources and Services Administration–funded Regional Public Health Training Centers, focus on topics including economic evaluation, policy evaluation, program evaluation, and training evaluation (National Network of Public Health Institutes [NNPHI], 2021).

Evaluation has been defined several ways in professional literature. Simply put, evaluation is a systematic approach to collecting and analyzing data to determine whether the strategy, campaign, program, approach, policy, activity, or other evaluation is making progress toward its intended result (CDC, n.d.-c). As discussed in Chapter 7, evaluation is a critical, but often forgotten, part of the policy process. For health education specialists, evaluation and research are such important skills that they has been delineated as a unique area of responsibility (Knowlden et al., 2020). Though evaluation and research are listed as Area IV, after assessment, planning, and implementation, it becomes clear while reviewing these professional standards that aspects of evaluation can be found in many other areas as well, including, as discussed in this chapter, advocacy. Advocacy activities, like other public health promotion efforts, need evaluation to be their best. In this chapter, you'll learn more about why evaluation is a critical element of public health programs, advocacy, and policy change, as well as what strategies you can use to plan and implement evaluation.

POLICY, PROGRAM, AND ADVOCACY EVALUATION
Policy Evaluation

The CDC defines **policy evaluation** as the "systematic collection and analysis of information to make judgements about contexts, activities, characteristics, or outcomes of one or more of the domains of the Policy Process" (Office of the Associate Director for Policy and Strategy [OADPS], 2019b). The policy process, as illustrated in the policy process wheel in Figure 13.2, was developed to foster common language and understanding around policy and the process by which policy is conceptualized, developed, adopted, implemented, and evaluated. It "provides a systematic way to develop policies to address public health problems and has 5 primary domains" (OADPS, 2019b).

Domain 1 of the policy process is focused on problem identification and is centered on clarifying and framing the problem or issue in terms of health effects and outcomes. During this phase, public health practitioners are focused on collecting, analyzing, summarizing, and interpreting data and other scientifically based information relevant to the frequency and severity of injuries and their consequences and describing the problem in clear, compelling ways, including groups that are affected (CDC, n.d.). Domain 2 is agenda setting and is focused on identifying different policy options to address the identified issue. In this phase, quantitative and qualitative methods should be used to determine the most effective, efficient, and feasible policy option. The health education advocacy experience case study, which appears at the end of this chapter, provides a salient example of how Domains 1 and 2 are operationalized in practice and offers perspectives on how an issue and possible policy options might be identified and researched. In addition, legal epidemiology might also prove helpful during Domain 2 of the policy process, when the goal is to evaluate laws. As described in Box 13.1, legal epidemiology is defined as the scientific study of the impact of law, as a specific policy tool, on health.

Domain 3 is about strategy and policy formulation. Here, the aim is to identify a strategy for getting the policy adopted and a plan for how the policy will operate. Domain 4 is focused on policy adoption and includes following internal or external

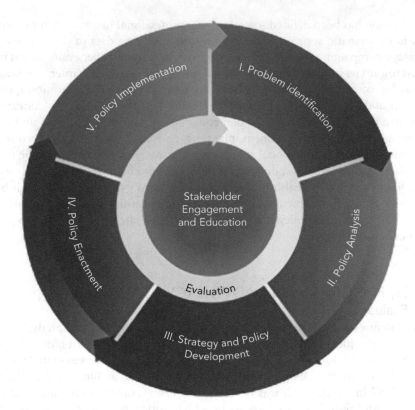

FIGURE 13.2 Centers for Disease Control and Prevention policy process.

procedures for getting the policy enacted or passed. The final domain, Domain 5, is focused on policy implementation and efforts to translate the enacted policy into action, monitor uptake, and ensure full implementation. The policy process also contemplates two overarching domains: stakeholder engagement and education and evaluation (OADPS, 2019a).

Until recently, in many models of policymaking, the evaluation stage was presented as the last step of the policymaking process, taking place after implementation of the policy, and focusing evaluation primarily on the outcome of said implementation (Giest & Howlett, 2015). However, the policy process recognizes that including evaluation as an overarching domain improves its potential to inform and guide all domains of the policy process. Embedding evaluation throughout each domain also provides opportunities to connect policies, outcomes, policymakers' decisions, and stakeholders at each stage of the policy development process; ensures progress toward stated health goals; and fosters "sound public governance" and governmental accountability. The next section explores the domains of the policy process in turn through the lens of policy evaluation.

When applied to Domain 1 of the policy process, the problem identification phase, evaluation can be used to identify the context and the cause of the problem. An evaluation study could also describe the extent that the identified problem lends itself to potential policy solution and action. These findings should provide a clear

What Is Legal Epidemiology?

Legal epidemiology is defined as the scientific study of law as a factor in the cause, distribution, and prevention of disease and injury, and it is centered on generating, analyzing, and communicating information about law and policy through quantitative and qualitative analysis (Culp & Silverman, 2021). It is an emerging field that merges the practice of developing and implementing public health laws with the evaluation of how laws can affect health. It involves studying complex laws that address public health issues and quantifying legal data that can then be linked with health-related datasets (Culp & Silverman, 2021).

Legal epidemiology data might prove specifically helpful in Domain 2, during the policy identification phase of the policy process. Legal epidemiology is grounded in the idea that laws and regulations must be both quantified and measured in terms of outcomes to understand its impact on health and health outcomes. Legal epidemiology data can offer an opportunity to compare language in the law across jurisdictions and the health impact of those laws. In the policy process, these data can be used to help prioritize which policy option might best address the problem identified.

Legal epidemiology has been used to study the following:

- the use of law to characterize states' prior authorization policies regarding medication used to treat attention-deficit/hyperactivity disorder (Ramanathan et al., 2017)
- the prevalence of state and local laws intended to encourage population access to reduced-sodium food products (Sloan et al., 2020)
- the degree of high school written concussion policy compliance with the respective state law and examination if the relationship between concussion policy compliance and school-level implementation of concussion laws (Sullivan et al., 2020)
- how state telehealth laws intersect with the opioid overdose epidemic (Pepin et al., 2020)
- state laws supporting hurricane evacuation in eight southern coastal states (Kruger et al., 2018)
- state laws that are related to structural racism for health equity research and practice (Agéno, et al, 2021)

picture of the issue and inform the identification of potential policy options to address the issue.

Evaluation findings associated with the agenda-setting domain, Domain 2, may be used to inform policy identification, development, enactment, and implementation by providing a clear picture of potential public health impacts, political and operational feasibility, and economic and budgetary impacts. This information can be used to drive decisions about policy content and roles and responsibilities related to enactment and implementation. Evaluation also proves critical in Domains 3, 4, and 5 when formulating, adopting, and implementing the chosen policy solution. When identifying, analyzing, and prioritizing the potential policy solutions, evaluation efforts should focus on gaining clarity about how policy options were analyzed, including contextual support or opposition, and potential public health and economic and budgetary impacts. At this stage, evaluation might focus on assessing the content of the policy, including how the policy will operate, how it will be enforced, and any mechanisms for monitoring implementation and measuring success, what policy actors (e.g., decision makers) were included, and how these stakeholders were engaged. Evaluation efforts might also assess whether jurisdictional and organizational context is reflected in the policy and the potential resources that will be necessary for enactment and implementation. Evaluation should also include examining the overall, short-, and long-term impact of the policy on health outcomes as it moves through implementation and enforcement.

Program Evaluation

McKenzie and colleagues (2017) explained that **program evaluation** is "the process of determining the value or worth of a health promotion program or any of its components based on predetermined criteria or standards of success identified by stakeholders" (p. 352). This includes **formative evaluation** as far as information and data collected and reviewed before or during program implementation to judge quality, as well as **summative evaluation** looking at effects or what results from or is associated with exposure to a program (Green & Lewis, 1986). Weiss (1972) also made the distinction that evaluation contributes to decisions about the program going forward.

As summarized by Issel and Wells (2018), the history of program evaluation is more recent than program planning and can be thought of as having four generations. Guba and Lincoln (1989) referred to the first generation as "measurement," meaning that it was science based and outcome focused. This type of evaluation focuses on systematic testing and estimating the effect of an intervention. Issel and Wells (2018) referred to the second generation as "descriptive" and focused on goals and objectives. This type of evaluation shifts the focus to determining the worth of programs. This generation of evaluation was associated with the growth in federal social services and the need to look for the cost-effectiveness of those resources. The 1980s saw the emergence of a third "responsiveness" generation of evaluation with a focus on the needs of those involved in the evaluation. Several pedigrees are part of this generation of evaluation, including utilization and participatory, which may partly account for the great range of approaches to evaluation used today. Finally, Issel and Wells (2018) mentioned a fourth generation of program evaluation: meta-evaluation. Like a meta-analysis of several research studies to determine more robust indicators of effect, this is basically an evaluation of several program evaluations conducted to look at proposed relationships and arrive at recommendations that are evidence based.

Advocacy Evaluation

Advocacy evaluation is the process of measuring progress made by an advocacy effort (Organizational Research Services, 2007). Like program and policy evaluation, the purpose of advocacy evaluation is to identify what works and what doesn't, as far as processes and impact, and to improve future activities. Like all evaluation efforts, advocacy evaluation data can be used to inform strategy and decision-making, build the capacity of advocacy stakeholders, or catalyze programmatic or societal change. However, as a field, advocacy evaluation is relatively nascent, having only gathered strength in the early 2000s (Innovation Network, 2009).

UNIVERSAL PRINCIPLES OF EVALUATION

The important takeaway here is that there are principles of evaluation design and practice that apply universally to program, policy, and advocacy evaluation. For example, all evaluators conduct systematic and database inquiries. Those inquiries can be quantitative or qualitative and typically use a set of methods, such as interviews and surveys. All evaluators employ tools such as logic models, affect theories, or theories of change. All evaluators should also be driven by a similar purpose of aiming to provide high-quality information that has significance or value for whom or what they are evaluating.

From the perspective of maximizing the likelihood of evaluation being both manageable and useful, evaluation objectives can also be especially helpful. Creating objectives for the program, policy, or advocacy evaluation being conducted can help ensure evaluation efforts are focused and that data are collected for specific reasons. While evaluators have choices in the kinds of data they produce and how they position that data for use, those choices are similar across program, policy, and advocacy evaluation. In terms of these core evaluation principles, then, the evaluation of policies, programs, and advocacy campaigns are not significantly different from all other evaluations. They can serve similar purposes and draw on the same basic evaluation design.

Integrating Health Equity

Another key principle that needs to be applied universally—across all evaluation efforts—is health equity. In fact, evaluators are increasingly being called on to integrate health equity considerations into **each** step of the evaluation process to ensure a more accurate interpretation of evaluation findings and to catalyze the development of more focused interventions (CDC, n.d.-b). As CDC noted:

> Without a focus on health equity in evaluation efforts, the effects of an intervention on addressing health disparities and inequities can go unnoticed. For example, an evaluation may reveal overall improvements in health, but overlook the fact that health disparities or inequities are widening. Health equity-oriented evaluations can be designed to understand what works, for whom, under what conditions, and reveal whether health inequities have decreased, increased or remained the same. (CDC, n.d.-b, p. 1).

Box 13.2 offers eight ideas on how to do this, as described in CDC's *Health Equity Guide*.

Evaluation Purposes and Questions

Capwell et al. (2000) provided six motivations for why people with a vested interest in a program may want it evaluated, including to determine whether objectives have been achieved, to improve implementation, and to provide accountability and generate support. These motives are also relevant to policy and advocacy evaluation. It is important to remember that there is a range of stakeholders as it comes to evaluation, such as funders or decision makers, community leaders, community members, and program participants, as well as the people who develop, implement, and evaluate policy, programs, and advocacy campaigns. The reasons mentioned above for *why* to evaluate also pose the question of *how* to best evaluate, including determining quality and effectiveness. For part of that answer, Fitzpatrick and colleagues (2004) pointed to a range of ways to interpret data related to evaluation, including seeing whether needs have been addressed, considering results within the context of procedures and professional standards, comparing actual to expected performance, and positioning findings relative to similar initiatives.

| ADVOCACY IN ACTION BOX 13.2 | Eight Ways to Integrate Health Equity in Evaluation Efforts |

1. Develop a logic model that includes health equity activities and goals.
2. Incorporate health equity into evaluation questions and design.
3. Identify appropriate variables to track populations experiencing inequities.
4. Use culturally appropriate tools and methodologies.

5. Use multiple approaches to understand an intervention's effect on health inequities.
6. Include health equity indicators in performance-monitoring systems.
7. Use process and outcome evaluations to understand the effect on health inequities.
8. Widely disseminate the results of equity-oriented evaluations.

From CDC, n.d.-b.

It may take great effort, but it is important to limit doing things that are not essential to the purpose of evaluation. It is hard not to get sucked into pursuing a variety of interventions and evaluation when you realize how many things are truly important to your ultimate goals. Just as in the case with much of public health research, evaluation efforts should be explicitly positioned within the context of delimitations (boundaries set by the investigator), limitations (things that are beyond the control of the investigator that could impact findings), and assumptions (things that are assumed to be true but cannot be verified, often in the context of limitations) (Cottrell & McKenzie, 2011). Further, the purpose and processes for evaluation of advocacy efforts can be established by considering who will do the evaluation, what the focus will be, when evaluation will take place, and the evaluation methodology (Center for Evaluation Innovation, 2009).

Planning an Evaluation

As previously pointed out for the policy process, the thought of what questions you want to answer through evaluation should constantly be considered as you go through assessment, planning, and implementation. It is important to remember that to be able to ask the right questions, one must know the problem. In fact, it may not be a problem that you need to understand; it could just as easily be thought of as a situation or for that matter an answer. From the perspective of program evaluation standards, evaluation that is useful, feasible, ethical, accurate, and accountable requires several fundamental steps of program planning (Yarbrough et al., 2011). The same is true for the evaluation of advocacy efforts; it is dependent on a range of interests, experiences, needs, and perspectives as the foundation for a variety of questions that may be useful. It can also be considered best practices to incorporate various stakeholders in the planning, execution, and reporting of evaluation results, whether one is dealing with a health education program or advocacy for public health as discussed in Chapter 5. Organizing and performing advocacy and policy evaluation work this way may help in correctly identifying questions or concerns through stakeholder participation and quality of information shared. It may also help build community capacity and promote sustainability of efforts (PolicyLink, 2012).

Following a program-planning model is a great way to maximize the likelihood that many relevant questions are asked as far as what to evaluate, why, and how in an advocacy campaign or other type of public health intervention. Several program-planning models explicitly prescribe questions around evaluation, as far as what to evaluate and how, be developed as a part of the assessment and planning phases. In other words, your evaluation plan is developed much earlier than when it is implemented, and much of the data to make determinations around quality and effectiveness are generated at various stages from planning through evaluation. As far as choosing the "right" model to follow, as it comes to program evaluation, McKenzie and colleagues (2017) suggested a consideration of the three Fs: fluidity (sequential steps of a model), flexibility (ability to adapt to the needs of stakeholders), and functionality (that planning leads to improved health). A good model should also meet the needs of large populations and recognize the ecological nature of influences on health of individuals and groups of people.

In the spirit of Benjamin Franklin often being credited with the saying "if you fail to plan, you plan to fail," McKenzie and colleagues (2017) summarized several barriers to effective program evaluation, including the use of an inappropriate evaluation design, inadequate evaluation resources, inconsistent intervention strategies, environmental restrictions, and a mismatch in perceptions of the value of evaluation between various stakeholders. Many of the same concerns have been discussed in the professional literature specifically for advocacy evaluation, and there is an emphasis on the value of varied and innovative approaches (International Initiative for Impact Evaluation, 2017; Teles & Schmitt, 2011). Another way to better understand how high-quality evaluation is dependent on work that takes place much earlier than at the end of a program and extends past collecting and analyzing data is to review the "Framework for Program Evaluation in Public Health" (CDC, 1999). This structure contains six steps and starts with "engaging stakeholders" early in the planning process to understand and account for how they will judge program success. This engagement will help prevent any later misunderstandings as far as what should have been accomplished, how, and why. The last step of the framework is to ensure use and share lessons learned. In this step, often referred to as the evaluation feedback loop, results are disseminated to make determinations around program continuation. This is also when the evidence base on a certain topic has a chance to expand or solidify because of how data are made available to professionals in the field. For advocacy in public health, similar frameworks have been proposed that make it clear that high-quality evaluation is dependent on early initiation and the incorporation of findings into future efforts (Innovation Network, 2009).

FORMATIVE AND SUMMATIVE EVALUATION

With the backdrop of the ever-ongoing and cyclical nature of evaluation, it is important to consider how to operationalize collection of data that allows for assessment and reporting of results. Like previously stated, evaluation can further be separated into two types: formative and summative. **Process evaluation** is often identified as a part of formative evaluation, while **impact** and **outcome evaluation** fit into the more general term of summative (McKenzie et al., 2017). The campus-wide needs assessments that you and the Healthy Vending Machine work group conducted in our hypothetical example in the beginning of the chapter would be considered a type of formative evaluation. In fact, much of what has been referred to up to this point as far as planning for evaluation deals with formative evaluation, such as having and using findings of a needs assessment, working to have stakeholder interests addressed, having an initiative tailored to the needs of the priority population, and having community partners represented in the programming process.

Process Evaluation

Process evaluation assesses to what extent a program was implemented as intended, including getting members of the priority population to take part in the program and considering factors that may have influenced the effects of your intervention (McKenzie et al., 2017). One way that this can be done is by assessing to what extent objectives, often written to be SMART (specific, measurable, achievable, relevant, time bound) (CDC, n.d.-a), set as part of the program or advocacy campaign planning, were achieved. Process objectives, as far as how each one is written and how one is connected to another, can be thought of as the recipe for success built from a list of ingredients. Knowing everything that goes into a program or advocacy campaign to be successful, as that is defined, is not enough to reach that success. We must know the *why* and *how* of the order and format of efforts. The why and how in this case come from all the data and theory reviewed and interpreted as part of assessment and planning. For example, self-efficacy may be something to improve through a program because you know that it is important in increasing the likelihood of changing a health behavior. You may also understand that knowledge and practicing skills are important elements for generating self-efficacy. However, if you do not know how and in what order knowledge and skills should be used as building blocks for self-efficacy, then a program may not have as much of a positive impact as possible or expected. Process objectives allow facilitators to identify and pursue specific steps that, in theory and based on previous work, should allow for the achievement of the desired impact. Case in point, note that the main change in Year 4 of the Health Education Advocacy Experience, described in the case study at the end of the chapter, was the intentional incorporation of theory into their tools and processes to better align data with standardized frameworks to support future changes and to make it easier to share findings.

Process evaluation and the ability to adjust efforts based on formative data may be particularly useful for evaluating advocacy campaigns because of how long it often takes for the type of impact you are looking for to occur as well as the existence of complex relationships, leading to an emphasis on contribution versus attribution. In fact, the term **developmental evaluation** has been applied in the professional literature specifically as it comes to advocacy evaluation because efforts are so multifaceted and ever changing, and there is an aim for continuous intentional improvement (Patton, 2006). Further, as stated by Loscalzo (2014), failure should be celebrated and embraced for its potential for learning. In the case of the discussion in this section of the chapter, failure is a process not happening as planned or expected. However, if evaluation allows you to realize what did not happen and why, then you should be able to adjust processes, which theoretically should increase the likelihood of longer term success. As it comes to health education or promotion programs, to aim for a reasonable amount of learning coming out of failures, it is beneficial if problems with implementation can be identified during pilot testing, which is basically trying out a program on a smaller scale, or as a program is phased in by limiting program offerings, participants, or location (McKenzie et al., 2017).

Impact and Outcome Evaluation

In policy and program evaluation, impact evaluation is often considered as focusing on more immediate measures, such as attitudes or knowledge, often from the perspective of learning, behavioral, or environmental objectives (CDC, n.d.-d). Outcome evaluation, on the other hand, can be thought of as looking at end-points of interest in the form of specific vital statistics (McKenzie et al., 2017). However, there are public health resources that flip these two terms, with outcomes being more immediate and impact considered long term (Issel & Wells, 2018). Both impact and outcome measures are useful when evaluating advocacy campaigns as there will be short-term impacts of the campaign, such as increased awareness of the issue, as well as long-term impacts such as the passage of legislation, as well as the impact on health measures because of the new policy.

As a reminder, the *what* and *how* of measurement for evaluation as well as the benchmarks (*how much*) that data will be compared to should be determined long before data are collected. Among other things, this will promote ethical conduct as it comes to data analysis and reporting. Knowing what your data show before or as you are setting targets may tempt you to align objectives with what you found in your study, not the phenomenon of interest as it may exist in a community based on needs assessment findings. As far as evaluation designs to look for program or advocacy campaign effects or associations, they can generally be split into nonexperimental (or pre-experimental), quasi-experimental, and experimental. While an evaluator may want to pursue a more advanced design to talk about cause and effect and to what extent results apply outside of your specific project, evaluation procedures should ultimately be driven by what is possible and what is needed to answer salient questions. The Health Education Advocacy Experience case study toward the end of this chapter certainly highlights this approach. Though more robust experimental or quasi-experimental designs can be applied to evaluate advocacy campaigns, the focus of such efforts is often on changing individual attitudes or behaviors and not on systems or policy (International Initiative for Impact Evaluation, 2017). At that point, it may be hard to get a good sense of significant differences between a health education program and an advocacy campaign.

QUALITATIVE AND QUANTITATIVE PROCEDURES AND ANALYSIS

Procedures that are fully or partly qualitative that can be part of formative evaluation by providing a rich description of the phenomenon of interest include focus groups, interviews, and observations. Evaluation procedures that have the potential to generate quantitative data include surveys and checklists. As far as quantitative data, it is important to emphasize that just because you *can* engage in sophisticated statistical analyses does not mean that you automatically *should*. There are a range of data characteristics that should be met for certain statistical procedures, many of which are hard to ensure when working with a select, small group of subjects. Many times, stakeholders who review your findings will find just as much or even greater use for descriptive quantitative findings and qualitative examples. It is also important to point out that one type of data is not in itself *better* than another. What really matters is the purpose of your evaluation and what questions you want your evaluation to answer. The Health Education Advocacy Experience case study below offers an example of a reasonable approach to data analysis because of considerations around sampling procedures and sample size. It also shows the value that may come from qualitative data in improving practices and increasing the likelihood of success.

Though summative evaluation is often considered from the perspective of quantitative data from program surveys or vital statistics pointing to some type of relationship between an intervention and results, it can be a good idea to plan for a mixed-methods approach to evaluation with multiple collection efforts of a range of data both before and after an intervention. Like the change to online surveys between Year 1 and Year 2 in the case study that follows, data collection efforts should also be set up in a way that enables as many and as varied responses as possible. Further, there are procedures that can be employed to try to ensure that tools and processes in fact measure the issue of interest and do so consistently. Even with well-planned and well-executed evaluation designs, it is often difficult for the evaluator to answer *how* and *why* to go with the more numerical considerations such as *what* and *who*. That is where the qualitative elements may come in handy, at least as far as being able to speculate why certain results were found. Also, an in-depth rich description of a phenomenon of interest may help explain or persuade partners or stakeholders of the value of your work. For advocacy specifically, a case study design has been presented as an example of evaluation that can achieve this hard-to-reach balance (Center for Evaluation Innovation, 2009; International Initiative for Impact Evaluation, 2017).

As it comes to process evaluation, having participants complete a survey to gather information during or immediately after the intervention can help quantitatively establish fidelity, or to what extent a program was implemented as intended (McKenzie et al., 2017). This, in turn, should help public health practitioners judge to what extent process objectives that were established as part of the planning phase were achieved. The same can be said about checklists completed by evaluators, as far as determining whether or to what extent an intervention was completed as planned. It may be important to point out that you should be careful or at least intentional with what you expect participants to contribute as it comes to judging whether process objectives were reached. As it comes to both quantitative and qualitative data, it is probably a good idea to ask participants to indicate what was done, how well, or to what extent. But it is also important to remember that many factors outside of program quality may influence these data. Just as it is recommended to have several evaluators provide data through checklists to be able to consider how consistently measures are indicated between raters, comparing participant and evaluator data may allow for the identification of situations where responses do not reflect program quality or effectiveness. This was much of the reason for asking for data from both students and legislative offices in Year 4 of the Health Education Advocacy Experience case study below. This is certainly also applicable advice for advocacy efforts in general where it is not that uncommon that the advocates believe and feel quite differently about the issue than decision makers or funders.

A CASE STUDY ON ADVOCACY EVALUATION: THE UNIVERSITY OF WISCONSIN–LA CROSSE HEALTH EDUCATION ADVOCACY EXPERIENCE

To allow students to engage in experiential learning to best develop professional competencies, the Public Health–Community Health Education Program at the University of Wisconsin–La Crosse implements an annual advocacy experience. Students, faculty, and community partners travel to Madison, Wisconsin, for a 3-day event where a public health issue is explored in depth, and students are trained and engage in state-level legislative advocacy.

Though the public health program advises on the process and facilitates logistics, part of what makes this work as an example of community organizing and engagement with a range of interested parties is the fact that it is set up through the local Eta Sigma Gamma chapter. A range of stakeholders is also involved in the selection of the advocacy issue each year partly based on within and between policy evaluation and community and legislative context. Community partners that are experts on some aspect of the issue or the practice of advocacy are invited to be part of the training that students go through during 2 days of workshops, leading into a third day of visits with legislative offices.

Over the course of 4 years, the evaluation approach for this event evolved. Though you could make the case that this constitutes regular educational efforts, since work took place outside the classroom, sometimes included data from subjects other than students, and had the potential to be professionally disseminated, the university institutional review board approved data collection processes and tools each year.

Year 1: Data were collected through hard-copy surveys to evaluate the educational sessions students participated in as part of advocacy training and preparation. Students were also asked to take part in a focus group to qualitatively debrief on the advocacy experience about 1 week after returning to campus, with discussions recorded, transcribed, and coded for important themes.

Year 2: The event was restructured to include additional time off campus as part of the training. The main reason for this was findings from the debrief focus group that was conducted at the end of the Year 1 experience. The same two evaluation processes were completed again but with session evaluations being issued electronically through a survey platform to students to ease completion and improve response rates. Students were also asked to complete an online pre–post test on advocacy confidence based on professional competencies. This additional piece was added after a review of Year 1 data revealed a need to combine qualitative and quantitative data more intentionally to better be able to answer a range of interesting questions as far as this experience helping to prepare students for the public health field. In addition, staff and elected officials were emailed a survey after meeting with students; the survey asked questions about the advocacy issue, the quality of advocacy by students, and the usefulness of this type of advocacy interaction. Data collected as part of this survey allowed for a comparison of offices, as well as what was reported by students versus staff and elected officials.

Year 3: All the same evaluation measures were again applied as Year 2, with the survey for legislative offices slightly modified to assess changes over time in perceptions and knowledge of the advocacy issue. The reason for this change was again tied to the desire to be able to evaluate the impact of our advocacy work on students as well as legislative offices. This year was also the first time a more robust evaluation design was applied. Instead of a nonexperimental design with only attendees completing the pre-post test, a quasi-experimental design was utilized, with the survey issued to all public health students at the University of Wisconsin–La Crosse. Using a comparison group of nonattendees provided an opportunity to more distinctly isolate unique effects of the experience on advocacy knowledge, confidence, and intentions.

Year 4: The same general evaluation approach was again applied as in Years 2 and 3. However, the survey sent to legislative offices to evaluate meetings was significantly modified to better assess important aspects of advocacy from a theoretical perspective. This change was made as there was a need to better align data with standardized frameworks to support future changes and to make it easier to share processes and findings. Also, key items from this survey were used to create a hard-copy form that students and faculty mentors completed immediately after each meeting. This was helpful in investigating a direct correlation between the perceived quality of advocacy interactions between a specific legislative office and students and faculty, as well as factors that may influence that type of relationship.

Moving forward, the ideal next steps will include implementing this project with a true experimental evaluation design with public health students from multiple schools as the sampling frame. However, that type of development would require careful consideration of several challenges as it comes to logistics and data analyses. If long-term maintained improvements can be determined for participants, it is also possible that any control group could be scheduled to receive the intervention the next year. This approach would be ethical and may allow for the best assessment to date for cause and effect as it comes to the impact of this type of experiential learning on public health competencies.

CONCLUSION

This chapter is meant to serve as a reminder that it is essential that evaluation is not merely an afterthought as health programs, advocacy campaigns, or policies are planned and implemented. Instead, evaluation should be a fundamental piece in each step of the life cycle of an intervention. It is also clear that there is a range of practices that may be appropriate to apply depending on what you are evaluating and being able to determine *why* something happened may be just as important as *what*. At the end of the day, as discussed by Capwell and colleagues (2000), the most critical consideration of effective evaluation may be to establish why stakeholders want an initiative evaluated. Understanding to what extent such aims as determining the achievement of objectives, improving implementation, and providing accountability and information are the reasons for why you evaluate will go a long way in informing effective evaluation practices.

Finally, it is important to emphasize that it is unlikely that evaluation should or will stay consistent over a long period of time. Though everything within your power should be done to plan high-quality evaluation and you want to be able to compare "apples to apples" over time and between efforts, as can be seen in the case study of the Health Education Advocacy Experience conducted by the University of Wisconsin–La Crosse, there are always things that change or are better understood after implementation.

Evaluation must be responsive to such findings and must evolve in step with the purpose and structure of a policy, program, or advocacy campaign. An example of this is that evaluation can only be truly effective if results are used, and quality control and quality assurance are key to ensuring the right things are evaluated the right ways. Further, standards play a principal role in quality assurance of processes. Other quality control mechanisms, such as peer review, systematic reviews, and competency requirements for evaluators, are also relatively common (Bonturi, 2020). All these formative elements will ensure there is documentation of the development and implementation process, an assessment of support and compliance with the existing environment, and demonstration of the potential impacts and value of an advocacy program. An effective advocacy evaluation can inform the evidence base, inform future advocacy approaches, and provide accountability for the time and resources invested. As such, evaluation is central to supporting evidence-based public health advocacy efforts at all levels and critical to understanding the impact of policies on community- and individual-level behavior changes (Brownson et al., 2009).

REFERENCES

Agénor, M., Perkins, C., Stamoulis, C., Hall, R. D., Samnaliev, M., Berland, S., & Bryn Austin, S. (2021). Developing a database of structural racism-related state laws for health equity research and practice in the United States. *Public Health Reports (Washington, D.C.: 1974)*, *136*(4), 428–440. https://doi.org/10.1177/0033354920984168

Center for Evaluation Innovation. (2009). *Overview of current advocacy evaluation practice.* https://nyshealthfoundation.org/wp-content/uploads/2019/02/overview_current_eval_practice.pdf

Capwell, E. M., Butterfoss, F., & Francisco, V. T. (2000). Why evaluate? *Health Promotion Practice, 1*(1), 15–20. https://doi.org/10.1177/152483990000100103

Centers for Disease Control and Prevention. (n.d.-a). Evaluation guide: Writing SMART objectives. https://www.cdc.gov/dhdsp/docs/smart_objectives.pdf

Centers for Disease Control and Prevention. (n.d.-b). Introduction to program evaluation for public health programs. https://www.cdc.gov/eval/guide/cdcevalmanual.pdf

Centers for Disease Control and Prevention. (n.d.-c). *A practitioner's guide to advancing health equity: Community strategies for preventing chronic disease, section 1: Addressing health equity in evaluation efforts.*

Centers for Disease Control and Prevention. (n.d.-d) Step by step—Evaluating violence and injury prevention policies. Brief 5: Evaluating policy impact. https://www.cdc.gov/injury/pdfs/policy/Brief%205-a.pdf

Centers for Disease Control and Prevention. (1999). Framework for program evaluation in public health. *MMWR Morbidity and Mortality Weekly Report, 48*(RR-11), 1–40.

Cottrell, R. R., & McKenzie, J. F. (2011). *Health promotion and education research methods: Using the five-chapter thesis/dissertation model* (2nd ed.). Jones and Bartlett Publishers.

Culp, L., & Silverman, R. (2021) An introduction to legal epidemiology. In M. Ransom & L. Valladares (Eds.), *Public health law: Concepts and case studies.* Springer Publishing.

Fitzpatrick, J. L., Sanders, J. R., & Worthen, B. R. (2004). *Program evaluation: Alternative approaches and practical guidelines* (3rd ed.). Pearson.

Green, L. W., & Lewis, F. M. (1986). *Measurement and evaluation in health education and health promotion.* Mayfield.

Guba, E. G., & Lincoln, Y. S. (1989). *Fourth generation evaluation.* Sage Publications.

Innovation Network. (2009, January 1). Pathfinder: A practical guide to advocacy evaluation. http://www.pointk.org/client_docs/File/advocacy/pathfinder_advocate_web.pdf

International Initiative for Impact Evaluation. (2017, December). Evaluating advocacy: An exploration of evidence and tools to understand what works and why. https://

www.3ieimpact.org/sites/default/files/2019-01/wp29-advocacy.pdf

Issel, L. M., & Wells, R. (2018). *Health program planning and evaluation: A practical, systematic approach for community health*. Jones & Bartlett Learning.

Knowlden, A. P., Cottrell, R. R., Henderson, J., Allison, K., Auld, M. E., Kusorgbor-Narh, C. S., Lysoby, L., & McKenzie, J. F. (2020). Health education specialist practice analysis II 2020: Processes and outcomes. *Health Education & Behavior, 47*(4), 642–651. https://doi.org/10.1177/1090198120926923

Kruger, J., Smith, M. J., Chen, B., et al. (2020). Hurricane evacuation laws in eight southern U.S. coastal states—December 2018. *MMWR Morbidity and Mortality Weekly Report, 69*, 1233–1237. https://doi.org/10.15585/mmwr.mm6936a1

Loscalzo, J. (2014). A celebration of failure. *Circulation, 129*(9), 953–955. https://doi.org/10.1161/CIRCULATIONAHA.114.009220

McKenzie, J. F., Neiger, B. L., & Thackeray, R. (2017). *Planning, implementing, and evaluating health promotion programs: A primer* (7th ed.). Pearson.

Mid Atlantic Regional Public Health Training Center. (2017). *Public health training needs assessment: Report on Maryland Department of Health and Mental Hygiene*. https://health.maryland.gov/pophealth/Documents/Accreditation/Training%20Needs%20Assessment%20Report%20-%20Maryland%20DHMH.pdf

National Network of Public Health Institutes. (2021). *Public health learning navigator*. https://www.phlearningnavigator.org/

Organizational Research Services. (2007). *A guide to measuring advocacy and policy*. http://www.pointk.org/resources/files/Guide_to_measuring_advocacy_and_policy.pdf

Patton, M. Q. (2006). Evaluation for the way we work. *Nonprofit Quarterly, 13*(1), 28–33.

Pepin, D., Hulkower, R., & McCord, R. F. (2020). How are telehealth laws intersecting with laws addressing the opioid overdose epidemic? *Journal of Public Health Management and Practice: JPHMP, 26*(3), 227–231. https://doi.org/10.1097/PHH.0000000000001036

PolicyLink. (2012). Community-based participatory research: A strategy for building healthy communities and promoting health through policy change. https://www.policylink.org/sites/default/files/CBPR.pdf

Ramanathan, T., Hulkower, R., Holbrook, J., & Penn, M. (2017). Legal epidemiology: The science of law. *Journal of Law, Medicine & Ethics, 45*(1, Suppl.), 69–72. https://doi.org/10.1177/1073110517703329

Sloan, A. A., Keane, T., Pettie, J. R., Bhuiya, A. R., Taylor, L. N., Bates, M., Bernard, S., Akinleye, F., & Gilchrist, S. (2020). MPH mapping and analysis of US state and urban local sodium reduction laws. *Journal of Public Health Management and Practice, 26*, S62–S70. https://doi.org/10.1097/PHH.0000000000001124

Sullivan, L., Harvey, H. H., Smith, G. A., & Yang, J. (2020). MPH putting policy into practice: School-level compliance with and implementation of state concussion laws. *Journal of Public Health Management and Practice, 26*, S84–S92. https://doi.org/10.1097/PHH.0000000000001128

Teles, S., & Schmitt, M. (2011). The elusive craft of evaluating advocacy. *Stanford Social Innovation Review, 9*(3), 39–43.

Weiss, C. (1972). *Evaluation research: Methods for studying programs and policies*. Prentice Hall.

World Health Organization. (2008). Advocacy step 8: Monitoring and evaluation. In *Cancer control: Knowledge into action: WHO guide for effective programmes: Module 6: Policy and advocacy*. https://www.ncbi.nlm.nih.gov/books/NBK195428/

Yarbrough, D. B., Shulha, L. M., Hopson, R. K., & Caruthers, F. A. (2011). *The program evaluation standards: A guide for evaluators and evaluation users* (3rd ed.). Sage Publishers.

CHAPTER 13: END-OF-CHAPTER ACTIVITIES

DISCUSSION QUESTIONS

1. In small groups, discuss program evaluation you have been a part of developing or implementing. This could be something for your coursework, department, a student organization, or other activity on campus.

2. With a partner or in an online discussion, identify what the difference is between summative and formative evaluations. When would you use one over the other?

3. In a classroom discussion, explain the concept of universal evaluation and the similar methods used across all forms of evaluation, including program, policy, and advocacy evaluation.

APPLICATION ACTIVITIES

1. Create five small groups of students. Assign one domain to each group and have them brainstorm and explain that domain aligned with a health topic chosen by the facilitator or faculty. Allow each team 10–15 minutes to discuss, place their explanation on a large piece of paper or white board, and have one from each team share. Go in order of the domains.
   Domain 1 of the policy process is focused on problem identification.
   Domain 2 is agenda setting.
   Domain 3 is about strategy and policy formulation.
   Domain 4 is focused on policy adoption.
   Domain 5 is focused on policy implementation.

2. Create a program evaluation timeline on the wall, whiteboard, or, if taught on-line, use the whiteboard feature. Students identify the four generations of program evaluation and then identify examples in each.

   First generation—"measurement," meaning that it was science based and outcome focused. This type of evaluation focuses on systematic testing and estimating the effect of an intervention.

   Second generation—"descriptive" and focused on goals and objectives. This type of evaluation shifts the focus to determining the worth of programs. This generation of evaluation was associated with the growth in federal social services and the need to look for the cost-effectiveness of those resources.

   Third "responsiveness" generation of evaluation—focuses on the needs of those involved in the evaluation. Several pedigrees are part of this generation of evaluation, including utilization and participatory, which may partly account for the great range of approaches to evaluation used today.

   Fourth generation of program evaluation: meta-evaluation. Like a meta-analysis of several research studies to determine more robust indicators of effect, this is basically an evaluation of several program evaluations conducted to look at proposed relationships and arrive at recommendations that are evidence based.

ADDITIONAL RESOURCES

1. To expand your knowledge of program evaluation, visit https://www.phlearni ngnavigator.org/ and search for "Advanced Program Evaluation" in the search bar. Take the training. Then using one outcome question that was not chosen from the ShapeTracker app example, develop an additional short-term outcome and long-term outcome related to your chosen question for the logic model.

2. Visit https://www.phlearningnavigator.org/ and type "Economic Evaluation" in the search bar. Take the training. Then complete the Economic Evaluation Activity worksheet to test your knowledge for the two scenarios.

QUIZ QUESTIONS

1. _____ is "the process of determining the value or worth of a health promotion program or any of its components based on predetermined criteria or standards of success identified by stakeholders."
   a. Prescriptive procedure
   b. SWAT analysis
   c. Process evaluation
   d. Program evaluation

2. In reference to the concept of universal evaluation, there are similar methods used across all forms of evaluations, including program, policy, and advocacy evaluations. Which of the following is true?
   a. All evaluators should be driven by a similar purpose of providing high-quality information.
   b. All evaluators employ logic models, affect theories, or theories of change.
   c. All evaluators conduct systematic and database inquiries.
   d. All of the above.

3. Problem identification, agenda setting, strategy and policy formulation, policy adoption, and policy implementation are the five domains of the _____ process.
   a. CDC's policy
   b. summative evaluation
   c. universal evaluation
   d. national organization

4. _____ explore the effects or what results from or is associated with exposure to a program whereas _____ focus on the quality of a program by gathering information and data to review before or during program implementation.
   a. Formative evaluations; summative evaluations
   b. Summative evaluations; formative evaluations
   c. Process evaluations; economic evaluations
   d. Economic evaluations; process evaluations

5. _____ is often identified as a part of formative evaluation, while _____ _____ fits into the more general term of summative.
   a. Universal evaluation; public health policy
   b. Impact and outcome evaluation; process evaluation
   c. Process evaluation; impact and outcome evaluation
   d. SWAT analysis; prescriptive procedure

6. Which of the following generations of program evaluation is science based and outcome focused and focuses on systematic testing and estimating the effect of an intervention?
   a. meta-evaluations
   b. descriptive
   c. responsibleness
   d. measurement

7. The third "responsiveness" generation of evaluation focuses on
   a. the goals and objectives.
   b. the needs of those involved in the evaluation.
   c. proposed relationships between programs.
   d. cost-effectiveness of program utilization.

8. An effective advocacy evaluation can inform the evidence base, inform future advocacy approaches, and _____
   a. agenda marketing.
   b. provide accountability for the time and resources invested.
   c. analyzing the situation on where a program should not explore.
   d. collaboration, insinuation, and multiplication.

9. _____ guide professionals through a process of strategically assessing the needs of the priority population, carefully planning appropriate interventions, executing the planned interventions, modifying the plan if necessary, and evaluating the immediate, short-term, and long-term efficacy of the program.
   a. Program-planning models
   b. Policymaking agendas
   c. Education evaluation representatives
   d. State legislators' agendas

10. Which of the following is the first step in the CDC's Framework for Program Evaluation in Public Health?
    a. program description
    b. gathering credible evidence
    c. engaging the stakeholders
    d. reject conclusions

ANSWER KEY
   1. **D.** Program evaluation
   2. **D.** All of the above

3. **A.** CDC's policy
4. **B.** Summative evaluations; formative evaluations
5. **C.** Process evaluation; impact and outcome evaluation
6. **D.** Measurement
7. **B.** The needs of those involved in the evaluation
8. **B.** Provide accountability for the time and resources invested
9. **A.** Program-planning models
10. **D.** Reject conclusions

Advocacy for the Long Haul

JODY EARLY AND SELINA A. MOHAMMED

Take a long, hard look down the road you will have to travel once you have made a commitment to work for change. Know that this transformation will not happen right away. Change often takes time. It rarely happens all at once.

—FORMER REP. JOHN LEWIS, *Across That Bridge: Life Lessons and a Vision for Change* (2017)

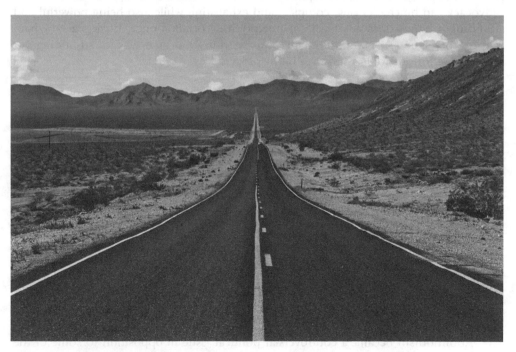

FIGURE 14.1 The long road ahead.

Jody Early and Selina A. Mohammed, *Advocacy for the Long Haul*. In: *Be the Change*. Edited by Keely S. Rees, Jody Early, and Cicily Hampton, Oxford University Press. © Oxford University Press 2023. DOI: 10.1093/oso/9780197570890.003.0014

INTRODUCTION

Those who seek careers in the health professions are often individuals guided by a strong sense of altruism and desire to help contribute to the health and well-being of individuals and society. It is this altruism that can drive us to go beyond addressing the needs and capacity of individuals to tackling the sociocultural, environmental, economic, and political factors that comprise unjust systems of exclusion and oppression. In doing so, our efforts have the potential to impact not only a few, but also thousands, or even millions. However, change rarely happens quickly. As we have discussed throughout this textbook, advocacy can be challenging, complex, and exhausting while also being powerful and fulfilling. Change does not usually happen quickly or all at once: It takes a long-haul approach (Figure 14.1). In this chapter, we provide some strategies for sustaining our advocacy efforts as well as ourselves in the process.

ADVOCACY NEVER ENDS

Progress is not always a straight line. In fact, it often "comes in fits and starts . . . and it's not always a smooth path" (Barack Obama, 2012; para 16). Let's use the Civil Rights Act of 1964 as an example. This landmark legislation prohibits discrimination on the basis of race, color, religion, sex, or national origin. The act also prohibits discrimination in public accommodations and federally funded programs, and it strengthened the enforcement of voting rights and the desegregation of schools. Even though many of its key events occurred in the 1950s and early 1960s, one could argue that the advocacy and history leading to the Civil Rights Act extended over a hundred years prior. The quest for equal rights under the law began long before the 1954 *Brown v. the Board of Education* decision outlawing segregation in schools, the Montgomery bus boycott of 1955, or the march on Washington in 1963 where Martin Luther King Jr. delivered his powerful "I have a Dream" speech (Figure 14.2). Movements, such as abolition, led to the fight for civil rights and emerged in the United States around 1830 from Great Britain.

Abolitionism became a controversial political issue in opposition to some of the "founding forces" that drove America, including power, capitalism, racism, and colonization. Abolitionists and critics often engaged in heated and—and even deadly—confrontations. The divisiveness and animosity fueled by the movement, along with other factors, led to the American Civil War and eventually to the passing of the

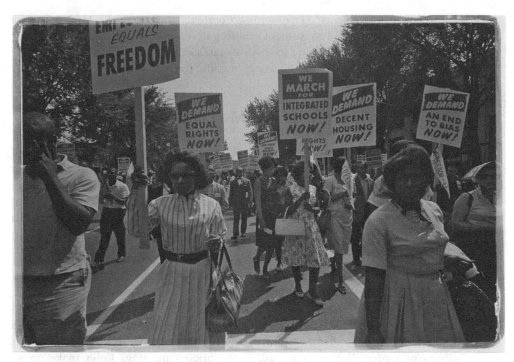

FIGURE 14.2 Civil Rights March on Washington, D.C., 1963.

Thirteenth Amendment, which ended legal slavery. A few years later, with the passing of the Fifteenth Amendment in 1869, African American men were theoretically granted the constitutional right to vote. Yet it took another 51 years for Black/African American women to obtain this legal right. However, in reality, it took much longer. Black men and women were effectively barred from voting from around 1870 until the passage of the Voting Rights Act of 1965. These victories were the result of decades, even centuries, of relentless advocacy by courageous and dedicated individuals and communities who may have spent their entire lives in the quest to protect civil liberties or bring about major change. Many did not live to see the fruits of their labor, yet their work paved the way for many of the U.S. freedoms we enjoy today.

However, the march for civil rights and equality is not over. For example, on June 15, 2020, in the case of *Bostock v. Clayton*, the Supreme Court of the United States ruled that protection against discrimination based on "sex" under Title VII of the Civil Rights act extends to those identifying as LGBTQ+ (lesbian, gay, bisexual, trans, queer, and others). Whether we are striving to protect LGBTQ+ rights, prevent voter suppression, or achieve equal pay for all genders, the destructive forces of exclusion, exploitation, and discrimination that led to the Civil Rights Act are still deeply entrenched in our society and have proven difficult to end. The future of civil rights, like its past, will be shaped largely by collective efforts and *movement building*. In the words of scholar, activist, and author Angela Y. Davis (2016): "No change has ever happened simply because the President chose to move in a more progressive direction. Every change that has happened has come as a result of mass movements" (*Freedom Is a Constant Struggle*, p. 35). Understanding that the work of advocacy and movement building never ends will help you manage expectations and the process over time so that you can sustain momentum for the work as well as yourself. Below we offer some advice for going the distance.

TACTICS TO SUSTAIN LONG-TERM ADVOCACY
Get Organized

If you are launching a long-term advocacy effort, you will need a clear structure and more formal organization to sustain it. Structure is the framework around which your group is organized, the parts of your organization that keep your work moving forward. Organizational structure is not one size fits all. The best structure for any organization or initiative will depend on its size, how many people are involved, what the setting is, and its stage of development. Regardless of the type, there are three common features within any organizational structure:

1. *Governance:* Who will make decisions within the organization (e.g., chief executive officer [CEO], executive director, cochairs, executive committee, etc.)?
2. *Rules by which the organization operates:* What rules and protocols will the organization use to operate? Establish rules by stating how formal and informal groups operate within the organization. For example, many committees use Robert's Rules of Order (Robert et al., 2020) to conduct meetings Rules make up an organization's culture. A small organization or group that is formed to resolve a single issue may not need a formal structure, but large groups typically need clear guidelines to minimize confusion and set expectations on things such as collegiality, respect, and ethical behavior.
3. *Distribution of work:* Inherent in any organizational structure is a distribution of work. The distribution and delegation of this work can be formal or informal, temporary or enduring, paid or volunteer, but every organization will have some type of division of labor.

Two examples of organizational structures for a large, statewide coalition and a small, newly formed nonprofit are depicted in Figure 14.3. The organizational structure you need for your group or organization might be simpler or more complex.

Create an Inspiring Vision and Strategic Plan

Fundamentally, organizations need to come to an understanding of why they exist. To determine this purpose, members first need to establish the overarching issue they are trying to address (i.e., the reason they are coalescing) and ascertain the myriad factors that contribute to that issue. Once these aspects are determined, they need to ask themselves what the hallmarks of "success" would be if they effectively tackled the problem (i.e., what does success look like?) and, importantly, what they will have to change in order to meet the ultimate resolution they seek. To answer these questions, organizations engage in **strategic planning**, a collective process that helps determine what an organization wants to achieve, how it will achieve those objectives, who will be involved, and a timeline for achieving milestones along the way. Part of strategic planning involves

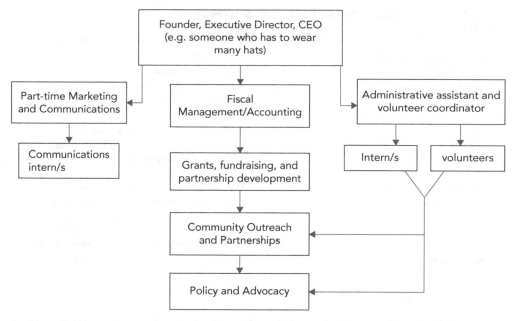

FIGURE 14.3 Organizational structure of a small, newly formed advocacy organization (nonprofit).

determining an organization's vision, mission, and values to guide the behaviors of people in that organization and ensure that, as a whole, they have a shared purpose and direction.

A **vision statement** (Table 14.1) is a clear and concise assertion that is broad in nature and encompasses an organization's aspirations of what it hopes to achieve or become. It is the desired end state resulting from the change that can ensue from an organization's work. The best vision statements are inspirational and memorable, are future oriented, and motivate people to contribute to their organization.

A **mission statement** describes what an organization is and what it needs to do to differentiate itself from similar organizations and achieve its vision. It answers the question of how a vision will be accomplished and is more actionable than a vision statement in that it describes what it will do to achieve that vision. Both the mission and vision of an organization function within a set of values that defines what members of an organization believe in and creates a code of ethics that they follow. These values serve as a moral compass for the organization, guiding and setting standards for behaviors, decision-making, and action.

When developing your organization's strategic plan, it is critical to know who the diverse stakeholders are for the type of advocacy work you are doing and that you work closely with them to co-create meaningful mission, vision, and value statements. It is a process that utilizes everyone's background experiences, knowledge, and skills and involves putting minds together to think creatively. Once you have identified these statements, the next step will be to determine how the mission will be used to achieve the vision. This can be done by constructing *strategies* to cohesively leverage the mission; *goals* that describe what needs to be accomplished to implement each strategy (i.e.,

TABLE 14.1 Examples of Organizational Vision Statements

Organization	Vision Statement
Human Rights Campaign	Equality for everyone
Feeding America	A hunger-free America
Alzheimer's Association	A world without Alzheimer's
Oxfam	A just world without poverty
National Multiple Sclerosis Society	A world free of MS
Habitat of Humanity	A world where everyone has a decent place to live
Dolores Huerta Foundation	To inspire and organize communities to build volunteer organizations empowered to pursue social justice
ASPCA (American Society for the Prevention of Cruelty to Animals)	That the United States is humane community in which all animals are treated with respect and kindness
Kiva	We envision a world where all people—even in the most remote areas of the globe—hold the power to create opportunity for themselves and for others
The Nature Conservatory	To leave a sustainable world for future generations

targets that you want to achieve); *objectives* that provide specific, quantifiable milestones and timelines for each goal (and keep you motivated!), and *action plans* that detail the specific steps that will be implemented to achieve a goal, within the frame of each objective. Creating this laddered approach makes your vision tangible.

By engaging multiple stakeholders in strategic planning, you have the potential to proactively achieve a greater understanding of your project's constraints, risks, assets, and opportunities. However, in addition to developing this organizational road map, you will need to determine how to evaluate and measure progress and how frequently that evaluation process will occur. If the strategic plan is not being used regularly or as the foundation for your advocacy work, an organization can lose sight of its direction and goals. At the very least, strategic plans should be reviewed every year to maintain accountability and monitor progress. Ask yourself what your organization accomplished in a year, whether or not you followed the plan you created, and if not, why you veered off track. Examine if what you are doing has been effective and, if not, what needs to change. It is vital to remember that the strategic plan is not static; it is a fluid, living document that will inevitably change over time. The assumptions, challenges, threats, and possibilities that your organization based its plan on may have changed within a year and will change again over time. Flexibility and continually working together to adapt and pivot are crucial. Remember, "Even reaching the ultimate goal doesn't mark the end of advocacy. New goals may arise, and, just as with earlier gains, the final goal has to be maintained" (Lock & Fine, 2016).

Form Strong Partnerships and Allies That Can Help Support You

A significant component of advocacy work is forming strong partnerships and alliances that can support and strengthen you and your work. Teamwork is essential to actualizing your vision. Using an analogy from the sport of cycling to illustrate this point, within

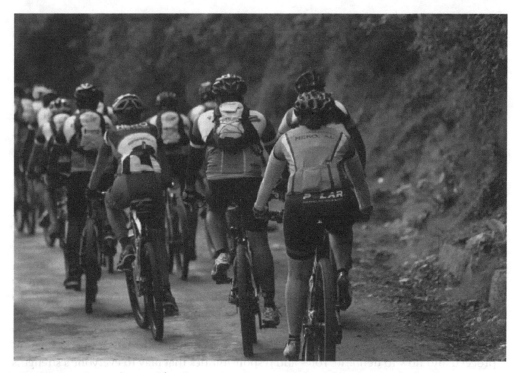

FIGURE 14.4 In a peloton, riders in a group save energy by riding close to each other.

cycling teams, one member serves as a team leader (the strongest cyclist), while the key function of the other team members is to do everything they can to help their team leader win the race (Figure 14.4).

These "domestiques," as they are called, use a strategy where they ride in front of the team leader to cut the wind and make it easier for that leader to pedal. This "drafting" saves the team leader energy in a long event. Various teams in a race tend to ride in a **peleton**, or tight group, with one cyclist who rides at the front of the group, setting the pace and pulling the pack along. The rider who is pulling tires more quickly, so after a short stint in front, they move to the back to let another rider take over. This allows team leaders to stay in back of the peleton while their teammates take turns out front, protecting them. By functioning as a cohesive unit, each team can engage in more advanced strategies that, depending on their need, quicken or slow the pace of the race, allow for attack runs by their team leader to win the race, and block rivals from mounting a chase. In this way, collectivism is balanced with individualism.

Central to this notion of collectivism is finding partners who can engage in teamwork to further your organization's mission (and theirs). Align with organizations that have similar missions, visions, and goals. Engage respected community members and stakeholders so that you can learn from their wisdom and experiences and achieve outcomes that are relevant and beneficial to them. Listen to your opponents so that you can embrace multiple perspectives, understand where others are coming from, create buy-in where possible, and work innovatively to bridge differences. Importantly, partner with local political leaders and policymakers to drive your advocacy issues forward. But, also remember that in order to get support, you need to give support. Determining who your allies are, how best to partner with them, and how to work efficiently and effectively together is fun, yet it is time consuming and challenging work.

Using principles of community-based participatory research (CBPR) can help you to establish strong collaborations and engage in collective work. CBPR is an orientation to research that focuses on the formation of equitable partnerships throughout all work phases, and it values co-learning and reciprocity, unpacking issues around power and privilege, long-term commitment, and centering local knowledge (Wallerstein & Duran, 2006). Shared decision-making and power, throughout all work phases and mutual ownership of products and achievements, is central to this approach. CBPR neutralizes power imbalances between partners and transforms the socially constructed roles of who is more or less "knowledgeable" to one where expertise is shared. Although this approach can extend to any type of partner-based work, utilizing CBPR is especially important when collaborating with marginalized communities that have been historically exploited and harmed by more one-sided paradigms. The collaborative, action-oriented, emancipative, and social justice dimensions of CBPR make it particularly relevant to advocates who are committed to engaging in ethical and community-driven work to dismantle inequities and promote positive social change. There are multiple ways to articulate CBPR; how you decide to operationalize these guiding principles will always be context dependent. Together, you and your partners can mutually determine how best to proceed and how to delineate roles and responsibilities that play to everyone's strengths and advance everyone's goals.

There are numerous examples of strong coalitions and partnerships that have successfully been built on foundations of CBPR. The Detroit Urban Research Center (URC) is a primary example of a community–academic partnership network that fosters CBPR to promote health equity, bidirectional capacity building, and policy change. The Detroit URC is composed of representatives from local community-based organizations, the Detroit Health Department and Henry Ford Health System, and faculty representatives from the University of Michigan Schools of Public Health, Social Work, and Nursing. Their mission

> is to enhance understanding of the relationship between the social and physical environmental determinants of health, and translate that knowledge into public health interventions, programs, and policies aimed at promoting health equity. The Detroit URC seeks to maintain an effective partnership that identifies problems affecting the health of residents in Detroit and promotes and conducts interdisciplinary, community-based participatory research which recognizes, builds upon and enhances the resources and strengths in the communities involved." (Detroit URC, n.d.)

Together, these partners determine organizational priorities and oversee the development of CBPR projects and activities.

Over the last 25 years, the Detroit URC has been instrumental in changing the health and social policy landscape of the city of Detroit. They have tackled intractable problems prevalent in city communities and engaged in action to reduce the impact of environmental triggers on childhood asthma; promote environmental justice; inform the strategic framework to guide the regeneration of Detroit; build community capacity to address intimate partner violence against Latina women; promote heart health; enhance health insurance literacy for community residents; and improve high school graduation rates and health, to name a few. In addition to the numerous positive outcomes that have resulted from their collaboration, the Detroit URC uses the knowledge gained through its projects to advance public health policy formulation, dissemination, and education at individual and system levels.

Identify and Secure the Resources You Need for the Journey

Advocacy for the long haul means that you will need resources to support your plan and advocacy strategies. The most basic of resources are people, money, and time. The people you need usually include paid staff and volunteers. How many volunteers may depend on your budget as well as the expertise and continuity you need to work your plan and achieve your objectives. The types of people you need might include a project coordinator director, researchers, outreach workers, fundraisers, grant writers, student interns, media contacts, and a volunteer coordinator. Having the right people be a part of your team and engaged in the cause is a key ingredient to long-term success and sustainability. According to the Center for Community Health and Development at the University of Kansas, "For a long-term advocacy effort, you have to make a special attempt to find staff, whether volunteer or paid, who have the passion for the issue that will compel them to stay with it for as long as it takes. Continuity is an important factor in successful long-term advocacy, and continuity comes from people" (Community Tool Box, n.d.-c).

Funding is a vital resource. Beyond volunteers and interns, as your campaign or organization grows, you may need to hire staff to manage the day-to-day operation and to keep continuity. This requires reliable funding streams. In addition to staff, there are supplies and office space to consider as well as phones, internet, computers, software, and other equipment. Transportation costs, marketing, and printing are also things you should write into your budget. Even if much of the materials and labor for your effort is donated, what's left can add up—money that you'll have to raise from donations, grants, or other sources. Many larger advocacy organizations either employ a part-time or full-time fundraiser ("development" staff) or contract with a fundraising organization to raise money for them. In smaller organizations, including most community-based and grassroots groups, fundraising may be part of everyone's job description or may be largely the job of the board. No matter who is involved, you will want to plan for a diverse portfolio of funding sources, such as state, federal, and/or foundation grants; private donations; sponsorships; in-kind donations from partners; sales from your campaign merchandise; or corporate donations. Relying too much on one funder may put your campaign or organization at risk if the funding source dries up.

ADVOCACY IN ACTION BOX 14.1	Examples of Short- and Long-Term Objectives
Long-term (outcome) objective: Reduce the rate of pregnancy-related deaths in King County by 50% before the end of 2035.	**Short-term (process) objective:** Implement a community-based peer pregnancy support program at five provider sites within King County to improve perinatal education and social support by the end of 2025.

Track Your Progress and Celebrate Small Gains Along the Way

After spending significant time and energy working toward a common goal, if people do not see signs of progress, energy and motivation will wane. That is why it is important to set short-term or intermediate objectives to accompany the long-term goal (Box 14.1). For example, let's say your organization is working on reducing deaths from childbirth and pregnancy in your county. A short-term objective could be to establish a community-based educational and outreach program within 12 months that includes trusted community peer health navigators that help connect those who are pregnant to midwives, doulas, nurse practitioners, or other health providers for free or low-cost perinatal support and care.

Communicating even the smallest achievements to your team, to your partners, to your funders or donors, and to the community plays an important role in helping people maintain motivation, persistence, and engagement for trying to achieve the longer term goals. If you allow yourself to think that you don't have to continue to remind policymakers and funders that your issue is important or that the work your constituency does is both socially and economically crucial, your organization may face funding cuts and a lack of interest from the stakeholders you are trying to keep engaged. Therefore, regular newsletters, blog posts, community events, social media messages, news, and human-interest stories can serve as vehicles to share good news and keep people informed of short-term achievements.

Research demonstrates that perceived progress is a significant predictor of motivation and happiness within an organization or workplace. This is known as the *progress principle*. Harvard researchers Amabile and Kramer (2011) surveyed 238 employees daily over 4 months and found that employees who felt the happiest and most satisfied with their work, their employer, and the work environment were those who felt they had accomplished even the smallest of tasks. Progress was the biggest motivator and mood elevator, no matter if the progress was small or great. So, applying this principle to health advocacy, it is important to celebrate every gain, small or large, collectively and individually, to keep yourself as well as others encouraged about achieving the long-term goal. In the words of former Georgia representative, activist, and Fair Fight founder Stacy Abrams: "I learned long ago that winning doesn't mean you get the prize. Sometimes you get progress, and that counts" (Our Time Is Now: Power, Purpose, and the Fight for a Fair America, p. 3).

Tracking progress can also help you and others reflect on what's working or what barriers are inhibiting the work moving forward. It might be that your objectives may need adjustment based on circumstances or new information or perhaps your expectations were too unrealistic to start.

Prepare for Setbacks and Adversity

Setbacks, or a single event or series of events that impedes progress, can sometimes leave you questioning why you are doing advocacy work at all. Perhaps your program funding wasn't renewed or a media story provides inaccurate information that threatens your organization's reputation. These are all setbacks that will require immediate action geared specifically to removing the obstacle or reversing the situation, whatever it is. What can you do to turn things around? Setbacks are usually limited by time. Once you deal with them, you can usually move ahead.

Adversity, on the other hand, is more likely to be an ongoing unfavorable condition. You might have ongoing problems with reaching the group you are trying to reach or perhaps another organization and community group has banded together to campaign against you. It can also be internal: a change in leadership that results in organizational distrust or nurtures a culture of fear and disrespect among employees: Adversity can break down individuals, partnerships, and organizations.

Leading yourself, an organization, or coalition through adversity calls for steadfastness, patience, and optimism. Think back to the struggle for civil rights past and present. What was achieved happened over decades with plenty of setbacks and adversity along the way. Endurance usually requires a longer, multifaceted approach, as well as "glass half-full" optimism. Dealing with adversity and setbacks are opportunities for true leadership and commitment to shine. If you can handle a difficult situation or condition and keep things on an even keel, your advocacy efforts will be more likely to roll on, and people will likely gain even more conviction to the cause and assurance in your credibility as a leader. Although setbacks and adversity may call for slightly different approaches, we offer some strategies below at the organizational level.

TIPS FOR DEALING WITH SETBACKS AND ADVERSITY

Assess the situation, then take action. First, it's important to look at why something did not work out the way you expected or hoped. Were you or the organization responsible for the situation? It is important to take accountability and to understand the root causes of the problem so you can try to address them in order to move forward. If your program proved ineffective, learn why. You have to be courageously honest when assessing the situation so that you can understand how to fix things. Understanding how you got into a situation is the best strategy for not getting into it again.

If the situation is beyond your control (e.g., if the state was in a financial crisis and cut funding), are there ways around it? Are there things you could do that would affect it? Try to analyze the situation so you can understand how to deal with it. Once you have a good understanding of what went wrong, develop a recovery plan that involves your whole team or organization, even if the setback or adverse circumstances only impact part of it. Even if you know the primary influence was out of your control (reduced state budget, e.g.), look for a way to take over control of that area of your work. If it is a funding issue, for instance, perhaps you can diversify your funding (i.e., find a variety of funding sources instead of depending on only one or a small number) so that a cut from any one source will not affect you seriously.

Accentuate the positive. When things seem to be falling apart, it's easy to only focus on the negative. However, that won't get you very far. To move forward, it's important to look at what's working or, at the very least, what you learned from the experience that can strengthen your organization or you. Emphasizing the positive will strengthen staff and/or volunteer morale and keep the organization heading in the right direction. How are challenges presenting new opportunities? Shannon Watts, activist and founder of the grassroots movement Moms Demand Action for Gun Sense in America, wrote about the "upside of losing" in her book, *Fight Like a Mother*:

I had always known that America's gun laws wouldn't happen overnight, but . . . I hadn't completely understood that we needed to dig in for the grueling, years-long process of incremental progress. In any kind of advocacy, you're going to encounter losses and setbacks. In order to have the mental wherewithal, we had to redefine success and accept that while we couldn't always win, we could make every loss count by losing forward. (2019, p. 83)

Ask for help if you need it. After assessing the situation, you may determine that you need additional expertise to help improve the situation. Other advocates or leaders of nonprofits who have been through something similar, funders, academics, community partners, businesses—they might be able to help. The advantage of bringing in outside help is that, in addition to providing what the organization lacks, it can provide you with greater community understanding of your work and your needs and thus greater community support.

Focus on things within your direct control. This might come as a disappointment or surprise, but most aspects of the dynamic world we live in are beyond your individual control. You, alone, for example, cannot stop a pandemic. You cannot save the economy or prevent natural disasters from occurring. And, try as you might, you may not be able to change the course of a life-threatening illness that your friend or loved one is facing. While it can be tough to acknowledge, railing against events or circumstances outside your control will only drain you of energy and leave you feeling anxious and hopeless. Acceptance of things you cannot control can free you up to devote your energy to the things that you do have control over. Give yourself permission to stop worrying about what you cannot control and focus on the action you can take. For example, if you are unemployed, you cannot control whether the ideal job appears in the want ads or whether an employer will grant you an interview. But you can control how much time and effort you put into searching for work, what your résumé looks like, and brushing up on skills or learning new ones.

Deal with your problems one step at a time. If a problem is too big to deal with all at once, try breaking it down into smaller, more manageable steps. Paring down the expectations, and dealing with each issue one by one, can help you create success experiences and strategies that can help you deal with even greater challenges the next time you face them. According to psychologist Albert Bandura (originator of social cognitive theory), this approach to problem-solving can lead to greater self-efficacy and motivation.

Resilience and reflection go together. Look back at examples where you and/or your organization coped with uncertainty and change. Reflecting on your past experiences can help you accept your current situation and better understand your own resiliency. Examining your past, and what you were able to overcome, can help you see past the current crisis and derive some confidence and strength that (in the words made famous by legendary activist Dolores Huerta), "Sí se puede" (Yes, it can be done!).

Care for Yourself

When you are working to provide solutions for complex social issues and helping to dismantle oppressive systems, it is easy to burn out. For example, in a 2015 study, research fellows Chen and Gorski at the Center for the Advancement of Well-Being interviewed social justice advocates and activists. They discovered a disheartening pattern: Roughly half of those surveyed who experienced burnout did not take a break; they left their movements for good. Caring for yourself is a huge component of endurance and long-term success. It is not a luxury, as some may think, but an essential part of survival. Scholar, poet, and activist Audre Lorde wrote: "Caring for myself is not self-indulgence, it is self-preservation, and that is an act of political warfare" (Audre Lorde, Burst of Light, p. 118)

RECOGNIZING BURNOUT AND COMPASSION FATIGUE

According to the American Psychological Association, **burnout** is a condition that results from a cumulative process marked by emotional exhaustion and withdrawal associated with increased workload and institutional stress that has not been sufficiently managed (American Psychological Association, 2020). Burnout can result in depression and anxiety, physical and emotional exhaustion, less enjoyment of work, anger, and/or increased irritability. **Compassion fatigue** occurs when those in helping-related roles or occupations take on the suffering of individuals and/or communities they serve who have experienced extreme stress or trauma. According to Dr. Charles Figley, an expert and researcher on compassion fatigue, it is an occupational hazard and "the psychological cost of using your emotions and heart to help people heal" (Figley, 1995). The difference between burnout and compassion fatigue is that burnout is *not* trauma related, but usually coincides with the compassion fatigue experience. Table 14.2 differentiates between burnout and compassion fatigue providing common characteristics and symptoms.

TABLE 14.2 Common Symptoms of Burnout and Compassion Fatigue[a]

	Burnout	Compassion Fatigue
Differences	Not trauma related Develops over time Slower recovery	Vicarious traumatization More rapid onset May have quicker recovery than burnout
Symptoms	Excessive stress, anger, and irritability; feelings of detachment or apathy; fatigue; insomnia; sadness; inability to concentrate; feeling unmotivated and despondent; loss of creativity; forgetfulness; feeling a loss of control over work-related conditions; wanting to quit	Feelings of sadness and depression; loss of productivity; intrusive thoughts; jumpiness; tiredness; feelings of being on edge or trapped; inability to separate personal and professional life; loss of compassion satisfaction (e.g., the happiness, pride, and satisfaction derived from helping others)

[a] Note: Burnout usually coincides with compassion fatigue.

Created by J. Early based on "Symptoms of professional burnout: A review of the empirical evidence," APA PsycNET, American Psychological Association, 1998; and "Signs of caregiver stress and burnout," *Helpguide*, July 2018.

STRATEGIES FOR MANAGING AND PREVENTING BURNOUT

When you are burned out, problems seem insurmountable, everything can look bleak, and it may be difficult to muster up the energy to care, let alone take action to help yourself. However, taking action to manage it is the key to resolving it. The following are evidence-based steps you can take to prevent or manage burnout:

- *Reach out to others.* Social contact is nature's antidote to stress and talking face to face with a good listener is one of the fastest ways to calm your nervous system and relieve stress. The person you talk to doesn't have to be able to "fix" your stressors; they just have to be a good listener and listen attentively without becoming distracted or expressing judgment. Reach out to those closest to you whom you trust, such as your partner, family, and friends. Talk to them about how you are feeling and connect with them socially as well. Having strong ties in your workplace or part of your advocacy initiative can help reduce monotony and counter the effects of burnout. Having friends to chat and joke with during the day can help relieve stress from an unfulfilling or demanding job or task, improve performance, increase feelings of social support, and simply get you through a rough day.
- *Get to the root of it.* Feelings of burnout are usually caused by multiple factors, not just one. The source of your burnout may actually have little to do with your advocacy work. The stress that accompanies each factor in your burnout algorithm might be manageable on its own, but the combination can easily overwhelm you if you do not take steps to get support. Talking to a therapist or using mental health resources available can also help you get to the core of it and help you navigate through this period.
- *Get some rest.* You cannot pour from an empty cup. Arguably the most fundamental protective factor against burnout symptoms (e.g., cynicism, desensitization, and irritability) is rest. Rest includes whatever helps you reset; it could be physical rest (e.g., trying get more sleep) or doing anything that puts your mind, spirit, and body in a state of relaxation, such as checking in with friends, meditating, enjoying nature, exercising, engaging in a favorite hobby, and/or trying to limit your exposure to social media (see Box 14.2). Unchecked burnout can infiltrate every area of life, so hold fast to your boundaries.
- *Take time off.* If burnout seems inevitable, try to take a complete break from the work. Go on vacation, use up your sick days, ask for a temporary leave of absence—anything to remove yourself from the situation. Use the time away to recharge your batteries and pursue other methods of recovery.
- *Limit your contact with negative people.* Hanging out with negative-minded people who do nothing but complain will only drag down your mood and outlook. If you have to work with a negative person, try to limit the amount of time you spend together.
- *Say "No."* It's easy for service-driven people to become overextended. Being able to go the distance means learning to say no to everyone who comes to you with a request. If you find this difficult, remind yourself that saying no or "not right

ADVOCACY IN ACTION BOX 14.2	Different Forms of Rest
Taking time away from the workplace	Stepping away from the computer
Permitting yourself not to be helpful	Getting sleep
Being "unproductive"	Taking a break from worry
Connecting to art and to nature	Being still or meditating
Finding solitude to recharge	Doing something active that brings you joy
Taking a break from social media	Spending time with loved ones or friends
Being creative	Getting alone time
Being silly	Letting go of things weighing you down
Finding a "safe space"	Taking a break from technology

now," allows you to say "yes" to the commitments you already have—and focus your energy on fulfilling those to the best of your ability.

- *Find time to do something you enjoy that is unrelated to your work.* Creativity is a powerful antidote to burnout. Try something new, start a fun project, or resume a favorite hobby. Choose activities that have nothing to do with whatever is causing your stress.
- *Add some exercise.* Even though it may be the last thing you feel like doing when you're burned out, exercise is a powerful antidote to stress and burnout, and it produces dopamine and endorphins that help lift your mood. You do not have to exercise for long to reap the benefits. Aim to exercise for 30 minutes or more per day or break that up into short, 10-minute bursts of activity. Go outside if you can. Mother Nature can help you feel better. A 10-minute walk at lunch to get some air, for example, can reduce your stress, help improve your metabolism, and lift your spirits.
- *Eat for energy.* What you put in your body can have a huge impact on your mood and energy levels throughout the day. Minimize sugar and refined carbs, which can cause your mood and energy levels to crash. Also, pay attention to the amount of caffeine you might be consuming or foods with unhealthy fats and preservatives. Try to stick with whole foods that have not been processed. Include good sources of protein that can help you maintain your energy and respond to stress in positive ways.
- *Switch lanes.* Burnout can come not only from extending ourselves beyond what we can give but also from monotony. If you are predominantly introverted, but you have been out in front of the microphone or taking the lead on initiating community meetings, you might be expending even more energy than those for whom this type of activity might seem restful. It might be time to switch things up. Sustaining advocacy efforts requires a diverse mix of people and roles. Some very indispensable tasks do not require a bullhorn.
- *Normalize self-care.* According to the theory of reasoned action, your attitudes about self-care as well as the way you think others perceive it will impact your intentions to practice it. If you don't take it seriously, you pose a risk to yourself and to your team as well. Diminishing it or ignoring it can have a ripple

TABLE 14.3 Healthy Coping Strategies

Cognitive	Emotional	Behavioral
• Moderation • Write things down • Make small, daily decisions • See the decisions you are already making • Give yourself permission to ask for help • Plan for the future • Get the most information you can to help make decisions • Anticipate needs • Remember you have options • Review previous successes • Problem solve • Have a Plan "B" • Break large tasks into smaller ones • Practice, practice, practice	• Moderation • Allow yourself to experience what you feel • Label what you are experiencing • Give yourself permission to ask for help • Be assertive when necessary • Keep communication open with others • Remember you have options • Use your sense of humor • Have a buddy with whom you can vent • Use "positive" words and language • Practice, practice, practice	• Moderation • Spend time by yourself • Spend time with others • Limit demands on time and energy • Help others with tasks • Give yourself permission to ask for help • Do activities that you previously enjoyed • Take different routes to work or on trips • Remember you have options • Find new activities that are enjoyable and (mildly) challenging • Set goals, have a plan • Relax • Practice, practice, practice

Spiritual	Interpersonal	Physical
• Moderation • Discuss changed beliefs with spiritual leader • Meditation • Give yourself permission to ask for help • Practice rituals of your faith/belief • Spiritual retreats/workshops • Prayer • Remember you have options • Mindfulness • Find spiritual support • Read spiritual literature • Practice, practice, practice	• Moderation • Give yourself permission to ask for help • Take time to enjoy time with trusted friend/partner • Hugs • Healthy boundaries • Remember to use "I" statements • Use humor to diffuse tense conversations • Play together • Talk with trusted partner/friend • Apologize when stress causes irritable behavior or outbursts • Stage needs and wants as clearly as possible • Practice, practice, practice	• Moderation • Aerobic exercise • See doctor and dentist • Routine sleep patterns • Minimize caffeine, alcohol, and sugar • Give yourself permission to ask for help • Eat well-balanced, regular meals • Drink water • Wear comfortable clothes • Engage in physical luxuries: spa, massage, bath, personal trainer • Remember to breathe—deeply • Take minibreaks • Practice, practice, practice

Source: Figley, F. (2013). *The Basics of Compassion Fatigue Workbook*. Figley Institute. Available at http://www.figleyinstit ute.com/documents/Workbook_AMEDD_SanAntonio_2012July20_RevAugust2013.pdf

effect. Having conversations about self-care, checking in with each other, and making an organizational commitment and plan to address it will help you as well as the campaign or initiative keep momentum. Consider ways in which self-care can become a norm within your organization. Here is an example offered by activist Shannon Watts, founder and executive director of Moms Demand Action:

Self-care is so important that we've baked it into our organizational structure: we train volunteers on self-care and even host yoga classes, nature outings, and meditation seminars. One of the biggest things we emphasize in our self-care training is that everyone needs to know how and when to say, "no" and just as important, not to feel bad about it. To that end, we have a process that allows people to pass the baton when they need to. (Fight Like a Mother, 2019, p. 252)

- *Stay connected to your vision.* Over time, your passion for the issue you are trying to resolve or promote may wane if you are experiencing burnout. In addition to adopting some of the strategies for self-care mentioned above and in Table 14.3, reconnecting with your campaign or organization's vision and/or the people it serves can remind you why you are in the long haul and re-fuel you to keep you going.

CONCLUSION

The work of advocacy never really ends. A comprehensive view of advocacy as a long and complex process is important to both managing that process and keeping you going for the long term. Endurance requires persistence, optimism, and a good plan. It is important to have a clear and inspiring vision of what the community or the situation looks like when your advocacy goals are achieved. This vision is what may keep you motivated and ultimately what you think about when you are on the verge of quitting. Planning short-term objectives that are part of your long-term vision and goals will help you and your team experience small wins. Or, if what you gain are lessons rather than achievements, you can take a pause to recalibrate your plan and evaluate what's working or what's not. Ensuring you have the resources you need (e.g., people, money, and time) for the long haul is also a key part of sustainability. People and partnerships are vital to driving change. Be sure to communicate regularly with your staff, volunteers, and groups served as well as policymakers, donors, and other supporters.

Of course, there will be setbacks along the way. Expect these as part of the process and as part of life. Calibrate your expectations accordingly and remember that wisdom is gained through experience and challenge. Take it step by step, and remember to care for yourself. Promote others do the same and foster an environment where self-care is the norm, not the exception.

We hope that what you read in this book inspires and motivates you to engage in advocacy in whatever ways are best for you. Advocacy can be exhausting work, which might lead you to question, "Is it worth it?" Consider this: By helping to change policy, you are not just impacting one life, but multitudes. The work you are doing now can benefit generations to come. We need only to look to courageous advocates, living and gone, for wisdom and inspiration:

You are a light. You are the light. Never let anyone—any person or any force—dampen, dim or diminish your light. Study the path of others to make your way easier and more abundant. Lean toward the whispers of your own heart, discover the universal truth, and follow its dictates. . . . Choose confrontation wisely, but when it is your time don't be afraid to stand up, speak up, and speak out against injustice. And if you follow your truth down the road to peace and the affirmation of love, if you shine like a beacon for all to see, then the poetry of all the great dreamers and philosophers is yours to manifest in a nation, a world community, and a Beloved Community that is finally at peace with itself.

—John Lewis, *Across That Bridge: A Vision for Change and the Future of America* (2017)

REFERENCES

Abrams, S. (2020). Our time is now: Power, purpose, and the fight for a fair America.

Amabile, T. M., & Kramer, S. J. (2011). The power of small wins. *Harvard Business Review.* https://hbr.org/2011/05/the-power-of-small-wins

APA Dictionary of Psychology. (2020). Burnout. https://dictionary.apa.org/burnout

Chen, C. W., & Gorski, P. (2015). Burnout in social justice and human rights activists: Symptoms, causes and implications. *Journal of Human Rights Practice, 7*(3), 366–390. https://doi.org/10.1093/jhuman/huv011

Community Tool Box. (n.d.-a). Chapter 8, Section 1: An *overview of strategic planning or "VMOSA"* (*vision, mission, objectives, strategies, and action plans*). https://ctb.ku.edu/en/table-of-contents/structure/strategic-planning/vmosa/main

Community Tool Box. (n.d.-b). Chapter 30, Section 2: Survival *skills for advocates.* https://ctb.ku.edu/en/table-of-contents/advocacy/advocacy-principles/survival-skills/main

Community Tool Box. (n.d.-c). Chapter 33, Section 20: Advocacy over and for the long haul. https://ctb.ku.edu/en/table-of-contents/advocacy/direct-action/long-term-advocacy/main.

Davis, A. Y. (2016). *Freedom is a constant struggle: Ferguson, Palestine, and the foundations of a movement.* Haymarket Books.

Detroit Urban Community–Academic Research Center. (n.d.). *Home page.* https://detroiturc.org/

Engber, D. (2005). How do cycling teams work? What Lance Armstrong's "domestiques" do?

Slate. https://slate.com/news-and-politics/2005/07/how-do-cycling-teams-work.html

Figley, C. R. (1995). Compassion fatigue as secondary traumatic stress disorder: An overview. In: Figley CR, editor. Compassion fatigue: Coping with secondary traumatic stress disorder in those who treat the traumatized. Brunner-Routledge; New York.

Figley, C. R. (Ed.). (2013). *Treating compassion fatigue.* Brunner-Rutledge.

Israel, B. A., Schulz, A. J., Parker, E. A., Becker, A. B., Allen, A. J., III, & Guzman, J. R. (2003). Critical issues in developing and following community based participatory research principles. In M. Minkler & N. Wallerstein (Eds.), *Community-based participatory research for health* (pp. 53–76). Jossey-Bass.

Lewis, J. (2017). *Across that bridge: A vision for change and the future of America.* Hachette Books.

Lock, K., & Fine, M. (2016). What makes an effective advocacy organization? A framework for determining advocacy capacity. TCC Group. https://www.tccgrp.com/resource/what-makes-an-effective-advocacy-organization-a-framework-for-determining-advocacy-capacity/

Lorde, A. (1988). A burst of light. Firebrand Books.

Lumen Learning. (n.d.). Principles of management: Mission, vision, and values. https://courses.lumenlearning.com/wm-principlesofmanagement/chapter/reading-mission-vision-and-values/

Obama, B. (Nov. 7, 2020). *Remarks by the President on Election Night*. Obama Whitehouse Archives. https://obamawhitehouse.archives.gov/the-press-office/2012/11/07/remarks-president-election-night

Robert, H. R., Seabold, D., Honemann, D., Robert, H. M., III, Gerber, S., & Balch, T. (2020). Robert's Rules of Order Newly Revised, 12th edition. Public Affairs.

Wallerstein, N. B., & Duran, B. (2006). Using community-based participatory research to address health disparities. *Health Promotion Practice, 7*(3), 312–323.

Watts, S. (2019). *Fight like a mother*. Harper Collins.

CHAPTER 14: END-OF-CHAPTER ACTIVITIES

DISCUSSION QUESTIONS

1. Why is having a clear and inspiring vision so important for driving and sustaining advocacy efforts?

2. What are some key steps to planning and sustaining advocacy efforts for "the long haul"?

3. What is a historical example (internationally or in the United States) of a legislative victory that was hard won? How did advocacy play a role?

4. What are two or three strategies for dealing with advocacy setbacks and adversity?

5. What are signs of burnout, and what can individuals involved with advocacy do to prevent and/or address it?

APPLICATION ACTIVITIES

1. Interview someone locally, nationally, or globally who has been involved with advocacy efforts for at least 10 years or more. What keeps them engaged as an advocate? How do they manage burnout and setbacks along the way? What advice do they have for others who may be new to advocacy? What other questions do you have for them? Audio record or take notes of your interview. Write a summary of your interview based on the questions posed.

2. Explore a historical advocacy milestone, or movement, in the United States or globally, such as the passing of the U.S. Marriage Equality Act, Paris Climate Agreement, or the U.S. Rights Act of 1965, and how it came to pass. What can you learn about organizing and sustaining advocacy efforts from this historical example? Write a two-page summary and reflection paper that addresses this question.

3. Create your own burnout prevention plan for engaging in advocacy. What are strategies that you would include to help you engage in advocacy for the long haul?

ADDITIONAL RESOURCES

- Learn more about the Detroit Urban Community–Academic Research Center: Go to https://detroiturc.org/ to see examples of community–academic partnerships and projects rooted in CBPR.
- Figley Institute: Learn more about trainings and workshops relating to compassion fatigue, burnout, dealing with trauma, and managing self-care by going to http://www.figleyinstitute.com/
- "Why advocate?" Stand for Your Mission: Learn more about advocacy in action in the nonprofit sector and read case examples by visiting https://standforyourmission.org/advocacy-your-nonprofit/

- "Meaningfully Connecting With Communities in Advocacy and Policy Work": A downloadable PDF that provides a landscape scan exploring whether and how U.S. funders and nonprofits seek to meaningfully connect with the people and communities that their advocacy and policy work is intended to benefit. Visit Landscape Scan: Meaningfully Connecting with Communities in Advocacy and Policy Work for more information

QUIZ QUESTIONS

1. Abolitionism became a controversial political issue in opposition to some of the "founding forces" that drove America, including
   a. capitalism
   b. racism
   c. colonization
   d. all of the above

2. Which of the following is NOT a tactic to sustain long-term advocacy?
   a. creating an inspiring vision and strategic plan
   b. forming strong partnerships and allies for support
   c. identifying and securing resources you need
   d. saving celebrations until your long-term goal is achieved

3. Organizational structure is not a one-size fits all. The best structure for any organization or initiative will depend on
   a. its size, how many people are involved, what the setting is, and its stage of development.
   b. its size, how many people are involved, what the setting is, and funding.
   c. how many people are involved, what the setting is, funding, and how long it will take to achieve goals.
   d. what the setting is, funding, how long it will take to achieve goals, and type of advocacy.

4. There are three common features within any organizational structure. These are
   a. organizational democracy, systems of checks and balances, fixed timelines
   b. governance, rules by which the organization operates, distribution of work
   c. equal distribution of work, systems of checks and balances, organizational democracy
   d. governance, rules by which the organization operates, systems of checks and balances

5. Strategic planning is a collective process that helps determine
   a. what an organization wants to achieve
   b. how an organization will achieve its objectives and who will be involved
   c. a timeline for achieving milestones
   d. all of the above

6. Part of strategic planning involves determining an organization's vision, mission, and values. Which of the following is NOT correct about visions, missions, and values?
   a. They are created to guide the behaviors of people in that organization and ensure a shared purpose and direction.
   b. The best vision statements are inspirational, future oriented, and motivate people to contribute to their organization.
   c. The mission statement is less actionable than the vision statement.
   d. It reflects what an organization values.

7. Critical aspects of strategic planning include all of the following EXCEPT
   a. knowing your diverse stakeholders and working closely with them
   b. utilizing everyone's background experiences, knowledge, and skills, and putting minds together to think creatively
   c. creating a fixed road map and fixed timeline
   d. determining how the mission will be used to achieve the vision

8. Evaluation is a key component of the strategic planning process. At a minimum, how often should strategic plans be evaluated to maintain accountability and monitor progress?
   a. every 3 months
   b. every year
   c. every month
   d. every 5 years

9. Teamwork and strong partnerships are essential to actualizing advocacy work and an organization's vision. Which of the following is NOT true when working in partnerships?
   a. Collectivism is balanced with individualism.
   b. It is important to engage stakeholders to learn from their experiences and achieve outcomes that are beneficial to them.
   c. Tune out opponents who have different perspectives from your organization's.
   d. In order to get support, you'll need to give support.

10. Using principles of community-based participatory research (CBPR) can help you to establish strong collaborations and engage in collective work. Which of the following is TRUE about CBPR?
    a. CBPR involves striving to form equitable partnerships throughout all work phases and values colearning and reciprocity, unpacking issues around power and privilege, and centering local knowledge.
    b. CBPR focuses on short-term commitments to keep partnerships dynamic.
    c. CBPR is not as important to use when working with marginalized and historically exploited.
    d. CBPR is about individualism and autocracy.

11. Identifying and securing resources is an important part of advocacy work. Which of the following is NOT true, in terms of resources?
    a. The most basic of resources are people, money, and time.

b. Having the right people be a part of your team and engaged in the cause is a key ingredient to long-term success and sustainability.

c. It is important to plan for a diverse portfolio of funding sources.

d. High turnover in organization members is vital to keeping creativity flowing.

12. In advocacy work, why is it important to track progress and celebrate small gains along the way?

a. After spending significant time and energy working toward a common goal, if people do not see signs of progress, energy and motivation will wane.

b. If you don't continually remind policymakers and funders that your issue is important, your organization may face funding cuts and a lack of stakeholder interest.

c. Research demonstrates that perceived progress is a significant predictor of motivation and happiness within an organization or workplace.

d. All of the above.

13. Which of the following is NOT a recommended tip for dealing with setbacks and adversity?

a. Assess the situation, and then take action

b. Accentuate the positive

c. Focus on things you cannot control

d. Deal with problems one by one

14. Which of the following is a tip for preventing and dealing with burnout?

a. Forging ahead

b. Ignoring self-care

c. Eating highly processed "comfort foods" with lots of sugar

d. Taking a break from your usual routine to do something different

ANSWER KEY

1. **D.** All of the above
2. **D.** Saving celebrations until your long-term goal is achieved
3. **B.** Its size, how many people are involved, what the setting is, and funding
4. **B.** Governance, rules by which the organization operates, distribution of work
5. **D.** All of the above
6. **C.** The mission statement is less actionable than the vision statement
7. **C.** Creating a fixed road map and fixed timeline
8. **B.** Every year
9. **C.** Tune out opponents who have different perspectives from your organization's
10. **A.** CBPR involves striving to form equitable partnerships throughout all work phases, and values colearning and reciprocity, unpacking issues around power and privilege, and centering local knowledge
11. **D.** High turnover in organization members is vital to keeping creativity flowing
12. **D.** All of the above
13. **C.** Focus on things you cannot control
14. **D.** Taking a break from your usual routine to do something different

For the benefit of digital users, indexed terms that span two pages (e.g., 52–53) may, on occasion, appear on only one of those pages.

Tables, figures, and boxes are indicated by *t, f,* and *b* following the page number

Printed in the USA/Agawam, MA
March 28, 2023

807620.026